MEUINDIA

Medical Education Research

Theory, Practice, Publication and Scholarship

Editors

B V Adkoli
Amita Ray

notionpress.com

INDIA • SINGAPORE • MALAYSIA

ISBN 978-1-68586-606-8

डॉ. विनोद कुमार पॉल
सदस्य
Dr. Vinod K. Paul
MEMBER

सत्यमेव जयते

भारत सरकार
नीति आयोग, संसद मार्ग
नई दिल्ली–110 001
Government of India
NATIONAL INSTITUTION FOR TRANSFORMING INDIA
NITI Aayog, Parliament Street
New Delhi-110 001
Tele. : 23096809, 23096820, Fax : 23096810
E-mail : vinodk.paul@gov.in

14th September, 2021

FOREWORD

Universalization of health care and access to quality health care has been a foremost agenda for India. In order to meet the challenges, the Government of India has introduced game changing reforms in recent years. Opening new medical colleges across the country, increasing the number of UG/PG seats, augmenting National Board Examination system and constituting a National Medical Commission (NMC) are some of the major steps taken in this direction.

We need to look at medical education research (MER) from a much broader perspective. MER should be seen as a connecting link between patient care and education. The NMC concept of an Indian Medical Graduate revolves around patient care, team work, interpersonal communication, professionalism and life long learning. This requires an interprofessional approach to training of all health professionals which should be supported by faculty development based on best evidence medical education (BEME).

Internationally, there has been a phenomenal growth in Medical Education Research (MER) over the last 70 years. This is evident from huge increase in publications, specialized journals, professional networks/associations, international conferences, masters and doctoral courses, besides the establishment of Units/Centers of education. In contrast, our contribution to research has been very modest, in spite of our capacity to produce largest number of doctors in the world.

MER in India is still at a nascent stage of development. It is possibly due to factors such as faculty members' lack of awareness and motivation for research, lack of skills in conducting MER, preoccupation with patient care, and lack of clear job description linked with career progression. Absence of mentors and the supportive community of practice, shortage of books, journals and forums for professional growth are other factors that might have inhibited our faculty from reaching greater heights in this field.

Contd...

डॉ. विनोद कुमार पॉल
सदस्य
Dr. Vinod K. Paul
MEMBER

सत्यमेव जयते

भारत सरकार
नीति आयोग, संसद मार्ग
नई दिल्ली–110 001
Government of India
NATIONAL INSTITUTION FOR TRANSFORMING INDIA
NITI Aayog, Parliament Street
New Delhi-110 001
Tele. : 23096809, 23096820, Fax : 23096810
E-mail : vinodk.paul@gov.in

In this back drop, the present book on "Medical Education Research: Theory, Practice, Publication and Scholarship" edited by Dr BV Adkoli and Dr Amita Ray, is most welcome and timely initiative. It is welcome because of its focus on educational research in contrast with other books on medical education available in the market. It is timely because, all the regulators, especially the National Assessment and Accreditation Council (NAAC), have been emphasizing on research infrastructure, funding, and outcome as a major criteria for quality assurance and accreditation.

This book has several unique features. It is a pioneering effort grounded in the Indian context. Organized in to four parts, theory, practice, publication, and scholarship the book covers 30 chapters contributed by eminent authors from India and abroad. Besides core issues in MER, the book includes topics such as research applied to program evaluation, public health, integrative medicine and medical humanities. The last part on scholarship addresses Scholarship of Teaching Learning (SoTL), its application to Intellectual Property Rights (IPR) and its integration with user- driven, patient centered approach. The editorial team with logistic support from MEU India have worked hard in bringing a uniform structure. The book has been published by Notion Press, Chennai, with a large distribution network to reach national and international community of readers.

On a final note, medical education research in India, is bound to grow as 'Scholarship in health professions education', which augurs well with the new agenda of India to develop a comprehensive research and innovation ecosystem. We need to ask new research questions, and explore new methodologies, driven by new technologies to address both specialization (depth) and integration (breadth). The educational research with its application of quantitative, qualitative and mixed methodology is ideally suited for achieving this daunting task. Our ultimate goal is to develop a seamless 'community of scholars' transcending the professional barriers and geographical borders, who can develop a shared vision, and undertake scholarly activities in a holistic manner. Hopefully, the National Medical Commission, along with other regulators will be working in concert, following a blueprint laid down by the National Education Policy 2020. Its proposed outfit 'National Research Foundation' is likely to play a key role in this process. Towards this end, this book is a small but solid contribution. I am sure, the scholars in health profession in India and abroad will derive immense benefit from this work.

(VINOD PAUL)
MD, PhD, FAMS, FNAsc, FASc, FNA

Preface

Writing a book is a tough job. Editing a book with multiple authors is even more demanding, especially while dealing with a new field. Medical Education Research (MER) in the Indian context is one such area. We dared to take up this challenge with courage and humility for three reasons. First, we were moved by the fact that MER has made significant stride at the international level, however, in contrast, the contribution from India has been minimal. Bringing out a book dedicated to MER is, therefore, the need of the hour. The second impetus came from the regulatory bodies. The National Medical Commission (NMC) has linked the promotion of faculty with the requirement of publications in indexed journals. On similar lines, the National Assessment and Accreditation Council (NAAC) has identified research and publication, innovations, and Intellectual Property Rights (IPR) as major criteria for assessment and accreditation. Ironically, these 'push' factors have also caused a high stress for the faculty to 'publish or perish'. We therefore thought this book will enhance research and publication skills among faculty.

The third stimulus for writing this book came from the revised MBBS curriculum (2019) which underlines Competency Based Medical Education (CBME) with several features, such as foundation course, early clinical exposure, integrated teaching, formative assessment and a longitudinal model of attitudes, ethics and communication (AETCOM) to develop Indian Medical Graduate (IMG). Each one of these interventions requires evidence for its efficacy, outcome, and impact. While new curriculum was being introduced, the COVID pandemic broke out and forced the medical colleges to come out with ad-hoc solutions such as emergency remote teaching (ERT) whose efficacy is not yet established. We, therefore, believe that a comprehensive book on MER would stimulate the faculty in evidence-based practice.

The scope of our book is not limited to MER. It addresses the needs of all faculty across the health professions education, besides administrators, researchers, and leaders in the field. The 30 chapters written by renowned authors have been organized in four parts: Theory, Practice, Publication and Scholarship, which are interlinked. Theory informs practice. Practice leads to publication. Both contribute to scholarship. We have highlighted the role of scholarship as an overarching concept in lieu of research.

Besides dealing with the conventional core topics in research, we have addressed diverse issues such as program evaluation, research in public health, integrative medicine, and medical humanities. Ethical issues pertaining to research and publication in health professions education have been discussed in detail. The last part on Scholarship covers Scholarship of Teaching and Learning (SoTL), the governance issues, Intellectual Property Rights (IPR) and user - driven, patient centered approach in bringing scholarship of integration. The book concludes with a final chapter showing the way forward.

Another unique feature you will find in this book is a uniform template called ABCD-SER© developed by the editor [A - Assess Need, B – Brief, C – Contextualize, D – Describe, S – Summarize, E – Evaluate, and R - Road ahead/Reference]. We believe that this format makes the book interesting and user-friendly.

We are fortunate to have received contributions from eminent scholars in the field. Some of them are the leaders associated with the international networks such as SEARAME, WFME and AMEE. They have contributed willingly, in a spirit of international cooperation. On the top of everything, **Dr. Vinod Paul**, member, NITI Aayog, an eminent leader in health profession has written foreword to this book.

In summary, this book is a combined effort of several individuals who have tirelessly contributed in several ways as authors, members of the editorial board, and peer reviewers. This project would not have materialized without the strong logistics support extended by **Dr. Sanjay Bedi**, CEO, MEU INDIA. Our thanks are due to the Notion Press, Chennai for publishing this book in the present form. We sincerely acknowledge the contribution of **Dr. Angelina Bedi** for her editorial support and liaising with the publisher throughout this project.

We hope, the readers will draw fullest benefit from our work. We shall be obliged to receive comments, criticism and feedback which will help us in improving our work. Our ultimate aim is to raise a community of scholars in HPE who will nurture evidence-based practice to make a small difference to the health care and wellbeing of the mankind.

B.V. Adkoli (Editor)
Amita Ray (Co-Editor)

Acknowledgments

This book is a collective work of several individuals who contributed in various ways. We sincerely thank Dr. Vinod Paul, Member, NITI Aayog for writing a fitting foreword to our book. The role played by Dr. Sanjay Bedi, CEO, MEUINDIA in launching a Certificate Course on Medical Education Research and Publication (MERP) for the first time in India, gave us the much-needed stimulus to start this project in January 2021. The Resource Faculty of this course, viz., Drs Medha Joshi, Nirmala Rege, Chinmay Shah, Harshal Sabane and Sanjay Bedi worked along with us as a core team and supported us throughout this project. The contribution made by Dr. Angelina Bedi in compiling the manuscripts, designing the layout, formatting of the chapters, designing cover page, besides, liaising with the publishing team is highly appreciated. We are grateful to our editorial team comprising Drs Annie Sheeba, Jasmine Rayapudi, Jananni M, and Jayanthi S., who worked hard in language enhancement and polishing the drafts.

While initiating this project, we received immense support and guidance from the Editorial Advisory Committee consisting of Drs Avinash Supe, Thomas V Chacko, Amol Dongre, Anshu, Vishnu Bhat, Zayapragassarazzan, and Rakesh Biswas. They helped us not only in deriving the Table of Contents (TOC), but also in identifying lead authors from India and abroad, which is highly appreciated. Dr. Rashmi Kusurkar with her international standing and experience in MER, happily contributed chapters on Scholarship Development, and further helped us in peer reviewing a few chapters dealing with the current trends in international literature in MER.

Peer review is the hallmark of quality in scientific paper writing. While some of the authors themselves willingly came forward do this arduous work, a number of others also joined the team of reviewers. We sincerely thank them all.

We thank Notion Press, Chennai and their publication team led by Ms. Hema Priyadarshini and Jason Philip for designing, and printing this book facing the hardship caused by heavy rains in Tamil Nadu, which disrupted the work for a while.

Finally, we thank Sri Balaji Vidyapeeth (Deemed to be University), Pondicherry, Academy of Health Professions Educators (AHPE) and several leaders in medical education who supported indirectly in completing this task.

B.V. Adkoli, Editor
Amita Ray, Co-Editor

Table of Contents

List of Contributors

AMITA RAY
MS, FAIMER Fellow MSc MHPE
Professor and Head
Department of Obstetrics and Gynecology
Rajshree Medical Research Institute
Bareilly, Uttar Pradesh - 243501, India
amitarays@gmail.com

AMOL R DONGRE
MD, MPS, MHPE
Head,
Department of Extension Programmes,
Pramukhswami Medical College, Bhaikaka
University, Karamsad, Gujarat
23, Jaiprabhu Society, Manish Nagar,
Nagpur - 440015, India
amolrdongre@gmail.com

AMY PRICE
MSc MA MSc DPhil
Senior Research Scientist Stanford School of
Medicine, Research Editor The BMJ, Center for
Evidence Based Health Care Oxford Fellow
2065 NW 15TH PL Delray Beach USA 33445
amyprice@stanford.edu

ANANTHAKRISHNAN N
MS., DNBE., FRCS (Eng., Edin., Glasg.,) FACS., FICS.,
FACG., FIMSA., FAMS.
Dean of Faculty, Sri Balaji Vidyapeeth
2A, Vairam Enclave, Sithananda Nagar,
Pondicherry - 605005, India
n.ananthk@gmail.com

ANSHU
MD, DNB, MNAMS, MSc (HPE)
Professor,
Department of Pathology, Mahatma
Gandhi Institute of Medical Sciences, Sevagram,
Wardha, Maharashtra 442102
6 New MLK Colony, MGIMS Sevagram, Wardha,
Maharashtra - 442102, India
dr.anshu@gmail.com

ARIN KAR
Master of Population Studies
Karnataka Health Promotion Trust
1st main, ex-servicemen colony, R T Nagar,
Bangalore, Karnataka - 560032, India
kar_arin@rediffmail.com

AVINASH SUPE
MS DNBE MHPE
Emeritus Professor, Surgical Gastroenterology and
Medical Education
602, Sixth Floor, Sangeeta Towers, Vijay Vihar
society, Off Sion Trombay Road, Chembur,
Mumbai - 400071, India
avisupe@gmail.com

BALLAMBETTU VISHNU BHAT
MD, DHA, DDE
Director-Medical research, Professor of Pediatrics
and Neonatology, AVMC &Hospital, Vinayaka
Mission's Research Foundation Kirumampakkam,
Pondicherry - 607403, India
drvishnubhat@yahoo.com

BHAGYAJYOTI PRIYADARSHINI
MBBS, 3rd year
Saheed Laxman Nayak Medical College and Hospital, Koraput, Odisha
Room no. 31, Girls Hostel, SLN MCH, Koraput, Odisha- 764020, India
luckybhagyajyoti@gmail.com

B V ADKOLI
M Sc, M Ed, Ph D, MMedEd PhD Educator ATLS
Director, Centre for Health Professions Education, and Professor of Medical Education Sri Balaji Vidyapeeth, Puducherry - 607402, India
bvadkoli@gmail.com

CHINMAY SHAH
MBBS, MD, PhD., PGDHPE, PGDHM, FAIIMER Fellow
Government Medical College, Bhavnagar
A-201, Vrusha Residency, Atabhai Chowk, Bhavnagar, Gujarat - 364001, India
chinmay.ffri@gmail.com

G G GANGADHARAN
Ayurvedacharya, Master of Management, PhD
Ramaiah Indic Specialty Ayurveda Restoration Hospital, MSRIT Post, New BEL Road, Mathikere, Bangalore - 560 054, India
vaidyaggganga@gmail.com

GOMINDA PONNAMPERUMA
MBBS, Dip. Psychology, MMEd, PhD
Faculty of Medicine, University of Colombo, Sri Lanka
Professor and Head, Department of Medical Education, Faculty of Medicine, University of Colombo, Sri Lanka, 00800
16/5 (18/10), Quarry Road, Mirihana, Nugegoda, Sri Lanka
gominda@medarc.cmb.ac.lk

HARSHAL SABANE
MBBS, MD, FAIMER Fellow
Associate Professor and Head, Department of Community Medicine, SSR Medical College, Belle Rive, Mauritius
drsabane@gmail.com

HENAL SHAH
MD, MSc (HPE)
Professor (Additional)
Department of Psychiatry, TNMC & BYL Nair Charitable Hospital, Co-Director GSMC FRI
47 Khotachi Wadi, Girgaum, Mumbai - 400004, India
drhenal@gmail.com

IAN G WILSON
MBBS, FRACGP, PhD, FAMEE
International Medical University Bukit Jalil, Kuala Lumpur - 5700, Malaysia
ianwilson1@internode.on.net

INDIKA KARUNATILAKE
MBBS, MMedEd, FCGP, FHEA, FRCP
Head, WHO Collaborating Centre For Medical Education, Faculty of Medicine, University of Colombo - 00800, Sri Lanka
indika@medarc.cmb.ac.lk

JYOTSNA S.
BDS, MDS, FAIMER Fellow, (MHPE)
Reader, Department of Public Health Dentistry
D A Pandu Memorial RV Dental College
63, Sri Shankara Krupa, 3rd main 7th cross, Akshayanagar, West Bengaluru - 560058, India
drsjyotsna@gmail.com

KRISHNAMURTHY JAYANNA
MBBS MD; Professor: Public Health & Dean: Faculty of Life and Allied Health Sciences
M S Ramaiah University of Applied Sciences
University House, New BEL Road, Bangalore - 560098, India
krishnamurthyjayanna@gmail.com

LARRY D. GRUPPEN, PHD
Professor and Director, Master of Health Professions Education Program
219 Victor Vaughan House,1111 E. Catherine Str, University of Michigan Medical School Ann Arbor, MI 48109
lgruppen@umich.edu

LATHA RAVICHANDRAN
MBBS, DCH, DNB, FAIMER Fellow, IFME
Professor of Paediatrics and Associate Dean Education, Sri Ramachandra Institute of Higher Education and Research,
Chennai, Tamil Nadu - 600116, India
latha@sriramachandra.edu.in

L V SIMHACHALAM KUTIKUPPALA
MBBS
Intern, Konaseema Institute of Medical Sciences and Research Foundation (KIMS&RF), Amalapuram, Andhra Pradesh - 533201, India
simhachalam.kutikuppala@gmail.com

MADALENA PATRICIO
PhD
Faculty of Medicine, University of Lisbon, Department of Medical
AV. PROFESSOR EGAS MONIZ 1649-028 LISBOA,
patricio@medicina.ulisboa.pt

MALU MOHAN
MDS, PhD
Consultant- II, Basic Course in Biomedical Research (BCBR),
Indian Council of Medical Research - National Institute of Epidemiology (ICMR - NIE), Ayapakkam, Chennai, Tamil Nadu - 600077, India
dr.malumohan@gmail.com

MANOJ KUMAR PATI
PhD
Karnataka Health Promotion Trust
KHPT # 5 5th Floor IT Park Rajaji Nagar Industrial Area, Bengaluru - 560044, India
manojkumar.pati@khpt.org

MEDHA A. JOSHI
M.D., M.H.P.E., ECFMG, IFME
Consultant, Health Professions Education
K 43, Shriram Sadhana Apartments, M.S. Ramaiah Road, Gokul, Bangalore - 560054, India
medhajoshi11@gmail.com

MEGHAN MCCONNELL
PhD
Associate Professor, Department of Innovation in Medical Education and Department of Anesthesiology and Pain Medicine, University of Ottawa
850 Peter Morand Crescent, Ottawa, ON, K1G 5Z3
meghan.mcconnell@uottawa.ca

MOHAMMED NAJJAR
MD, MHPE
Nationwide Children's Hospital/ Ohio State University
7013 Post Preserve blvd, Dublin, OH 43016
Mohammed.Najjar@nationwidechildrens.org

MONA HMOUD ALSHEIKH
MBBS, Ph.D. Neurophysiology,
MHPE, FAIMER Fellow
Department of Physiology, College of Medicine,
Imam Abdulrahman Bin Faisal University.
Khozama, Azizia, 3066 Al Khobar 34719, Saudi Arabia.
monaalsheikh@gmail.com; msheikh@iau.edu.sa

M. SENTHIL
MDS - Public Health Dentistry, PGDHPE,
CCEPC, PGDIPR
Professor and Team Leader, Indira Gandhi Institute of Dental Sciences,
Sri Balaji Vidyapeeth, Pilliyarkuppam,
Pondicherry – 607402, India
senthilm@igids.ac.in

NARASIMMAN SWAMINATHAN
MPTh (Cardio-Pulmonary), FAIMER Fellow
Professor Physiotherapy, Vice Principal, Faculty of Allied Health Sciences, Sri Ramachandra Institute of Higher Education and Research,
Chennai, Tamil Nadu - 600116, India
naraswamin2001@gmail.com

NIRMALA NARAYAN REGE
MD, DNB, PhD, FAIMER Fellow
Professor Emeritus, Dept of Pharmacology & Therapeutics, Seth GS Medical College & KEM Hospital, Mumbai
B-10, Kamdar Vaibhav Coop Hsg Society, Gokhale Road (South), Dadar (West), Mumbai - 400028, India
nimarege@gmail.com

PATHIYIL RAVI SHANKAR
MBBS, MD, FAIMER Fellow, MAoME
International Medical University,
Malaysia Jalan Jalil Perkasa 19, Bukit Jalil,
Kuala Lumpur - 57000, Malaysia
ravi.dr.shankar@gmail.com

PAYAL BANSAL
MBBS, MS, MHPE, FAIMER Fellow, PGDHE
Professor, Medical Education & Director, University Centre for Professional Education & Faculty Development, Dr. D.Y. Patil Vidyapeeth, Pune, India
payal.bansal@dpu.edu.in; payalkbansal@gmail.com

PNINA WEISS
MD, MHPE,
Associate Professor of Pediatrics
Yale School of Medicine
333 Cedar Street, PO Box 208064,
New Haven, CT, 06520-064
pnina.weiss@yale.edu

PREMANATH KOTUR.
MBBS, MD, PhD (Med Edn), FICA.
Dean & Professor of Anaesthesiology,
AVMC, Pondicherry – 607402, India
dean@avmc.edu.in

PUSHPA KOTUR
MBBS, MD, PhD
Professor of Obstetrics and Gynaecology,
AVMC, Pondicherry – 607402, India
pushpakotur@gmail.com

PUSHPANJALI KRISHNAPPA
BDS, MDS, PhD, PGDHHM, FAIMER Fellow, MHPE
Professor, Department of Public Health Dentistry, Faculty of Dental Sciences, M S Ramaiah University of Applied Sciences, Bengaluru - 560054, India
drpushpa14@gmail.com

P.V. VIJAYARAGHAVAN,
MCh., DNB, FRCS FAOI, FAIMER Fellow,
Fulbright Scholar
Vice Chancellor & Professor of Orthopaedics
Sri Ramachandra Institute of Higher Education and Research (DU)
Porur, Chennai – 600 116, India
drpvv53@gmail.com

RAKESH BISWAS
MBBS, MD
Professor Department of Medicine, Kamineni Institute of Medical sciences, Narketpally,
Hyderabad – 508254, India
rakesh7biswas@gmail.com

RASHMI KUSURKAR
MBBS, MD, PhD, FAMEE
Amsterdam UMC, Research in Education, Faculty of Medicine Vrije Universiteit Amsterdam,
P.O. Box 7057, 1007 MB Amsterdam, the Netherlands
R.Kusurkar@amsterdamumc.nl

RENATE KAHLKE
PhD
Assistant Professor, Division of Education & Innovation, Department of Medicine and Scientist, McMaster Education Research, Innovation and Theory Program, McMaster University
1280 Main St West, Hamilton, Ontario,
Canada, L8S 4L8,
kahlkerm@mcmaster.c

RAVIKUMAR SAMBANDAM
PhD
Associate Professor, Multi-disciplinary Centre for Biomedical Research, AVMC and Hospital, Vinayaka Missions Research Foundation, Kirumampakkam,
Puducherry - 607 403, India
ravikumar.sambandam@avmc.edu.in

SADHNA SHARMA
MD(Med), DOMS, PGDG, DGM, FACP
Professor of Medicine, NRI Medical College
3/2/13, NRI Staff Quarters, Chinakakani,
Namburu PO Guntur AP - 522508, India
drsadhnasharma@hotmail.com

SAI BABA M
PhD
MS Ramaiah University of Applied Sciences & National Institute of Advanced Studies,
Gnanagangothri Campus, New BEL Road,
Bengaluru, Karnataka - 560054, India
msaibaba@msruas.ac.in

SANJAY BEDI
MBBS, MD, FAIMER Fellow
CEO MEU INDIA
366 Green Avenue, Amritsar, Punjab - 143001, India
drsanjaybedi@gmail.com

SARANYA MUKHERJEE
MBBS final year
Kamineni Institute of Medical sciences, Narketpally, Telangana - 508254, India
saranyaroshni09@gmail.com

SATENDRA SINGH,
MD
Professor of Physiology, University College of Medical Sciences, Delhi
A5-303, Olive County, Sector-5, Vasundhara, Ghaziabad (U.P) - 201012, India
dr.satendra@gmail.com

SATYANARAYANA RAMANAIK
PhD
Karnataka Health Promotion Trust IT Park, 5th Floor, 1-4, Rajajinagar Industrial Area, Rajajinagar, Bengaluru - 560044, India
satya@khpt.org

SAVITA RAVINDRA
B. Sc, M. Sc, FAIMER Fellow
Professor & Head, Department of Physiotherapy, M S Ramaiah Medical College & Hospitals, MSRIT Post, Bengaluru - 560054, India
savitaravi@gmail.com

SHANTHI ANANTHAKRISHNAN
MD., DCH., PhD
Professor of Pediatrics, Mahatma Gandhi Medical College and Research Institute, Pondicherry.
2A, Vairam Enclave, Sithananda Nagar, Pondicherry - 605 005, India
shanthiak79@gmail.com

SHANTHAN JODAVULA
BAMS, MS (Ayu)
Consultant Ayurveda Physician
S.L Diagnostics, Windsor Plaza, Hyderabad
LIG B-77, Lane Beside Bajaj Electronics, Dr. A S Rao Nagar, Hyderabad - 500062, India
shantanjodavula@gmail.com

SHITAL BHANDARY
MSc, MPhil, FAIMER Fellow
Associate Professor
Department of Community Health Sciences, School of Medicine and School of Public Health, Patan Academy of Health Sciences, Lagankhel, Lalitpur Metropolitan City-5, Bagmati Province, Nepal - 44702
335/16 Charmati Marg, Chabahil, Kathmandu Metropolitan City-7, Bagmati Province, Nepal - 44602
shitalbhandary@pahs.edu.np

SUCHETA DANDEKAR
PhD, MHPE
Professor of Biochemistry, Era's Lucknow Medical College, Lucknow
Adjunct Faculty, Manipal Academy of Health Education, Manipal
3/1 Haji Ali Park, Off K. Khadye Marg, Mumbai - 400034, India
sucheta.dandekar@gmail.com

SWAROOP N
MBBS MD
Thematic Lead-Comprehensive Primary Health Care, Karnataka Health Promotion Trust
IT Park, 5th Floor, 1-4, Rajajinagar Industrial Area, Behind Kssidc Admin Office, Rajajinagar, Bengaluru, Karnataka - 560044, India
swaroop.n@khpt.org

SUPTENDRA NATH SARBADHIKARI
MBBS, PhD, FIAHSI, FAIMER Fellow,
Distinguished Fellow, HITLAB
Professor – Department of Digital Research
Santiniketan Medical College
Bolpur – 731 204, India
supten@gmail.com

TEJASWINI
BDS MDS
Assistant Professor
Faculty of Life and Allied Health Sciences, MS Ramaiah University of Applied Health Sciences, Gnanagagothri Campus, New BEL Road, Bengaluru - 560054, India
tejaswini.ah.ls@msruas.ac.in

THOMAS V CHACKO
MBBS, MD, IFME, FAIMER Fellow and Founder Director PSG FAIMER Regional Institute Coimbatore, Dean Medical Education, Believers Medical College, Kuttapuzha, Thiruvalla, Kerala - 689103, India
drthomasvchacko@gmail.com

UPREET DHALIWAL
MS, FAIMER Fellow
Former Director-Professor, University College of Medical Sciences, University of Delhi
A61 Govindpuram, Ghaziabad 201013, UP, India
upreetdhaliwal@gmail.com

VAMSI KRISHNA
MBBS MD (Student)
Kamineni Institute of Medical Sciences Narketpally
Telangana - 508254, India
vamsikrishna1996.vk@gmail.com

VINOD RAMANI
MBBS, MD, MPH, Associate Professor, Public Health
Ramaiah University of Applied Sciences
Gnanagagothri Campus, New BEL Road,
Bengaluru -560054, India
vinodramani77@gmail.com

Glossary

AAMC	Association of American Medical Colleges
AHPE	Academy of Health Profession Educators
AI	Artificial Intelligence
AMEE	Association for Medical Education in Europe
AR	Action Research
AYUSH	Ayurveda, Yoga and Naturopathy, Unani, Siddha and Homeopathy
BEME	Best Evidence Medical Education
BMD	Bone Mineral Density
BSE	*Boswellia serrata* Gum Extract
CAM	Complementary & Alternative Medicine’
CAQDA	Computer Assisted Qualitative Data Analysis
CASDAS	Computer Assisted Qualitative Data Analysis
CASP	Critical Appraisal Skills Program
CBBLE	Case-Based Blended Learning Ecosystem
CBME	Competency Based Medical Education
CBR	Clinical Benefit Rate
CBR	Case Based Reasoning
CBT	Consensus Based Technique
CDC	Center for Disease Control and Prevention
CEBM	Center for Evidence Based Medicine
CFR	Code of Federal Regulations
CME/CNE	Continuing Medical Education / Continuing Nursing Education
COPE	Committee on Publication Ethics
CSAS	Communication Skills Attitude Scale
CT	Chemotherapy/ Computerized Tomography

CTRI	Clinical Trials Registry India
CVD	Cardio-Vascular Diseases
DBER	Discipline Based Education Research
DCR	Disease Control Rate
DM	Diabetes Mellitus
DOPS	Direct Observation of Procedural Skills
DREEM	Dundee Ready Educational Environment Measure
EB / EBP	Evidence Based /Evidence Based Practice
EBM	Evidence Based Medicine
EBME	Evidence Based Medical Education
ER	Educational Research
ERIC	Education Resources Information Center
ESR	Erythrocyte Sedimentation Rate
ETQS	Evaluation Tool for Qualitative Studies
FAIMER	Foundation for Advancement of International Medical Education and Research
FDP	Faculty Development Program
FGD	Focus Group Discussion
FIC- SoTL	Facilitating Institutional Conversations about Scholarship of Teaching and Learning
FLW	Front Line Workers
GATE	General Architecture for Text Engineering
HPER	Health Professions Education Research
HPEU	Health Professions Education Unit
HRT	Hormone Replacement Therapy
ICMJE	International Committee of Medical Journal Editors
ICMR	Indian Council of Medical Research
IDI	In-Depth Interviews
IFME	International Fellowship in Medical Education
IMR	Integrative Medicine Research
IMRAD	Introduction, Methods, Results and Discussion
IRB /IEC	Institutional Review Board/Institutional Ethics Committees
IRTTC	International Regional Teacher Training Center
JBI	Joanna Briggs Institute
JC	Journal Club
JSPE	Jefferson Scale of Physician Empathy
KAP	Knowledge, Practice and Attitudes
KMC	Kangaroo Mother Care

LBW	Low Birth Weight
LMS	Learning Management System
MER	Medical Education Research
MeSH	Medical Subject Headings
MEU	Medical Education Unit
Mini-CEX	Mini-Clinical Evaluation Exercise
MKD	*MauktikYuktaKamdudha*
MMI	Multiple Mini-Interview
MMR	Mixed Methods Research
MPP	*MauktikYuktaPravalPanchamruta*
NAAC	National Assessment and Accreditation Council
NBE	National Board of Examination
NCD	Non-Communicable Diseases
NEP	National Education Policy
NGT	Nominal Group Technique
NMC	National Medical Commission
NTTC	National Teachers Training Centre
NVMO	Netherlands Association for Medical Education
OA	Open Access
OSCE/OSPE	Objective Structured Clinical Examination/Objective Structured Practical Examination
PBL	Problem Based Learning
PE	Program Evaluation
PMC	PubMed Central
PPE	Personal Protective Equipment
QDA	Qualitative Data Analysis
QES	Quality Evidence Synthesis
RBCs	Red Blood Cells
RIS Format	Reference In Specific Format
RTTC	Regional Teacher Training Center
SBD Formulation	*Suvarnabhasmadi* Formulation
SCI	Sciences Citation Index
SDLRS	Self-Directed Learning Readiness Scale
SERM	Selective Estrogen Receptor Modulator
SLBSP	Solid Lipid *Boswellia serrata* Particles
SOI	Scholarship of Integration
SoTL	Scholarship of Teaching and Learning

S-PEST	Structured Physical Examination Skills Training
UDHC	User-Driven Health Care
UPHC	Urban Primary Health Centre
USIEF	United States-India Educational Foundation
WFME	World Federation for Medical Education
WHO	World Health Organization

Section I

Theory

Chapter 1

Medical Education Research from an International Perspective

Pnina Weiss, Mohammed Najjar, Payal Bansal, Larry D. Gruppen

ABSTRACT

In many countries, the field of medical education is at a nascent stage of development and poorly understood. Medical education research (MER) is key to making medical education a scholarly field of study and more than just a domain of practice. Medical education research draws from many other disciplines for its research methods, theoretical frameworks, and analytics tools. It draws these together to form a scholarly body of knowledge that is rich and complex and which needs to reflect the diversity of settings and problems reflected in the international character of medical education. Medical education research balances applied and theoretical approaches to a wide range of problems and phenomena. It benefits from a wide array of researcher perspectives and training. This chapter contains several suggestions including the importance of international research collaborations. These are essential for identifying shared knowledge and localized contexts that together can prepare a global force of physicians who can address the healthcare needs of individuals and cultures.

Key Words: medical education, research, international collaboration, methods, theory

ASSESS NEED

Medical Education Research (MER) is a relatively young field, emerging in the 1950s (in North America and Europe) as the application of educational and social sciences to medical education. Medical education research is an essential component of medical education. It provides the evidence for making educational decisions and the criteria for making informed educational decisions.

The growth of MER has been considerable in the last three decades, fostered in part by more journals, conferences, faculty development, and educational innovations, both at national and international levels.

As MER has grown, it becomes more apparent that we need to foster international discussion on research goals and establish many more international collaborations to actually study these phenomena.

A disproportionate share of the research literature has come from Europe and North America. This imbalance introduces biases in the research evidence, the research questions asked, and the studies that are performed. We cannot assume that research from one culture or nation applies automatically to another. Such generalizability needs to be demonstrated and documented through research, which will require much more interaction among international colleagues and international research collaborations. Capacity building in educational research has implications for global health equity as it empowers faculty across boundaries to align educational decisions and practices to solve health problems in their own contexts in an evidence-based manner.

BRIEF

- Medical Education Research is a relatively young field, emerging in the 1950s (in North America and Europe) as the application of educational and social sciences to medical education.
- A disproportionate share of the research literature comes from Europe and North America, which introduces biases in the research evidence, the research questions asked, and the studies that are performed.
- Globalization of medical education research is necessary to ensure that a world-view is achieved to guide curricular reform, international standardization of competencies, and translation of knowledge for under-represented regions to ensure that the needs of local patient populations and healthcare needs are met.
- Collaborating within and across communities in medical education research enables the sharing of resources and expertise in various domains (teaching methods, curriculum development, decision making, psychometrics, research methods, etc.).
- International collaboration in medical education research is complex and while inequality in resources is unavoidable, care must be taken to ensure that the intellectual contributions to the studies are equitable.

CONTEXTUALIZE

The developing world has a larger disease burden and more medical and allied health institutions when compared to the developed world. Yet, these "non-western" countries are under represented in health and medical research, referred to as the 10/90 divide. This gap is also evident in medical education research (ten Cate 2021). The inequity needs to be addressed through conscious international collaborative efforts to mentor, support and strengthen medical education research productivity and quality, creating more opportunities and avenues for publication of the work therefrom.

For MER to be impactful it must be relevant. How can MER guide "under-resourced countries" help improve or develop curricula relevant to their context? Can we conduct research that reverses 'brain drain' and converts it to 'brain gain'? Research themes or areas need to be chosen with care with the overall goal of improving/informing the curriculum process such as needs assessment, evaluation research, assessment for measuring outcome attainment in specific contexts and a focus on quality of research.

Do countries with well-established MER recognize and understand the needs of their collaborators? Can MER tackle these problems alone or do research collaborations need to be more inclusive of allied health professions as well? Additionally, how can MER address the challenges presented by the COVID-19 pandemic, such as the need for virtual teaching and healthcare delivery and massive disruptions in the surrounding society and culture.

DESCRIBE

Medical education research (MER) plays a pivotal role in generating information that educators need to understand and advance teaching and learning to improve healthcare practice, patient care and patient outcomes. Medical education research advances the skills, knowledge and professionalism of health professional students by understanding and evaluating educational ecosystems. Furthermore, it provides the evidence and criteria for making informed educational decisions.

Origin and Development of MER

The need for the reform and clarification of the objectives of medical education led to the formation of national organizations such as the Association of American Medical Colleges (AAMC) in the United States in 1876 (Figure 1) and institutional offices within medical schools to provide oversight of education. In 1910 the Flexner report established the biomedical model as the gold standard of medical training. Medical education research arose in 1950s as a result of the increasing emphasis on advancing knowledge and scientific research, the explosive growth of scientific and medical information which required increasingly complex and lengthy curricula, the emergence of funding for MER, and the increased need for public accountability of medical education in the global North regions such as the United States, Europe and Canada (Kuper, Albert, et al. 2010; Norman 2011; Ten Cate 2021). In response to the increasing number of newly independent countries and part of its mission to improve health services for all, the World Health Organization (WHO) led a number of initiatives to improve medical education and expand faculty development, which led to the birth of the Association for Medical Education in Europe (AMEE) in 1972. Additionally, WHO established two sites in the US as International Regional Teacher Training Centers (IRTTCs) in 1969. Educational specialists trained in these IRTTCs later established Regional Teacher Training Centers (RTTCs), which then collaborated to establish National Teacher Training Centres (NTTCs) with the objective of training teachers who could then establish medical education units (MEUs) within colleges in their respective countries (Srinivas and Adkoli 2009). In India, faculty development in medical education arose in the 1970s and flourished as a result of the establishment of NTTCs, MEUs, the Consortium of Medical Institutions for the Reform of Medical Education, and initiatives supported by the Foundation for Advancement in International Medical Education and Research (FAIMER). Medical education continues to evolve, however, the Lancet Commissions Report (Frenk, Chen et al. 2010) in the centenary year of the Flexner report highlights inequity in healthcare and quality of education and advocates for educational reforms to address these gaps.

There has been a dramatic increase in the number of publications on MER, but the geographic representation of authors and articles is uneven (Buffone, Djuana et al. 2020). The most common themes of research from the English literature include student assessment, clinical skills training and clerkships, problem-based learning, community-based training, clinical competence assessment, teaching clinical sciences, communication skills training, student characteristics and objective structured clinical exams (Rotgans 2012). There is marked geographic variability in both problem content and trends.

Globalization of medical education and research is necessary to ensure that a world-view is achieved to guide curricular reform, international standardization of competencies, and translation of knowledge for under-represented regions to ensure that the needs of local patient populations and healthcare needs are met.

Medical Education as Science

Education is a field of study; the learners, educators, curricula, systems of education and healthcare are part of the ecosystem which provides raw material for inquiry, allowing it to be approached and analyzed from a diverse array of viewpoints and disciplines (Ringsted, Hodges et al. 2011; Hodges and Kuper 2012).

The complexity of medical education allows a variety of scholarship traditions and perspectives. One set of contrasting traditions is research on teaching and learning (the practice of medical education) vs. research on fundamental mechanisms and phenomena with the goal of building theory. While each aims to understand learning experiences, they differ somewhat in methods and applications (Crites, Gaines et al. 2014). Research on the practice of medical education draws upon experiential learning and the investigator often serves as teacher, integrated with the process of learning. In contrast, the educational research tradition is based upon the scientific method with the investigator remaining objective and separate from the teaching experience. A related distinction in scientific perspective is made by Albert, et al. (Albert, Hodges et al. 2007) between "service" to the educational mission of the institution and "science" or the generalized understanding of educational principle and phenomena.

Medical Education as Research

Conducting research in medical education reflects a variety of methodologies but can be approached in a stepwise manner (Beckman and Cook 2007). Medical education research can utilize quantitative methods, similar to those used in clinical research, or qualitative methods. Quantitative methods measure the associations and causal relationships between variables, while qualitative studies aim to understand the circumstances from the viewpoint of the study participants, which may generate a deeper understanding of phenomena by uncovering unanticipated findings.

The outcomes and influences in medical education are generally intangible and difficult to define, to say nothing of assessing them. Constructs such as motivation, knowledge, skilled performance, expertise, identity, professionalism and hundreds more are all important variables but to study them, we must have ways of measuring them. There is a sizable body of tools that already exist, including knowledge tests, attitude surveys, performance assessments, standardized patients, and many others, but there is always a need for new and better assessments, especially of new constructs. One very important form of scholarship in MER is the development of assessment procedures and gathering validity evidence for these methods.

Improving Medical Education Research from an International Perspective

Theory and conceptual frameworks. A common complaint of MER is that too many studies lack a conceptual framework, which is a way to think about a problem or complex relationships (Bordage 2009). Too often MER lacks the formulation of models and theories and does not build upon previous results (Cook, Bordage et al. 2008). Many MER studies describe "what was done," or "Did it work?" However, MER should go beyond and should strive to answer the "how" and "why" of a phenomenon or intervention. Medical education research should generate new hypotheses, which can move the field forward. For example, most studies on problem-based learning focus on comparing its effectiveness to more traditional teaching methods such as lecture. However, few studies have addressed the mechanisms by which it works.

Medical education research naturally uses educational theories, but it would benefit from broadening its scope to include sociological, ecological, economical and systems theories. Integration of diverse disciplines and viewpoints is important and can enhance pedagogy and health care system design. Medical education research would benefit from incorporating more elements of the scientific approach, characterized by iterative cycles of observation, hypothesis formulation, prediction of results based on the hypothesis and experimentation, which would result in expanding the field of knowledge. The present emphasis on competency-based education is an example of a broad educational framework that incorporates theories from systems and implementation science, evaluation research, psychology, and educational technologies to guide the development of hypothesis-driven and exploratory research efforts to improve the practice of medical education.

Grounding in the literature. One important way to improve the theoretical foundation on which MER rests is to carefully examine the existing research literature. However, accessing the literature in MER is costly and often challenging. Medical education research literature databases are not identical to biomedical literature databases. PubMed is not sufficient, although it covers the majority of medical education journals. Many educational problems in the health professions require literature from disciplines outside of medicine. Unfortunately, databases such as PsychInfo, ERIC, and others are seldom provided in many medical libraries. For example, research on burnout and wellness illustrates that, although there is a substantial literature in medicine on these topics, the fundamental theory, principles, and interventions come from other disciplines, such as psychology, human resources, and business.

"Convenience" research vs problem-oriented research. It is common for medical educators to find that they have access to large amounts of data on learners, curricula, and educational outcomes. It is natural that scholars explore these data and often find some interesting results and subsequently, want to publish them. These studies are typically post hoc in nature, rarely have a clear theoretical foundation, and tend not to link well with existing knowledge of the chosen problem. These studies are "convenient" because the data are already collected and the study can be done without having to design an experiment or develop a measurement tool.

Such studies are common in the medical education literature and are not without value, but they do not make as great a contribution to the field of MER as do studies that are designed with a specific research question in mind. Problem-oriented research is designed to provide an answer to a significant problem in the field, often with hard work and deep consideration of innovative studies that contribute to important questions. This is not to say that retrospective studies of existing data are inappropriate or flawed, but scholars need to engage in all the steps of scholarship (deep thinking about a problem, developing a rigorous research question, designing a study to address the research question with validity, selecting or creating measurement procedures, and careful analysis of the results). Examples of convenience research are common in connection with various survey instruments, e.g., learning environment questionnaires, which are often administered to a convenient sample of learners and then reported in a descriptive manner that doesn't advance our broader knowledge or theory on the topic.

Disseminating Medical Education Research

There is a growing number of national and international outlets for scholarly work. These include international journals like Academic Medicine, Medical Education, Teaching & Learning in Medicine, Advances in Health Sciences Education, Medical Teacher, The Network: TUFH journal- Education for Health, etc. Additionally, a growing number of new, online-only journals have become available, such as BMC Medical Education, Medical Education Online, International Journal of Medical Education, and others. Scholars must beware of predatory journals that charge very high publication fees but provide limited distribution of or access to the accepted articles (Garanayak and Ramaiah 2019, Patwardhan 2019). These are often heralded by unsolicited mass emails to physicians and researchers. Limited peer review of these journals results in publication of poor quality scholarship with irreproducible results. One must also be wary of journals with very quick turnaround time as the peer review process is likely to be absent or poor. Regardless of the publication or presentation outlet, it is important for MER to meet quality metrics and essential elements that culminate in scholarship (Glassick, 2000; Cleland, Jamieson, et al. 2021).

Faculty Development in Medical Education Research

Medical education research is a field of specialized knowledge and practice and may require additional training for those seeking to enter. However, many faculty development programs are of short duration, focused on teaching improvement or assessment and do not include development of research capabilities in education. Too often MER has little or no demarcated resource allocation and is under-valued as a faculty pursuit. Still, opportunities for and access to advanced training in MER have increased. International faculty development initiatives such as Centres of Medical Education, established by the WHO, United States-India Educational Foundation (USIEF), Foundation for Advancement of International, Medical Education and Research (FAIMER), The Network: TUFH and several other institutional level initiatives have promoted project-based skill development in education and leadership in medical education through fellowships, with emphasis on converting the project work into educational scholarship – full time as well as part-time/online.

There are a growing number of faculty development offerings for international scholars from organizations such as AMEE or the Asia Pacific Medical education conference. Opportunities are offered locally at medical schools, national specialty and educational societies. Training in research methods, writing and publication, research team function, etc. supports higher quality research, productivity and effective use of research resources. Mentoring in research skills is another important strategy for promoting MER. Funding for faculty from developing countries to pursue training in medical education in institutions abroad has resulted in many of them returning home and developing programs in their home countries (Drendall and Norcini 2019).

Collaborating in Medical Education Research

Medical Education Research seeks to improve both educational practice and theoretical knowledge. Collaborative research is valuable to both goals. International collaborations can leverage these benefits and add to them the power of being able to generalize more fully the impact of the findings of a study that shows similar dynamics and outcomes across international boundaries. Conversely, the collaboration may reveal critical cultural differences that alter these dynamics and outcomes and enrich our theoretical understanding of the phenomenon under study.

Collaborating within and across communities enables the sharing of such resources as expertise in various domains (teaching methods, curriculum development, decision making, psychometrics, research methods, etc.). Specialized knowledge is not evenly distributed and forming collaborations is an important strategy for investigators to acquire that expertise. Similarly, research infrastructure resources can also be shared within a collaboration. Computing and data analysis software, survey development and administration, specialized simulation equipment, and other necessities for research can provide incentives for building collaborations.

However, the sharing of resources and expertise that makes international collaborations attractive can lead to challenges in administration and the relationships among the investigators if there is imbalance in resource contributions. Such resource imbalances may be necessary but care must be taken to prevent them from becoming imbalances in intellectual contributions to the study. All partners in the collaboration should have equal rights to designing the study, interpreting the data, and writing the manuscript. Similarly, authorship should not be determined by who contributed the most resources to the collaboration but by intellectual and scholarly contribution. The complexity of such collaborations is shown in Table 1 based on the work by Larkan et al., (Larkan, Uduma et al. 2016) which shows core concepts (e.g., focus, values, equity, benefit, communication, leadership and resolution) and associated attributes that contribute to successful global MER partnerships.

Such international collaborations have grown in number over the past decade. One example is the collaborative effort of the Maharashtra University of the Health Sciences (MUHS) and the University of Michigan to jointly develop a competency-based master's degree program in health professions education. The collaboration focused on defining educational competencies that were salient to both cultures, educational research being a major one, and operational principles that addressed shared and unique characteristics of the educational institutions. The collaboration was supported by a grant from the United States-India Educational Foundation, which enabled teams from each institution to visit the other institution to develop the blueprint for the program. An important part of this collaboration was that experts from both India and the U.S. were equally engaged in the development process, and mutually shared resources and ideas. Both institutions ultimately were able to establish their particular version of the shared program.

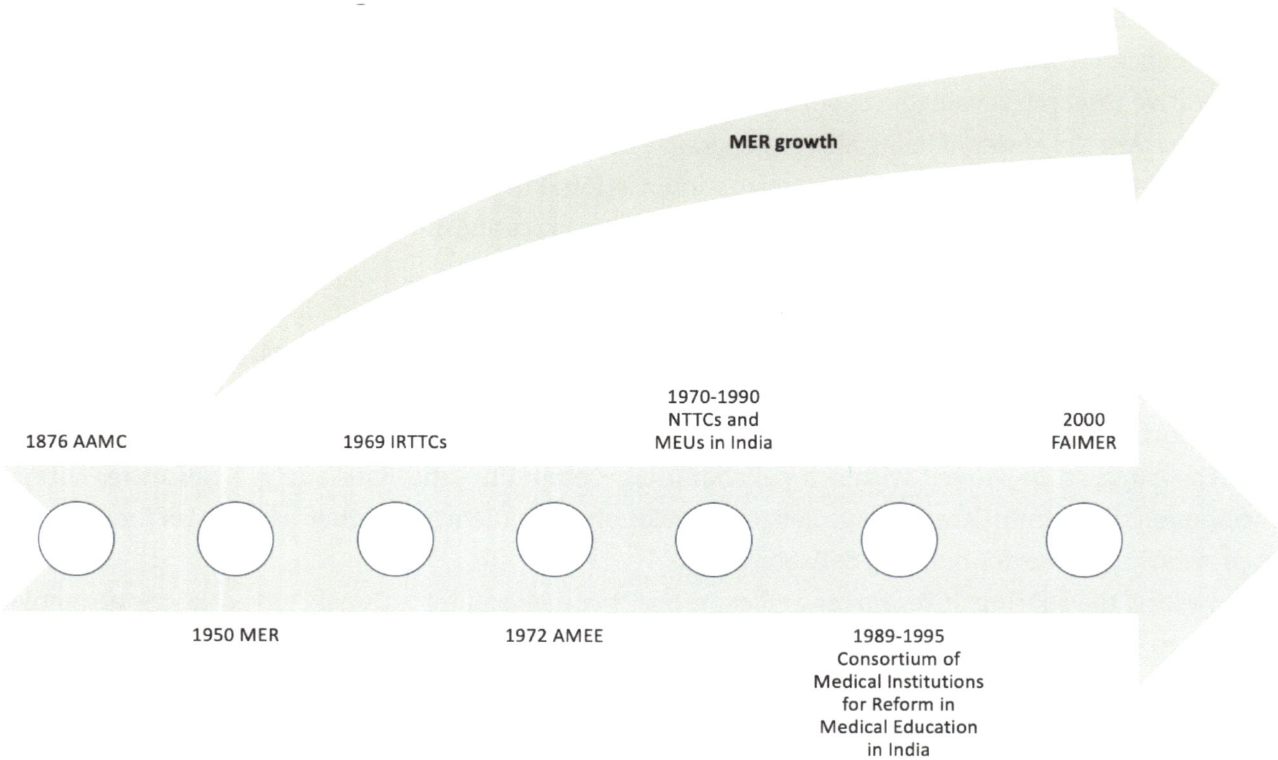

MER: Medical Education Research, AAMC: Association of American Medical Colleges, AMEE: Association for Medical Education in Europe, IRTTCs: International Regional Teacher Training Centers, NRTTCs: National Teacher Training Centers, MEUs: Medical Education Units, FAIMER: Foundation for Advancement in International Medical Education and Research,

Figure 1: Timeline for Development of Medical Education Research and the Organizations That Supported Its Growth

Table 1: Core Concepts and Attributes Necessary for Successful Global Mer Partnerships (derived from Larkan, Uduma et al. 2016)

Core concepts	Attributes
Focus	Common goals, shared interest, vision.
Values	Culture, societal norms, trust, commitment.
Equity	Recognition, respect for different capacities, sharing resources, inclusion.
Benefit	Reciprocal, mutually beneficial, skills generation, rewarding experience, knowledge exchange.
Communication	Transparent, open, honest, consistent, effective.
Leadership	Delegation of roles, responsibilities, accountability, balance, diplomacy.
Resolution	Resolve, perseverance, determination, mediation, conflict resolution.

Conclusion

Medical education research is essential to developing better educational programs and understanding the complexities of medical competence. It addresses both practical and theoretical concerns but, at present, it does not represent an even examination of the diverse contexts in which medical education is conducted worldwide. Much more attention and effort need to be devoted to research efforts by international collaborations that seek a broader sampling of settings and cultures. Only with a truly international body of research evidence will we be able to make wise judgments about improving medical education and practice in local and global settings.

SUMMARIZE

- Medical education research (MER) is a multidisciplinary and complex domain of study which provides the evidence and criteria for making informed educational decisions.
- MER includes research on teaching and learning (the practice of medical education) and on fundamental mechanisms and phenomena with the goal of building theory.
- MER is often based on educational theories, however, integration of diverse disciplines is important and can enhance pedagogy and health care system design.
- MER often lacks the formulation of models and theories and does not build upon previous results; both replication and innovation are critical in MER
- There are various types of MER - quantitative, qualitative and mixed methods.
- Reviewing the existing research literature is key to building a theoretical foundation, however accessing it may be costly and challenging.
- "Convenience" studies, which are retrospective studies of existing data, do not make as great a contribution to the field of MER as do studies with a specific research question in mind.
- Opportunities for and access to advanced training in MER have increased through international and national organizations, including subspecialty societies.
- Collaborating within and across communities enables the sharing of resources
- MER benefits from international collaborations which ensure that a world-view is achieved to guide curricular reform, international standardization of competencies, and that the needs of local patient populations and healthcare are met.
- Resource imbalances within international collaborations may be unavoidable, however, care must be taken to ensure that the intellectual contributions to the study are equitable.

EVALUATE

Considering the points raised in this chapter, what would be a research question relevant to your context that would be of possible interest to medical educators in a different country or culture?

How would you seek to find these international collaborators? Where would you look?

How would you set up a collaboration? What areas of strength would you bring to the collaboration and what areas of support would you need from collaborators?

How could your national, regional, or cultural medical education community develop more organizational support for MER and collaboration? What can you do to support those organizations?

ROAD AHEAD

Medical education research continues to grow in quantity and quality, but there are many challenges confronting it. Funding, faculty development, research resources, and collaborations have all been identified above. Additional challenges are emerging. Medical education research has typically been driven by educational theories and perspectives, but there are alternatives that may merge with MER, such as systems research, quality improvement studies, and clinical outcomes assessment. The world's health care needs and resources are becoming more entangled - witness the impact of the COVID pandemic. The other health professions are advancing their own research efforts and outlets, which should receive a welcoming embrace by medical education researchers. Finally, there is the continuous turnover of senior investigators and scholars to be replaced by junior colleagues with innovative ideas and enthusiasm. We believe the future of MER is rich and dynamic and we hope that it will evolve to reflect the needs of the global health care system.

REFERENCES

Albert, M., B. Hodges and G. Regehr (2007). "Research in medical education: balancing service and science." *Adv Health Sci Educ Theory Pract* **12**(1): 103-115.

Beckman, T. J. and D. A. Cook (2007). "Developing scholarly projects in education: a primer for medical teachers." *Med Teach* **29**(2-3): 210-218.

Bordage, G. (2009). "Conceptual frameworks to illuminate and magnify." *Med Educ* **43**(4): 312-319.

Buffone, B., I. Djuana, K. Yang, K. J. Wilby, M. S. El Hajj and K. Wilbur (2020). "Diversity in health professional education scholarship: a document analysis of international author representation in leading journals." *BMJ Open* **10**(11): e043970.

Cleland, J.A., S. Jamieson, R.A. Kusurkar, S. Ramani, T.J. Wilkinson, S. van Schalkwyk (2021). Redefining scholarship for health professions education: AMEE Guide No. 142. *Med Teach* 1-15.

Cook, D. A., G. Bordage and H. G. Schmidt (2008). "Description, justification and clarification: a framework for classifying the purposes of research in medical education." *Med Educ* **42**(2): 128-133.

Crites, G. E., J. K. Gaines, S. Cottrell, S. Kalishman, M. Gusic, B. Mavis and S. J. Durning (2014). "Medical education scholarship: an introductory guide: AMEE Guide No. 89." *Med Teach* **36**(8): 657-674.

Drendall, J. and J.J. Norcini (2019). "FAIMER fellowship programs: An international, project-centred approach to improving health through health professions education." *The Asia-Pacific Scholar: Medical and Health Professions Education* 4(1): 1-3.

Frenk, J., L. Chen, Z.A. Bhutta, J. Cohen, N. Crisp, T. Evans, H. Fineberg, P. Garcia, Y. Ke, P. Kelley, B. Kistnasamy, A. Meleis, D. Naylor, A. Pablos-Mendez, S. Reddy, S. Scrimshaw, J. Sepulveda, D. Serwadda, and H. Zurayk (2010). "Health professionals for a new century: transforming education to strengthen health systems in an interdependent world. *Lancet* **376**(9756): 1923-1958.

Garanayak, S. and C.K. Ramaiah (2019). "Predatory Journals Publishing Trend in India: A Study." University News. **57**(38): 11-18.

Glassick, C. E. (2000). "Boyer's expanded definitions of scholarship, the standards for assessing scholarship, and the elusiveness of the scholarship of teaching." *Acad Med* **75**(9): 877-880.

Hodges, B. D. and A. Kuper (2012). "Theory and practice in the design and conduct of graduate medical education." *Acad Med* **87**(1): 25-33.

Kuper, A., M. Albert and B. D. Hodges (2010). "The origins of the field of medical education research." *Acad Med* **85**(8): 1347-1353.

Larkan, F., O. Uduma, S. A. Lawal and B. van Bavel (2016). "Developing a framework for successful research partnerships in global health." *Global Health* **12**(1): 17.

Norman, G. (2011). "Fifty years of medical education research: waves of migration." *Med Educ* **45**(8): 785-791.

Patwardhan, B. (2019). "India strikes back against predatory journals." *Nature* 571:7.

Ringsted, C., B. Hodges and A. Scherpbier (2011). "'The research compass': an introduction to research in medical education: *AMEE Guide no. 56.*" *Med Teach* **33**(9): 695-709.

Rotgans, J. I. (2012). "The themes, institutions, and people of medical education research 1988-2010: content analysis of abstracts from six journals." *Adv Health Sci Educ Theory Pract* **17**(4): 515-527.

Srinivas, D. K. and B.V. Adkoli (2009). "Faculty development in medical education in India: The need of the day." *Al Ameen J Med Sci* 2(1): 6-13.

Ten Cate, O. (2021). "Health professions education scholarship: The emergence, current status, and future of a discipline in its own right." *FASEB Bioadv* **3**(7): 510-522.

ADDITIONAL INFORMATION

Opportunities for Networking and Collaboration

Many medical education organizations with international representation focus on networking for faculty development in medical education and on creating collaborative opportunities for medical educators and researchers around the globe. The Foundation for Advancement of International Medical Education and Research (FAIMER), the Association of American Medical Colleges (AAMC), the Association for Medical Education in Europe (AMEE), and The Network: Towards Unity for Health (TUFH) will be presented in this online version of the chapter. To learn more about other medical education organizations and collaboration opportunities use the following link *https://www.omed.pitt.edu/medical-education-organizations.*

The Foundation for Advancement of International Medical Education and Research (FAIMER)

The Foundation for Advancement of International Medical Education and Research (FAIMER) was established in 2000 by the Educational Commission for Foreign Medical Graduate (ECFMG) as a non-profit organization to improve the health of communities by cultivating international medical education through curriculum development and the support for research *https://www.faimer.org.*

The strategic goal for FAIMER focuses on three thematic areas: creating educational opportunities for medical educators; discovering patterns and disseminating knowledge; and developing data resources. The geographic focus of the organization is on under-resourced areas like South Asia, Africa, and Latin America.

Create Educational Opportunities for Medical Educators

FAIMER has two fellowship programs to train medical educators: the *International FAIMER Institute* that prepares health profession educators as leaders and curriculum developers in their home institutions and *FAIMER Regional Institute* that focuses on improving medical education in developing regions in Asia, Africa and Latin America through advancing FAIMER's regional centers of improvement in local medical education systems. To graduate from the fellowship programs, participants are expected to submit a proposal for educational change in their home institutions.

Discover Patterns and Disseminate Knowledge

FAIMER supports Medical Education Research initiatives and collaborations between medical educators. It focuses on three main areas: *International Migration of Physicians*, *United States Physician Workforce Issues*, *International Medical Education Programs.* The scale of this effort helps inform policy makers in government, academia, and various other interested organizations.

Develop Data Resources

FAIMER attempts to collect and present valuable medical education data and resources for international medical schools and their graduates. To achieve this goal the organization developed and maintained different directories: the Directory of Organizations that Recognizes and Accredits medical schools (*DORA*), the Directory of *Master's* and *Ph.D* programs in Health Profession Education worldwide, and the *World Directory of Medical Schools* that was established in association with the World Federation for Medical Education (WFME) to provide a comprehensive collection of accurate and up-to-date information of Medical Schools in the world.

The Association of American Medical Colleges (AAMC)

The AAMC was established in 1876 when deans and faculty from 22 colleges met at the Jefferson Medical college in Philadelphia "to consider all matters relating to reform in medical college work." The work then was focused on regulating medical education in order to improve trust between medical schools. AAMC annual meetings were then used as a platform for medical school deans to discuss medical education issues and regulations. Presently, the association is known for its major role in helping medical colleges select applicants for medical schools and residency. AAMC develops and regulates the Medical College Admission Test (MCAT©), the American Medical College Application Service (AMCAS) and the Electronic Residency Application Service (ERAS).

AAMC currently includes 172 accredited medical colleges in the United States and Canada with more than 400 teaching hospitals and health systems. Its mission focuses on achieving excellence in four areas: medical education, patient care, medical research, and diversity, inclusion and equity in health care.

The organization provides knowledge, resources and counselling for pre-medical students, medical students and residents through AAMC students and residents web page, *https://students-residents.aamc.org/*; and forms affinity groups to provide its members with access to professional growth, leadership development, networking and collaborations opportunities, *https://www.aamc.org/professional-development/affinity-groups.*

Group on Educational Affairs (GEA)

Since 1969, passionate medical educators have collaborated to form the GEA affinity group to improve medical education in North America through faculty development, curriculum development, educational research, and assessment in undergraduate, graduate, and continuing medical education. The GEA has four regions: Central GEA (CGEA), North eastern GEA (NEGEA), Southern GEA (SGEA), and Western GEA (WGEA). GEA regions form special interest groups to provide opportunities for members to collaborate in order to advance specific areas in medical education (i.e., Educational Leadership, Faculty Development, Interprofessional Education, Libraries in Medical Education, etc.).

The GEA has four sections to encompass the continuum of medical education, Undergraduate Medical Education to promote education of medical students from selection to graduation; Graduate Medical Education (GME) to promote education of physicians during residency training; Continuing Professional Development (CPD) to promote education for physicians throughout their careers; Medical Education Scholarship Research and Evaluation (MESRE) that focuses on improving the quality of research in medical education and its application to educational practice.

To accomplish its mission, MESRE creates collaborating opportunities through different GEA regions in the following areas: improving the quality of medical education scholarship, research, and evaluation; fostering the professional development of medical educators who seek to contribute to scholarship, research, and evaluation; building awareness and discourse in medical education scholarship to promote social justice and address health inequities; facilitating the exchange of new knowledge and research findings; and disseminating the results of novel scholarship, research, and evaluation and encouraging their application to educational practice in multiple contexts.

Additionally, MESRE publishes an annotated Bibliography of Journals for Educational Scholarship. It has detailed information about topics, types of manuscripts, and audiences for more than 60 journals that publish medical education manuscripts (*link*).

Conferences

AAMC facilitates yearly regional affinity groups meetings, however, *Learn Serve and Lead* is the signature learning and networking event, where professionals from all over North America gather to discover new ideas, discuss emerging innovations, and share experience *https://www.aamc.org/professional-development/events/learn-serve-lead*.

Funding

AAMC receives grants from the US federal government and private organizations for the work on different areas relevant to the mission of AAMC *https://www.aamc.org/what-we-do/grants-and-awards-received*.

Journals

Academic Medicine is the official, peer-reviewed journal of the AAMC. Its main focus is on the following areas: education and training issues; health and science policy; institutional policy, management, and values; research practice; and clinical practice in academic settings.

The Association for Medical Education in Europe (AMEE)

The AMEE was established in 1972 to facilitate communications among medical educators and to strengthen national associations for medical education throughout Europe. It is the European regional association of the World Federation for Medical Education (EFME) and a member of the WFME Executive Council. Over the last 10 years, AMEE expanded its influence and activities to become an international association with members from more than 90 countries worldwide.

The Association for Medical Education in Europe (AMEE) is a membership organization that assists teachers, physicians, researchers, administrators, curriculum developers, assessors and students stay up to date with the rapidly changing health professions education in the world through educational activities: annual conferences, publications, face-to-face courses, online courses, AMEE for students, webinars and other initiatives *https://amee.org/home.*

AMEE is led by an executive committee consisting of a leader, general/treasury secretary, six members, two nominated students, the president of WFME and the immediate WFME past president. One of AMEE main objective strategies is to be the foremost global community of health education stakeholders through encouraging diverse and collaborative global community, building strategies for international engagement of medical education stakeholders at individual and institutional levels, create communities of practice that include specialists in regional challenges in medical education and use AMEE conferences as means for global networking and knowledge sharing in medical education.

Conferences

The AMEE annual conference provides an opportunity for international collaboration and networking with others of similar interest in addition to the chance to learn from experts in medical education, and through variable workshops, teaching conferences, courses and seminars. It is held usually late August/mid-September every year.

The Ottawa Conference focuses on the assessment of competence in medical education. It provides an assembly for medical educators to network, share ideas and knowledge relevant to assessment of competence throughout the continuum of education.

Journal

Medical Teacher is the official monthly peer reviewed journal for the AMEE medical-teacher. Other journals include MedEdPublish, AMEE guide and Best Evidence Medical Education (BEME) guide.

Courses and Master Classes

AMEE offers different opportunities for face-to-face and online Essential Skills in Medical Education (ESME) courses and master classes. The aim for these courses is to provide educators with fundamental principles and updates on current best practice for medical education. They target different aspects like (medical education research, assessment, feedback, clinical teaching, leadership and management, etc.) *https://amee.org/what-is-amee/courses.*

Initiatives

AMEE has initiative programs to highlight and support specific yet essential aspects in medical education.

- askAMEE (*https://www.askamee.org/*) is an online tool that provides evidence-based and readily available answers to common questions relating to medical education hot topics such as feedback, Entrustable Professional activities (EPAs), lectures, Problem-Based Learning (PBL), etc.
- ASPIRE-to-Excellence initiative (*https://www.aspire-to-excellence.org/*) is a program to recognize and reward medical, dental and veterinary schools and institutions with excellent educational initiatives in different areas like assessment of students, curriculum development, faculty development, simulation, etc.
- Best Evidence Medical Education (BEME) (*http://www.bemecollaboration.org/*) is an international group of medical educators, universities and organizations committed to the advancement of evidence-based educational practices in medical education through: creating a culture of evidence-based education among individuals and institutions; publishing systematic review articles for best evidence/practice to be made available for the public; supporting individual medical educators and institutions to adopt best evidence in their educational practice.
- AMEE MedEdWorld (*https://www.mededworld.org/Home.aspx*) is an international online HP education community that shares expertise to advance education. Its website and monthly newsletter provide updates on the latest developments from organizations and individuals in the medical education field; details of education courses and conferences worldwide; information about emerging learning technologies; access to a range of education resources; and a variety of recommended publications and resources relevant to health professionals.

The Network: Towards Unity for Health

The Network: Toward Unity for Health (TUFH) was created in 1979 by the World Health Organization (WHO) as a consortium of 18 medical schools invited from across the world - institutions that represent innovative models of health professions education for improved health, healthcare access and health care delivery. It has since played a significant role in promoting healthcare equity through community-based education, dynamic research, and dedicated rural service. Its three pillars of focus to address global and local health needs have been social accountability, innovative medical education pedagogy such as problem-based learning, integrated clerkships, interprofessional education and healthcare, etc. and communities at risk, including rural and indigenous communities, women and the elderly. It emphasizes social accountability, equity, relevance and cost effectiveness as core values for informing health policy. *https://thenetworktufh.org.*

In over 40 years since inception, it has endeavored to improve access and equity in health care, trying to help build community-oriented medical schools, encompassing academic- community partnerships. The collaborating schools from developed and developing countries have both learnt from and often adapted each other's innovative practices.

With expansion from institutional membership to include like-minded organizations, community health institutions, students, professionals and thought leaders as members, it has since evolved to become a global connector- "The Network of Networks"

Activities

The Network: TUFH has a Global Advisory Board, a Secretariat Consortium and various task forces: Social Accountability, Interprofessional Education and Practice, Women's Health Indigenous and Remote and Rural Health. The members engage in collaborative activities in alignment with the Network's mission such as student and faculty exchange as well as innovative projects in addition to the work done through the task forces. The Annual Conferences hosted by member organizations are opportunities for the task forces to meet, share experiences and learn from each other. An online community, Leadership Academies, Student Academies, and TUFH Institutes are new additions to its activities.

Journal

The Network has its own journal *Education for Health* that serves as an outlet for the innovations and research done by the member institutions. The journal is Medline-indexed and is in its 34th year of publication. It is an open-access journal that actively encourages submissions from international contributors and students and aims to bridge the publishing divide, giving universal access to high quality publications. *https://www.educationforhealth.net/aboutus.asp.*

The journal also publishes special issues related to conference themes and the overall mission of the Network. *Education for Health* has published 864 articles from 72 countries between 2000 – 2020 and has an equally diverse reviewer pool from over 40 countries.

Annual Conferences

The annual conferences of The Network: TUFH are hosted by member organizations and provide opportunities for students and health professionals to engage with each other to form an "intergenerational community" where "bidirectional learning occurs." The conferences are highly participatory. Site visits to local non-profit organizations, health care centres and local communities provide a glimpse of activities in the host country and an opportunity to experience the local cultures and practices. *https://thenetworktufh.org/tufh-conferences.*

There are different formats for participants to present their work:

- Interactive thematic oral poster presentations
- Moderated group discussions and brainstorming sessions
- Workshops often related to the Networks' themes
- TUFH Talks moderated by experts with interactive discussions.

Participants are also invited to attend, participate, and engage during the keynote speeches; task force meetings; regional meetings; solutions challenge; and the general assembly meeting.

Chapter 2

Medical Education Research in India: The Journey Through the Years

Anshu, Avinash Supe

ABSTRACT

Medical education has taken center stage in India over the last two decades. While the initial years of faculty development were spent in strengthening different facets of instructional design, assessment and curricular development, it is time for medical educationists to shift the focus to the next level, i.e., to educational research and scholarship.

At the moment, the kind of educational research being conducted by faculty in the health professions is basic, piecemeal, and not very robust. A cursory review of publications from this country will reveal that a number of measures will need to be taken to encourage the quality of research, which then eventually can create an impact on the educational environment.

Concerted efforts need to be taken to encourage credible research. Some of these measures are: training, mentoring, supervision, support, provision of educational grants, incentives, rewards etc. Large-scale collaborative research needs to be encouraged. Ultimately, research should inform and impact practice and policy.

Key Words: medical education, educational research, India, health professions education, scholarship

ASSESS NEED

In the last two decades, medical education has taken remarkable strides in the educational framework of India. From an unknown speciality it has gradually become a stand-alone discipline. Further, with the recent corona virus pandemic and the shift to competency-based medical education, the quality of medical education has come into the spotlight. Given that India produces the world's highest number of medical graduates from a country, it is only logical that faculty development and quality of training were uppermost on our minds. While there has been considerable thrust on training faculty in curriculum design, instructional methods, and assessment in the last two decades, an important arm of faculty development, educational research, is still relatively in its stage of infancy in India (Rege & Bhuiyan, 2015; Adkoli, 2020).

This chapter looks at the medical education research scenario in India, and explores how it has evolved over the last few decades. It then goes on to analyse the strengths, areas of concerns and challenges; and then outlines the way forward.

BRIEF

- In India, it is now time for medical educationists to shift the focus to educational research.
- Presently, the educational research studies conducted in this country are rather basic and lack methodological rigor. There is need to encourage credible and robust research through several supportive measures such as: training, mentoring, and provision of incentives.
- There is need to choose areas of research which are relevant to the educational context of the country.
- Educational research must eventually inform educational practice and alter policy.

CONTEXTUALIZE

One might question the need for health professions faculty to get into educational research. Before you read further, pause and reflect on these questions. Think, make notes and jot down your thoughts.

- If teachers are able to communicate well, deliver instruction to their students, and assess them, is there any need to venture into the area of research?
- Health professions faculty are already overworked handling the dual arms of providing clinical service and teaching. Is it worth expending extra energy and effort into research?
- Is it easier to conduct educational research compared to biomedical research? Are their methods different?
- Does publishing a paper based on educational research help in promotion or placement? Is it even counted as actual research by universities?
- Can research conducted at the workplace actually create an impact elsewhere? How can research improve one's practice or alter policy in our workplaces?

DESCRIBE

India has the world's largest number of medical schools and we produce the highest number of medical graduates each year (Supe & Burdick, 2006; Sood, 2008). Training such large numbers of medical students demands committed, enthusiastic, and well-trained faculty.

In the recent years, there has been a renewed interest in using formal and informal approaches to faculty development. Most of these are through mandatory courses in basic medical education technology conducted by the national regulatory bodies, such as the erstwhile Medical Council of India and the present National Medical Commission. Besides these, advanced courses in medical education, degree/

diploma courses in health professions education run by universities, and several fellowship programmes in educational leadership are available for capacity building of health professions faculty in India.

While the first phase of medical education interventions included training the faculty in educational methods and assessment techniques, the last decade has seen lots of activity in curriculum design and development. Now that we have seen satisfactory capacity building in the former areas, in the third phase, it is now time to strengthen the foundation of educational research.

Medical teachers expend a lot of their time and energy in instructional design, assessment and curricular development. These experiences can be converted into scholarship. In his seminal paper, Boyer (1991) described the "scholarship of discovery, application, integration and teaching". Elsewhere in this book you can find details of these concepts. However, the basic premise behind these concepts is to find avenues where one's daily work, is carefully assembled, analyzed, and studied in a systematic way, so as to derive conclusions that can be extrapolated to the larger scheme of things.

Health professions teachers need to be trained in converting their activities into scholarly work. The activity-scholarship double-helix model illustrates the process of converting routine educational activities into scholarship (Morahan & Fleetwood, 2008). By sharing their carefully designed resources, their expertise, and their experiences in a scientific manner, it is possible to feed into the cycle of continuous quality improvement, and alter the educational environment and ecology.

The Journey of Educational Research in India

Let us have a look at how educational research has progressed through the years in India.

National Teachers Training Course

One of the earliest forays which encouraged faculty to take up educational projects came from the National Teachers Training Centre (NTTC) at Pondicherry. Participants enrolled into a fortnight-long course. Towards the end of the course, they were encouraged to propose a short project that they would undertake at their parent institution. While many participants did conduct these studies, there was no rigorous follow-up to ensure their completion or to measure their impact (Adkoli, 2017). Some participants went on to publish their studies in the NTTC Bulletin published from this centre. With time, this process has got better. The NTTC Alumni Association, JIPMER (2020) has published an e-book on "Effective Educational Practices in Health Profession Education (A Collection of Educational Projects completed by NTTC Alumni from 2006 to 2013)". The collection features 42 projects from 2006-2013 on a wide range of topics. Some of these are on innovative topics such as cadaver ceremonies, 3D models to enhance clinical skills, gamification in pharmacology, and flipped classes in histology.

FAIMER Regional Institutes

A huge impetus to educational research came after the year 2005 when the Foundation for Advancement of International Medical Education and Research (FAIMER), USA started its educational regional fellowship programmes at three sites: KEM Hospital and Seth GS Medical College, Mumbai (2005), Christian Medical College Ludhiana (2006), PSG Institute of Medical Sciences Coimbatore (2007); followed by another institute in 2015, the MAHE-FAIMER International Institute for Leadership in Interprofessional Education, Manipal.

Fellows wishing to apply to these programmes had to submit an educational project as part of their application. Through the fellowship programme, fellows were first mentored on-site and taken through a process of refining their projects using the Theory of Change. This was followed by a year-long online follow-up process where fellows were encouraged to explore educational resources, and provided support and supervision (Anshu et al, 2008).

Fellows chose projects to be conducted at their parent institutions in a variety of subjects such as: curriculum design, teaching-learning methods, assessment, faculty development, community-based medical education, humanities etc. The pie-diagram below (Fig.1) shows a broad categorization of educational research projects (N=741) undertaken by fellows of these programmes. Data were obtained from the following years: GSMC-FAIMER (2005-2019), CMCL-FAIMER (2011-2020), PSG-FAIMER (2007-2019) and MAHE-FAIMER (2015-2020).

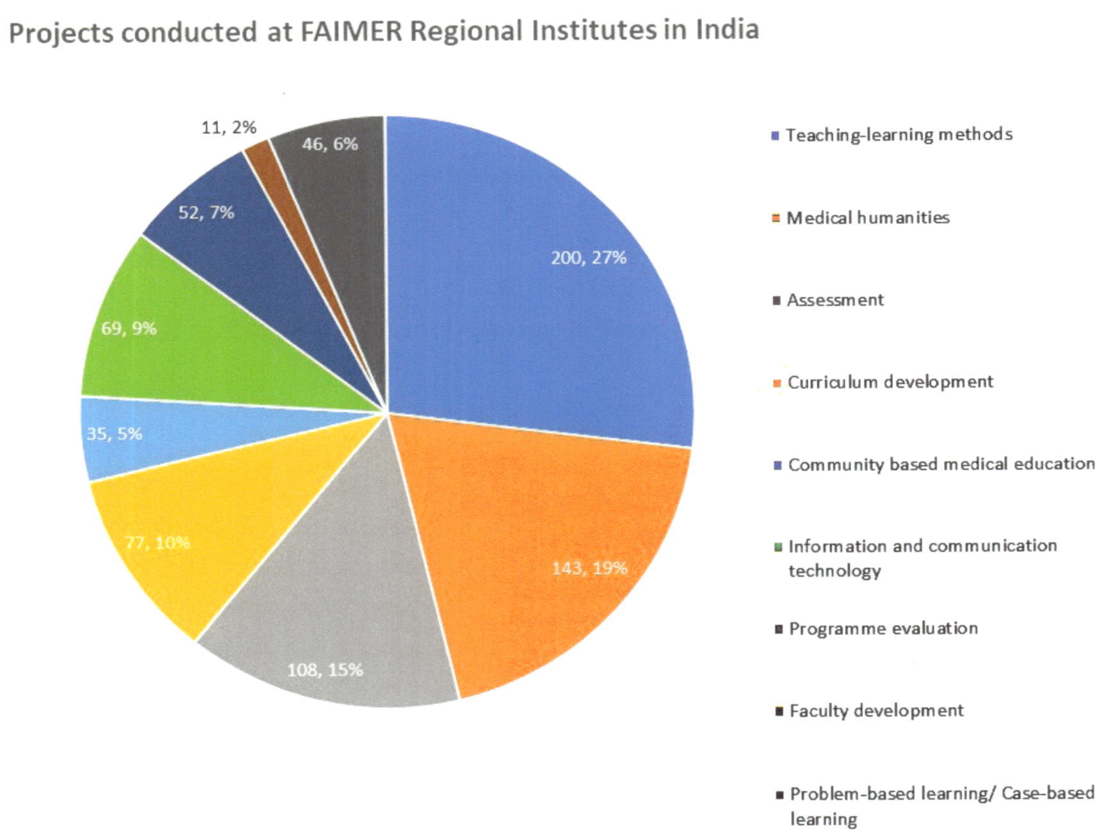

Courtesy: Directors of Regional FAIMER Institutes in India who shared this Data

What definitely worked in improving the quality of projects, was the inherent process of the fellowship programme, which encouraged fellows to explore and read educational literature. Structured online discussions helped to clarify issues and improve the robustness of study designs and study instruments. Peer and faculty feedback were provided as fellows worked in groups. Sharing of resources and ideas, as well as brain-storming sessions helped in refining the quality of the projects.

Throughout the year, fellows were required to submit phase-wise project progress reports online. This process culminated in the interactive presentation of a poster at the end of the fellowship before two batches of fellows and all faculty. In the second year of the project, fellows were mentored to write for publication. A large number of projects went on to be published in local, national and international journals.

With time, the process has become more robust and the quality of projects has improved. Since the Fellowship programme deals with elements of educational leadership, themes such as managing and implementing change are a part of the curriculum. The focus of these projects has now been moulded with more emphasis on sustainability of change in the institutions and beyond, once the initial project has been done. The design and the evaluation processes of these projects have been structured in an attempt to make a long-term impact beyond individual classrooms; either by their inclusion as departmental or institutional programmes or as university policy.

Advance Course in Medical Education

A combination of these processes was followed by the Medical Council of India in its Advance Course in Medical Education which was a year long course with on-site and online components. These courses were run by ten Nodal Centres across the country. Participants in these workshops were encouraged to present a study proposal towards the end of the first part of the workshop, submit progress reports, and present posters at the end of the second part of the workshop after a year. Almost 1800 faculty members who were participants completed their educational research projects under this programme and were awarded certification for the same. There will be useful to conduct a formal evaluation of all these projects to determine their sustainability and overall impact in the educational landscape of this country.

National Conferences in Health Professions Education

Since 2007, a series of National Conferences in Health Professions Education have been held across the country. These conferences have provided a platform for faculty to showcase their work. Slowly, through the years, the number and quality of abstracts and posters presented at these conferences has risen impressively. From small projects conducted in individual classrooms being presented in the early conferences, projects presented now show better study design and more frequent interdisciplinary collaboration. Since the faculty who attend these workshops come from all health professions specialities and across disciplines, this has encouraged collaboration between disciplines to some level. The overall interest in educational research has been encouraging and the snow-ball effect resulted in many peers taking up similar projects.

Current Trends in Publication of Educational Research

Initially not many journals in India accepted educational studies for publication. But now it is heartening to know that almost every speciality has its own medical education section, and the number of avenues for publication have increased. Concerted efforts through sessions on scholarship have helped faculty-researchers become more aware of where they can find a suitable audience for their work.

We explored the publications in educational research across the decades. Fig.2 depicts the Pubmed indexed publications from India in the area of medical education from 1941-2020.

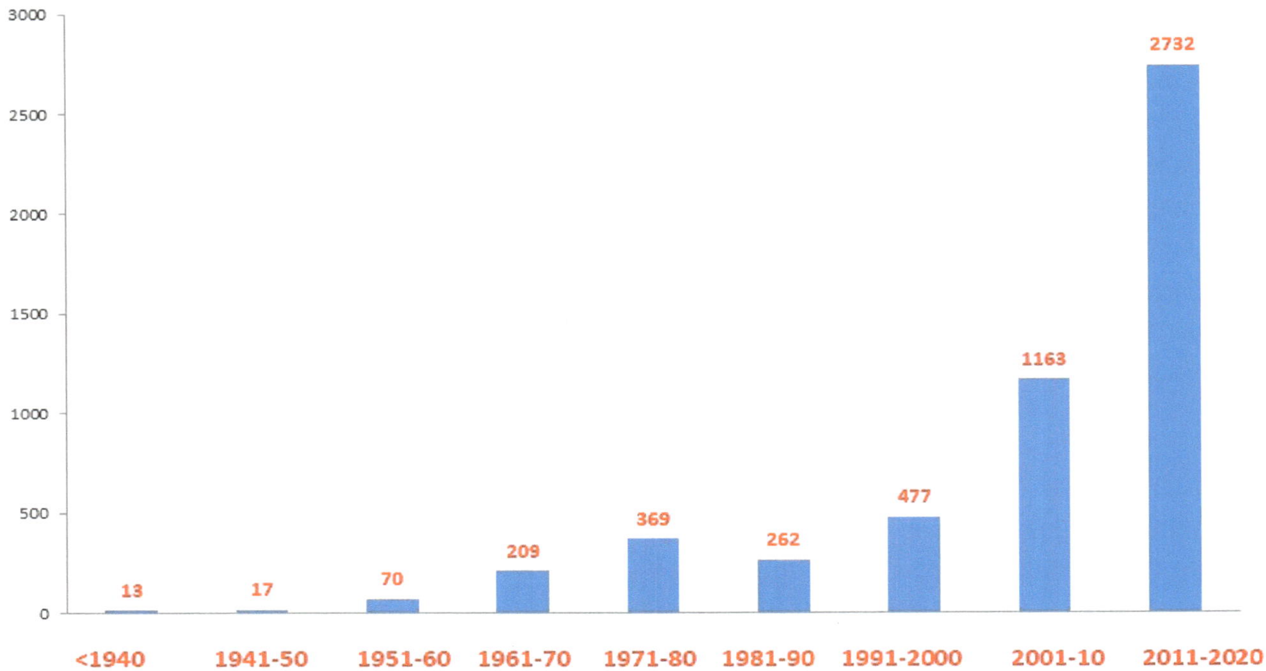

Figure 2: Publications in Medical Education from India (1941-2020)

(This data has been extracted from PubMed using a systematic process. The authors wish to thank Mrs. Vasumathi Sriganesh for her support and assistance)

There has been a substantial increase in the number of health professions faculty taking up educational research projects.

Dongre and Deshmukh (2019) carried out a systemic analysis of original papers in medical education published from India over a 10-year period (2006-14). Most studies were evaluations of undergraduate students. There was limited research on other target groups and stakeholders such as postgraduate students, interns or faculty. They found that of the 71 articles that were retrieved by them, 64.7% were evaluations of innovations at Kirkpatrick's level 1. The remaining 35.3% were surveys or research articles. Of them, 74.6% used quantitative methods, 18.3% used mixed methods and only 7% used qualitative methods. Almost 90% studies were conducted at a single site. Almost 23(32%) articles acknowledged support from FAIMER which is indicative of their impact on training faculty in educational research. Only 8.5% of the studies had received any form of financial support. Most studies only used Kirkpatrick's level 1 to evaluate learner satisfaction. The authors felt that the higher levels of Kirkpatrick's model will need to be explored to determine change in organizational practices and the consequent effect on patient outcomes. Predictive studies which can assess the validity of our student selection processes were also recommended.

Recognition of Educational Research By Regulatory Bodies in India

In 2009, the Medical Council of India released the teacher eligibility criteria for promotion of medical teachers to different levels, and one of the requirements was the number of research publications. It mandated that only research papers published in journals of national associations and societies of the concerned subject or speciality would count for this purpose (Medical Council of India, 2009). It was only in 2016, that the Academic Cell of the Medical Council of India released a clarification saying that "... publications in the field of medical education technology in indexed or national journal will be considered as valid and on par with publications in the concerned subject/speciality for placements and promotions..."(Medical Council of India notification, 2016). This was a step in the positive direction where educational research embedded within the specialty was given due recognition. However, this statement was further amended in a General Body Meeting the next year, where it was stated that "not more than one research publication in the field of medical educational technology in indexed or national journals shall be considered towards eligibility for promotion..." (Medical Council of India notification, 2017). While it is logical that subject-specific biomedical research is expected from faculty in their core disciplines, we feel that minimum number of publications in the core discipline could have been defined, rather than putting a cap on the number of medical education publications.

Concerns About Educational Research in India

The ultimate outcome of any kind of educational research is that it must inform practice and advance the quality of education. It is here that many of our research projects falter. Several projects are weakly designed, lack methodological rigour, and are often done with the purpose of adding another publication to a CV, rather than with the aims of either creating new knowledge or bringing about actual change in the workplace.

Educational research has the added issue of being conducted in a complex ecosystem where controlled conditions are not possible (Ringsted, Hodges & Scherpbier, 2011). Unlike biomedical research, stringent measurements for outcomes such as learning or performance cannot be made. Since most new entrants to this area are unfamiliar with these intricacies, studies are often found to have glaring deficiencies in study design. Poor study design cannot lead to practically useful research. Like any other research, the process of inquiry must be systematic and scientifically done. The robustness of study design and the planning that goes into conceptualizing a study cannot be undermined. In India, often researchers are seen to pay emphasis on gathering data and analysing it. However, the key step, which is the use of a theoretical framework, which is key to educational research, is often forgotten.

Projects which have been published are often simplistic and are usually conducted on one class of students. There is hardly any vision for follow-up and collaborative projects across institutions are not common. Projects with more meaningful outcomes which impact either practice or policy need to be promoted. We are in a stage of curricular upheaval where a new curricular model has been introduced. It is time to conduct regular research, monitoring and evaluation into how this change is impacting medical education. Results of these initiatives need to be fed into the curricular cycle to begin a rigorous cycle of quality improvement. Similarly, the impact of our selection processes should be evaluated based on the performance of our graduates in actual practice.

The Way Ahead

It is heartening to see the increasing number of health professions faculty in India showing an interest in pursuing research in education. Even through it appears to be propelled by promotion requirements defined by the regulatory bodies, hopefully, it will eventually find serious takers who will pursue quality research. One must remember that medical education research in India is in its stage of infancy. Fig.3 depicts some of the approaches that will encourage a cadre of faculty to take up educational research. These are explained below in detail.

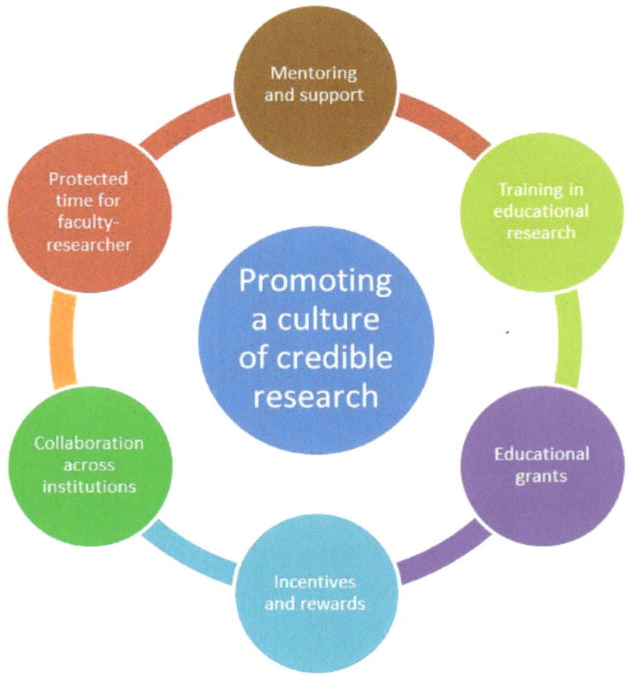

Figure 3: Approaches to Promote a Culture of Credible Research

(a) *Training in educational research*: Focused training workshops need to be initiated to train interested faculty in educational research. These can be conducted in a collaborative manner by the medical education units and the research units of institutes, depending on the available expertise. Educational researchers must be familiar with Glassick's standards for research. Getting participants to critically appraise existing literature can be a good way to familiarize them with the step-wise approach to designing, planning and implementing a research study.

While most are trained in biomedical research, qualitative approaches which are essential in social science research are not as familiar to the medical fraternity. These methods are useful in probing deeper and understanding the nuances in learning (Boet et al, 2012). Use of robust study design and approaches need to be advocated. The use of mixed methods in educational research should be encouraged.

It must be added that faculty members must be made aware of the need for ethics committee approvals and permissions before conduct of any educational research. In any kind of interventional study involving students or teacher, a formal approval from the institutional ethics committee is mandatory. This permission is also a requirement for document surveys and secondary data analysis. The 2017 guidelines of the Indian Council of Medical Research (ICMR) offer exemption for review for some routine educational activities such as comparison of instructional techniques, curricula, or classroom management methods, which have less than minimal risk and where there are no linked identifiers (Mathur, 2017).

(b) *Mentoring and support*: Most teachers want to undertake research and need support in conducting research as a part of their routine activities, rather than an add-on activity. The potential of research mentoring still lies untapped. There is need to develop a systematic process of hand-holding and mentoring as faculty initially delve into the process of doing educational research. This will need a group of experts trained in research methods who can volunteer their time for mentoring. Since the number of such experts are few compared to the number needed, there needs to be inter-institutional collaboration for this purpose. Merely organizing seminars or short-term coaching is unlikely to suffice. Research mentoring is a slow process and needs long-term commitment. It is a two-way synergistic learning process which benefits both the mentor and mentee (Fletcher, 2005)

(c) *Protected time for the faculty-researcher:* Teaching faculty in health professions education already wear multiple hats. They provide clinical service, are full time teachers and handle administrative roles. A new cadre of faculty-researchers needs to be established and given protected time to pursue research and compete for funding. These researchers must be given protection from clinical, teaching and administrative duties and allowed to spend dedicated time pursuing research, at least in the early years. Thereafter these researchers can be externally funded. These researchers need time to read literature, confer with colleagues, perform research, write grant applications and manage regulatory requirements (Barnard, 2015). This cadre can eventually serve as research mentors to other faculty.

(d) *Educational grants*: Large-scale projects which will make an actual impact to educational practice and policy require funding and manpower. These must be initiated at the government level in a competitive format, so as to encourage quality educational projects which make an impact on the educational scene.

(e) *Incentives and rewards*: Faculty who make inroads into research need to be encouraged with incentives and rewards just as any subject-specific clinical research would be. Educational research must be treated as par for purposes of tenure or promotion. It would be nice if there are journals dedicated to publishing quality educational research across the different disciplines in the Indian context.

(f) *Collaboration across institutes*: Studies done on a single batch of students with no follow-up usually have no meaning. To make an impact, there have to be large-scale, systematic, well-designed studies from which one can derive proper conclusions and change practice or policy. Collaborations across institutions or studies done within a university can give more insight into how educational practice needs to be altered for better outcomes. Usually a team of like-minded individuals with different strengths can collaborate across institutions and build up a body of work

Conclusion

The educational ecosystem needs to encourage health professional researchers to take up research. This process of nurturing a cadre of teacher-researchers is slow but rewarding. Overall, the way forward is to promote medical education research studies which have the potential to alter practice and policy. These will include studying the impact of different curricular models, teaching and assessment practices, faculty development initiatives, and selection processes on actual performance in practice. Findings of research need to be fed into the educational system so as to propel a cycle of quality improvement.

SUMMARIZE

Currently, faculty in India have just about begun to wet their feet into educational research. It is important to complement their enthusiasm with concrete plans such as training, mentoring, support and supervision in this journey. Collaborations across institutions or within the ambit of universities can help conduct large-scale studies from which meaningful conclusions can be drawn. The overall purpose is to encourage credible research which can impact practice and policy at the national level.

EVALUATE

Now that you know the value of educational research, we suggest you go online and look up some educational research papers from India. Critique them using some of the criteria that were mentioned in this chapter. First, is the topic of educational research relevant to our context? Next, is the study design robust? Are the conclusions correctly drawn? Will the study results be of use in actual practice?

Once you have evaluated 3-5 papers, consider the problems that are relevant to your own educational context. Which topics will be worth exploring further? Which area would you like to work in?

We hope you feel suitably charged enough to start thinking about the possibilities of delving into the world of educational research.

ROAD AHEAD

The reader is directed to the following articles which provide a guideline on how to critically appraise medical education literature. This exercise will be useful in understanding the concept of rigor in research.

Boet, S., Sharma, S., Goldman, J., & Reeves, S. (2012). Medical education research: an overview of methods. Canadian J Anesthesia. 59, 159-170.

Creswell JW. Educational Research: Planning, conducting, and evaluating quantitative and qualitative research. Delhi: PHI Learning Private Limited; 2014.

REFERENCES

Adkoli, B.V. (2017). Educational research in health sciences. *J EducTechnol Health Sci.* 4(2), 38-41.

Adkoli, B.V. (2020). Educational research: Much unexplored pathway to career enhancement of teachers in health sciences. *Annals of SBV.* 10.5005/jp-journals-10085-8120

Anshu, Bansal, P., Mennin, S.G., Burdick, W. P.& Singh, T. (2008). Online faculty development for medical educators: experience of a South Asian program. *Educ for Health*, 21 (3), 175.

Barnard, J.A. (2015). Protected time. J Pediatric Gastroenterology and Nutrition. 60 (3), 292-93.

Boet, S., Sharma, S., Goldman, J., & Reeves, S. (2012). Medical education research: an overview of methods. *Canadian J Anesthesia.* 59, 159-170.

Boyer, E. L. (1991). Scholarship Reconsidered: Priorities of the Professoriate. Princeton, NJ: The Carnegie Foundation for the Advancement. Metropolitan Universities.

Dongre, A.R. & Deshmukh, P.R. (2019). Current status of medical educational research in India and way forward. *Journal of Research in Medical Education and Ethics.* 9 (1), 73-78.

Fletcher, S. (2005). Research mentoring: The missing link in educational research. *Counterpoints.* 275, 177-189. Retrieved August 25, 2021, from http://www.jstor.org/stable/42978784

Mathur, R. (2017) National ethical guidelines for biomedical and health research involving human participants. Indian Council of Medical Research, Delhi, pp. 36.

Medical Council of India. No. MCI-12 (2)/2009- Med. Misc./56925. Published in the Gazette of India, Extraordinary, Part III, Section 4, No. 247, New Delhi, dated 15 Dec 2009.

Medical Council of India. No. MCI-6(2)/2016-Med/MCI General Body 7th session (continuing 143rd session). Minutes of meeting of the General Body dated 29th Mar 2017). Change in publication criteria for promotion. New Delhi.

Medical Council of India. Minutes of meeting of the Executive Committee, dated 16 Mar 2017 (item 16, page 5). Retrieved from: https://www.nmc.org.in/MCIRest/open/getDocument?path=%2FDocuments%2FPublic%2FPortal%2FMeetings%2FExecutive%20Committee%2F2017%2F03%2F16%2FECMN-16.03.2017.pdf (Accessed on 12 July 2021)

Morahan, P.S. & Fleetwood, J. (2008). The double helix of activity and scholarship: Building a medical education career with limited resources. *Medical Education*, 42 (1), 34-44.

Rege, N.N., & Bhuiyan, P.S. (2015). Educational research. In: Bhuiyan, P.S., Rege, N.N., & Supe, A. *The art of teaching medical students*. 3rd edn. New Delhi, Elsevier, 433-447.

Ringsted, C., Hodges, B., & Scherpbier, A. (2011). The research compass: An introduction to research in medical education: AMEE Guide No. 56. *Medical Teacher*. 33(9), 695-709.

Sood R. Medical education in India. (2008). *Medical Teacher*. 30, 585-591.

Supe, A. & Burdick, W.P. (2006). Challenges and issues in medical education in India. *Acad Med*. 81 (12), 1076-80

Chapter 3

Research Designs and Traditions in Medical Education Research: An Overview

Meghan M. McConnell, Renate Kahlke

ABSTRACT

Medical education research investigates a range of complex processes, outcomes, and systems using a variety of research methodologies. The goal of this chapter is to describe key characteristics of three research paradigms: quantitative, qualitative, and mixed methods. Quantitative research focuses on measuring and/or manipulating variables in order to test objective theories. Data from quantitative research are usually numbers gathered from standardized, validated instruments. Qualitative research focuses on exploring how individuals' or groups experience and ascribe meaning to social phenomena and on understanding the social processes behind their actions. Data from qualitative studies tend to take the form of words rather than numbers, and are often generated through observations, interviews, or documents. Quantitative and qualitative research paradigms are not discrete categories, but rather, belong on a continuum. Mixed methods research integrates elements of quantitative and qualitative approaches within a single study. There are several types of mixed methods research designs, which differ in how qualitative and quantitative data are integrated with one another. Whether a researcher should use a quantitative, qualitative, or mixed methods design depends on the nature of the research question. By familiarizing readers with a range of research methodologies, this chapter serves as a useful starting place for those interested in conducting, appraising, and publishing scholarly work in medical education.

Key Words: medical education, research design, research methodology, quantitative, qualitative, mixed methods

ASSESS NEED

Research in medical education, as with any other field of research, begins with a question that you would like to answer. This question may arise from a problem or concern encountered in your daily practice, a situation or practice that you think could be improved, or a topic that you would like to learn more about. This question is the pivotal first step of any research endeavour; it directs all subsequent research activities, including the choice of research methodology and the selection of data collection methods (Bezuidenhout & van Schalkwyk, 2015). But it is not enough to simply ask the right questions; you must also determine the best way to answer them. It is necessary for you select a research design that aligns appropriately with your research question.

Medical education has been described as a field of study, rather than an academic discipline (van Enk & Regehr, 2017). As such, it is able to draw insight from theoretical frameworks and methodological practices that are rooted in other disciplines, such as education, psychology, sociology, and anthropology. Each of these disciplines have their own set of concepts, assumptions, theories, and methodologies that inform the research process. Consequently, medical education researchers use a variety of research traditions and methods to investigate their research questions. Such theoretical and methodological diversity can be daunting, particularly to those new to educational research. This chapter describes various quantitative, qualitative and mixed methods research designs commonly used in medical education research. By doing so, we hope this chapter will help researchers select the most appropriate study design and, ultimately, improve the quality of medical education research, scholarship, and practice.

BRIEF

- There are a variety of different quantitative, qualitative, and mixed method research designs available to medical education researchers.
- It is important for researchers to ensure that their research methodology aligns with their proposed research question(s).
- Understanding key principles and practices of research methodology is crucial in conducting, appraising, and publishing medical education research and scholarship.

CONTEXTUALIZE

Dr. K runs an annual resuscitation skills workshop for medical students at her institution. She works hard to make the workshop fun, humorous and engaging for her students. Recently, however, she has been concerned that such an approach may not actually help students learn the course material. After all, resuscitation is not going to be "humorous" when the students have to do it in the real world!

This scenario presents an opportunity for educational scholarship and research. What are some potential research questions and methodologies available to Dr. K?

- Dr. K considers running an **experiment** to examine whether "fun" educational materials improve learning outcomes in her students. She asks: do students who receive humorous learning materials perform better on a resuscitation examination relative to students who receive non-humorous materials?

- Dr. K considers a **correlational study**. She wonders whether student engagement is related to a teachers' sense of humour. She wonders: Is there a relationship between an instructor's use of humour while teaching and learners' engagement with the learning materials.
- Dr. K may want to conduct a **survey** study to describe students' perceptions towards using humour as a teaching tool. She decides to ask: from the students' perspectives, what are the perceived effects of humour on learning, the preferred types of humour, and potential benefits and drawbacks of using humour when teaching clinical concepts?
- Dr. K could do a **constructivist grounded theory** study. Here, Dr. K thinks it would be useful to develop a theory to explain how learners engage with activities like hers. She asks: how do learners engage with "fun" educational experiences? What individual and social factors impact how they engage?
- Dr. K may be interested in shaping her study into an **ethnography**. She may what to know more about how learners interact with each other, with educators, and with her educational materials. She decides to ask: what is the learning culture in a non-mandatory resuscitation skills workshop?
- Dr. K may decide to take up **phenomenological** research questions. Dr. K decides that she would like to know: how do learners experience "fun" when engaging in educational activities? What role do they feel that "fun" educational activities play in their overall educational experience?
- Dr. K may want to use **action research** to look at this problem in a different way. She decides to work with her colleagues and students to explore the impact of fun on learning and develop a framework to help educators and learners integrate fun without sacrificing learning.
- Dr. K may want to conduct a **convergent mixed methods design** to explore how "fun" educational experiences influence students' engagement with learning activities. She gathers both quantitative (survey responses) and qualitative (semi-structured interviews) data in order to compare the findings. She wonders how these data sources converge and diverge from one another.
- Dr. may want to develop a survey that assesses student engagement. To do this, she considers using an **exploratory mixed methods design,** where she first conducts a grounded theory study develop a theory to examine cognitive, emotional, and social components of learner engagement. Dr. K uses these data to develop a survey that she distributes to the entire student body.
- Dr. K may perform an **explanatory mixed methods design** to examine whether students' cultural identity modulates the impact of humour on learning outcomes. Dr. K first conducts an experiment to see whether students' tests scores are influenced by the type of humour used (stories/anecdotes vs. dark humour). After running the experiment, Dr. K conducts an ethnographic study to understand how students' cultural background influences their attitudes towards and perceived value of these different types of humour.

DESCRIBE

Medical education is a field of study that examines the impact of individual, social, organizational, and/or instructional factors on educational experiences, processes, and outcomes. The field draws on a range of literatures, including education, sociology, anthropology, and psychology, all of which use different theories and methodologies to answer research questions. Selecting the most appropriate research design and methodology is an essential step in the research process. Inappropriate study designs will reduce the quality of research findings and can lead to inaccurate or incomplete conclusions.

Quantitative Research

Quantitative research is a theory-driven approach that examines relationships among variables (Creswell, 2014). These variables are measured using standardized, numerically-based instruments and analyzed using statistical procedures, in order to determine whether a theory explains or predicts the phenomenon of interest (Yilmaz, 2013). Quantitative research encompasses a broad spectrum of research designs, ranging from small-scale descriptive studies to complex, multicentric experimental studies. In the following section, we describe three quantitative traditions commonly used in medical education research – experimental, correlational, and survey (or descriptive) designs (Table 1).

Experimental Research. The purpose of experimental research is to examine potential cause-and-effect relationships between two (or more) variables. In a traditional experimental study, a researcher manipulates one or more variables (i.e., *independent variables*), and then measures the impact of this manipulation on an outcome variable (i.e., *dependent variable*).

A critical aspect of experimental design is that of a comparison, whereby the dependent variable is compared across individuals who receive different educational treatments or methods. For example, a researcher may compare test scores from a group of learners who received an educational intervention (i.e., intervention group) to learners who did not (i.e., control group).

Randomization is another important feature of experimentalism. In true experimental designs, participants are randomly assigned to the independent variable. Sometimes, however, randomization is not possible, as individuals belong to pre-existing groups (e.g., gender, medical specialty, etc.). Such cases are referred to as quasi-experimental designs, and are used to examine cause-and-effect relationships when it is not possible or practical to randomize individuals to different groups.

True experimental designs, while widely used in clinical research, are not as common in medical education research. There are several reasons for this. For example, randomization faces a unique set of challenges within educational contexts. There are ethical concerns with randomizing learners to different learning activities when one of these activities is presumed to be better than the other. Relatedly, it can be challenging to appropriately control for confounding variables in educational settings. The goal of experimentalism is to infer causality between experimenter-controlled independent variables and observed dependent variables (Norman & Eva, 2014). For this reason, a major focus for any researcher using experimental designs is control (Bell, 2009). However, the complexity of educational interventions do not often allow for such control. As Norman and Eva (2014) state, "it is well nigh impossible to identify what aspects of the workshop was the causal variable in inducing change, nor, for that matter, is it even likely that any single variable was causal for everyone in the workshop" (p. 305). Nonetheless, when used appropriately and rigorously, experimental designs can substantially deepen our understandings of the processes and mechanisms involved in learning.

Correlational Research. Correlational research is used to examine relationships among two or more variables. Unlike experimental research, variables are not manipulated or controlled by the researcher. There are two main purposes of correlational research (Fraenkel et al., 2015). In *exploratory studies*, the goal is to examine relationships among several variables. For example, a researcher may be interested in whether there is a relationship between physician burnout and the number of overtime hours worked. In *predictive studies*, the goal is to use scores from one variable to predict scores on another variable. For example, a researcher may want to determine whether students' scores on a practice examination can predict their performance on a national licensure examination.

Survey (Descriptive) Research. The purpose of survey research is to describe characteristics of a population. Researchers using survey designs typically want to determine how the members of a population distribute themselves on one or more variables (e.g., gender, specialty, attitudes, opinions, preferences, etc.) (Fraenkel et al., 2015). In this way, survey research methods are primary descriptive–information is collected from a group of people in order to *describe* certain aspects or characteristics of the population for which that group belongs (Cohen et al., 2011). For example, a researcher may want to describe medical students' perspectives on the impact of the COVID-19 pandemic on their medical training. To do so, surveys gather standardized information, meaning that participants receive the same instruments and questions, and this allows findings to be generalized to the larger population. In many surveys, participants are asked to quantify their experience (e.g., rate their level of satisfaction with or preparedness for an educational intervention). However, surveys also commonly integrate written responses and these are most often analyzed quantitatively (e.g., to count the number of participants who responded in a certain way) or used to inform analysis of the numerical scores (LaDonna et al., 2018).

Qualitative Research

Qualitative research is the rigorous study of people, cases, phenomena, social situations, and processes in their natural settings (Yilmaz, 2013). The aim of qualitative research is to gain a deep understanding of social phenomena by documenting experiences, using qualitative data generated from observations, interviews, or documents (Meadows, 2003). Qualitative research is most appropriate when the purpose of the research project is 1) to explore a topic on which little is known, 2) to make sense of complex and contextually-specific phenomena, 3) to understand how individuals experience a phenomenon, the meaning they apply to it, or how they interpret what they experience, 4) to construct a new theory or theoretical framework, and 5) to generate a deep understanding of a complex or multi-faceted phenomenon (Richards & Morse, 2013). Qualitative research covers a wide range of theoretical paradigms, methodologies, and research methods, all of which are designed to uncover different aspects of human experience and behaviour. In the following section, we describe four methodologies commonly used in medical education research – grounded theory, ethnography, phenomenology, and action research (Table 1).

Table 1: Description and Resources for Various Qualitative and Quantitative Research Methodologies

	Methodology	Purpose
Quantitative Research	Experimental	Examine cause-and-effect relationships between independent variable(s) and dependent variable(s).
	Correlation	Explore relationships between two or more variables.
	Survey (descriptive)	Describe characteristics of a population at a given point in time.
Qualitative Research	Grounded theory	Develop theory to explain social processes or situations.
	Ethnography	Describe how a culture functions through individual and shared beliefs, norms, and social practices.
	Phenomenology	Describe individuals' lived experience of a phenomenon.
	Action Research	Research and develop solutions to problems relevant to the researcher's practice.

Grounded Theory. Perhaps the most commonly used qualitative methodology in medical education, grounded theory is used to examine social processes or phenomena by documenting individuals' construction of shared meanings, and the ways in which those meanings shape their experiences and behaviours (Charmaz, 2014; Tavakol & Sandars, 2014). Early grounded theory methodologies took an objectivist perspective, assuming that the researcher is an objective observer in generating analyses (Glaser & Strauss, 1967); more recently, constructivist grounded theory has understood the researcher as having an active role in making decisions and interpretations (Charmaz, 2003).

Grounded theory methodology is marked by iterative study design, as researchers engage in concurrent data generation and analysis, and ongoing theoretical sampling based on analytic directions that they derive from their concurrent analyses (Kennedy & Lingard, 2006). Thus, results of the ongoing data analysis inform subsequent data collection, and, conversely, new data can then inform analyses (Lingard & Kennedy, 2010).

Sampling procedures in grounded theory are initially purposeful (i.e., researchers select participants and other data that will be most meaningful to the study), followed by theoretical sampling, in which researchers generate new data (often by recruiting new participants) in order to further develop their evolving analyses. Grounded theory uses a variety of qualitative data collection methods. Observations, interviews, and focus groups are most common in our field, though grounded theory can involve many types of data, including documents and other forms of text (Charmaz, 2014). Analyses are generated using a constant comparative approach through which researchers compare data to each other, and their analytic categories against the data, eventually resulting (as the name "grounded theory" suggests) in a new theorization of the phenomenon that is grounded in the data (Kennedy & Lingard, 2006).

Ethnography. Stemming from early anthropological research, ethnography is the study of culture, understood through the social interactions, behaviours, and perceptions of groups of people in a given social setting (Reeves et al., 2008). Originally, ethnography focused on objectively understanding a cultural group from the outside (i.e., an "etic" perspective). However, it has since evolved to appreciate that researchers always come to research with a perspective (Reeves et al., 2013). Today, there are many different approaches to ethnography, including institutional ethnography, which examines individuals' participation in larger institutions (Kearney et al., 2019; Smith, 2005), and auto-ethnography, where the researcher documents their own experiences (Chang, 2008; Farrell et al., 2015). Within medical education, ethnography has been used to study the cultures that inform teaching and learning in institutional settings across different levels of professional training (Atkinson & Pugsley, 2005), including the cultures of teams and organizations (Kearney et al., 2019).

The goal of ethnography is to provide rich, holistic insights into the practices of a specific cultural group, focusing on what people actually *do* in a culture. As such, a hallmark of ethnography is its emphasis on deep and often prolonged engagement with a culture, including observations and field notes that garner a rich picture of the practices and routines that drive everyday life (Bressers et al., 2020). However, ethnographic research rarely relies on a single source of data; ethnographers use other forms of data, such as interviews and documents, in order to view the same practices from multiple angles, and develop an appreciation of the ways in which participants interpret their practices and view their world (Reeves et al., 2013).

Phenomenology. Phenomenology seeks to explore a phenomenon from the perspective of those who have lived it (Teherani et al., 2015). There are many different approaches to phenomenology (e.g., transcendental, existential, hermeneutic, and linguistic), and each is informed by unique theoretical traditions. All phenomenological approaches seek to deeply describe the meanings individuals ascribe to their lived experiences, both in terms of *what* was experienced and *how* it was experienced (Neubauer et al., 2019). Phenomenology is most appropriate when the researcher is interested in investigating the meaning of a phenomenon or experience from a particular perspective or set of perspectives (Richards & Morse, 2013). For example, within medical education, phenomenology can be used to broaden our understanding of individuals lived experiences in the context of their learning and professional development (Neubauer et al., 2019).

To gain insights into participants understanding of their lived experiences, phenomenology generally relies on prolonged, in-depth interviews. However, phenomenology also employs other methods. Notably, researchers may incorporate participants' reflections through personal documents, such as diaries, e-portfolios, reflections, and observations.

Action Research. In action research, research is not conducted *on* participants, but, rather, is designed, conducted, and disseminated *by* professionals in the field *on* their own practice (McNiff, 2013). This type of research attempts to bridge the gap between research and practice, focusing on practical issues that have been identified as being problematic and developing practical research products that can support researchers and other stakeholders in improving their practice (Cohen et al., 2011; Koshy et al., 2011). For this reason, action research is a powerful tool for bringing about change and improving practice at the local level (Koshy et al., 2011). Developing findings that transfer beyond the specific setting is rarely the primary intent, since action research focuses on specific problems and issues within an organization or community (Patton, 2002). Action research is underutilized in medical education settings, but could be used very productively by professionals interested in making data-driven changes in their practice or larger organizational context.

Action research has been broken down in different ways by different theorists (McNiff, 2013; Williamson, 2012), but can be broadly understood as conducted through four phases: 1) Identification of an issue and setting up a project (reviewing the literature, focusing the topic, and formulating a research question); 2) Reflection (reflecting on practice as a group and as individuals); 3) Planning (e.g. developing an intervention, new practice, or educational strategy; developing research methods); 4) Evaluation of both process and products (Koshy et al., 2011). These phases are often cyclic and can overlap (Koshy et al., 2011). Action researchers can use quantitative or qualitative methods but tend to rely more heavily on qualitative methods, such as interviews, researcher journals, field notes, and documents, in order to explore the nuances of behaviours and interactions in practice (Koshy et al., 2011).

Mixed Methods Research

Often, quantitative and qualitative research are defined in opposition to one another—quantitative studies focus on deduction, confirmation, explanation, prediction, and theory-testing, while qualitative studies focus on induction, discovery, exploration, interpretation, and theory-generation (Johnson & Onwuegbuzie, 2004). Such polarization has resulted in a divide between quantitative and qualitative researchers, who often restrict themselves exclusively to either qualitative or quantitative designs (Onwuegbuzie & Leech, 2005b). Some researchers, however, have argued that qualitative and quantitative research are not contradictory to one another, but, rather, are complementary (Johnson & Onwuegbuzie, 2004; Onwuegbuzie & Leech, 2005a, 2005b). Proponents of this approach argue that combining qualitative and quantitative methods maximizes the strengths of both approaches, minimizes the weaknesses, and provides a more comprehensive understanding of a phenomenon (Johnson & Onwuegbuzie, 2004).

Mixed methods research is defined as a "class of research where the researcher mixes or combines quantitative and qualitative research techniques, methods, approaches, concepts or language into a single study" ((Johnson & Onwuegbuzie, 2004), p. 17). There are three main types of mixed methods designs: convergent, exploratory sequential, and explanatory sequential designs.

In *convergent designs*, quantitative and qualitative data are collected in parallel – separately but at roughly the same time. The results from each method are then integrated together in the final analysis (Fetters et al., 2013). The goal is to merge qualitative and quantitative data and describe whether there is convergence or divergence between the two data sources (Creswell, 2014). The assumption of this approach is that both qualitative and quantitative data provide different sources of information, and using both forms of data will allow for a more comprehensive understanding of the research problem (Creswell, 2014).

In *exploratory sequential designs*, researchers first collect and analyze qualitative data, and use the findings to inform subsequent quantitative data collection (Fetters et al., 2013). For example, a researcher may conduct semi-structured interviews to identify key concepts to be included in a new survey tool.

In *explanatory sequential designs*, researchers collect quantitative data, analyses the results, and then use qualitative data to help explain these results (Creswell, 2014). In this way, researchers' use the quantitative results to plan the qualitative follow up. For example, a researcher may first collect survey responses, and then conduct qualitative interviews to help explain and elaborate on any confusing or contradictory survey responses.

SUMMARIZE

As with any science, medical education research uses a variety of different research methodologies to answer questions relevant to the field. In this chapter, we described several quantitative, qualitative, and mixed methods designs. Their choice depends on several factors, such as the research question(s), the researcher's training and experience, and the overall purpose of the study. Quantitative studies focus on outcomes, generalization, predictions, and theory-testing using deductive reasoning, while qualitative studies focus on process, context, interpretation, meaning and theory-building using inductive reasoning (Yilmaz, 2013).

Mixed methods research integrates qualitative and quantitative methodologies in a single design in order to maximize strengths and minimize weaknesses. Understanding the principles and practices of these different research methodologies will help researchers select the most appropriate methodology to answer their research question and ensure that their research findings inform and advance educational theory and/or practices.

EVALUATE

- What are some of the key differences between qualitative and quantitative research designs? What are some of the similarities?
- Locate several research studies published in scholarly medical education journals and come up with a research question based on the results of each study. Discuss what methodological approach the authors used and why.
- Think about a topic within medical education that you would like to study. Using this topic, write down a research question that aligns to each of the quantitative, qualitative, and mixed method research designs described in this chapter.

ROAD AHEAD

Medical education is a field rife with complex, practical questions that have far-reaching impact on education and practice. While building effective studies to answer these questions can be a daunting task, it can also be incredibly rewarding and there are many resources available to support clinicians and other researchers in developing their research acumen. To get started, we suggest that new researchers:

- Decide on a question or type of research that most interests you, and begin to develop your knowledge base. Below, we suggest several entry-level research methods texts to get you started. It is also helpful to find ways to "join the conversation" on topics that interest you by participating in academic conferences, journal clubs, or other venues for sharing ideas.
- Find collaborators who you like working with and who have complementary expertise. It's a good idea to get feedback on your ideas early and often (Regehr, 2010). Some of these conversations may simply offer a new perspective or resources to guide you; others may lead to new collaborations of mutual interest.
- Build your mentorship network. You may find a single mentor who can guide you through your methodological decisions, professional development, and research processes specific to your context, or you may need to begin developing a broader mentorship network to meet your needs.

Resources

- For an overview of research methods: Creswell, J. W. (2017). *Research design: Qualitative, quantitative, and mixed methods approaches* (5th ed.). Sage.
- For an introduction to quantitative methodologies: Norman, G., & Eva, K. W. (2014). Quantitative research methods in medical education. In Tim Swanwick (Ed.), *Understanding medical education: evidence, theory and practice* (2nd ed., pp. 349–369). John Wiley & Sons
- For an introduction to qualitative methodologies: Richards, L., & Morse, J. M. (2013). *Readme first for a user's guide to qualitative methods* (3rd ed.). Sage.
- For an introduction to mixed-methods: Creswell, J. W. & Plano Clark, V. L. (2018). *Designing and conducting mixed methods research* (3rd ed.). Sage.
- Short primers on research methods in medical education:
    - Artino, A. R., Durning, S. J. & Boulet, J. R. (2011). AM last page: Generalizability in medical education research. *Academic Medicine, 86*(7), 917.
    - Artino, A. R., Durning, S. J. & Creel, A. H. (2010). AM last page: reliability and validity in educational measurement. *Academic Medicine, 85*(9), 1545.

- Bergman, E., de Feijter, J., Frambach, J., Godefrooij, M., Slootweg, I., Stalmeijer, R., & van der Zwet, J. (2012). AM last page: A guide to research paradigms relevant to medical education. *Academic Medicine*, *87*(4), 545.
- Castillo-Page, L. Bodilly, S. & Bunton, S. L. (2012). AM last page: Understanding qualitative and quantitative research paradigms in academic medicine. *Academic Medicine, 87*(3), 386.
- Dine, J. C. Shea, J. A. & Kogan, J. R. (2016). Generating good research questions in health professions education. *Academic Medicine, 91*(12),
- Frambach, J. M., van der Veluten, C. P. M. & Durning, S. J. (2013). AM last page: Quality criteria in qualitative and quantitative research. *Academic Medicine, 88*(4), 552.
- Paradis, E. (2016). AM last page: The tools of the qualitative research trade. *Academic Medicine, 91*(12), e17.
- Ringsted, C., Hodges, B., & Scherpbier, A. (2011). 'The research compass': an introduction to research in medical education: AMEE Guide no. 56. *Medical teacher*, *33*(9), 695–709.

REFERENCES

Atkinson, P., & Pugsley, L. (2005). Making sense of ethnography and medical education. *Medical Education*, *39*, 228–234.

Bell, S. (2009). Experimental design. In R. Kitchin & N. Thrift (Eds.), *International Encyclopedia of Human Geography* (pp. 672–675). Elsevier Ltd.

Bezuidenhout, J., & van Schalkwyk, S. (2015). Developing the research question: Setting the course for your research travels. In J. Cleland & S. Durning (Eds.), *Researching Medical Education* (pp. 35–41). Wiley Blackwell.

Bressers, G., Brydges, M., & Paradis, E. (2020). Ethnography in health professions education: slowing down and thinking deeply. *Medical Education*, *October 2019*, 1–9. https://doi.org/10.1111/medu.14033

Bryman, A., Becker, S., & Sempik, J. (2008). Quality criteria for quantitative, qualitative and mixed methods research: A view from social policy. *International Journal of Social Research Methodology*, *11*(4), 261–276. https://doi.org/10.1080/13645570701401644

Chang, H. (2008). *Autoethnography as method*. Routledge.

Charmaz, K. (2003). Grounded theory: Objectivist and constructivist methods. In N. K. Denzin & Y. S. Lincoln (Eds.), *Strategies for qualitative inquiry* (pp. 249–291). Sage.

Charmaz, K. (2014). *Constructing grounded theory* (2nd ed.). Sage.

Cohen, L., Manion, L., & Morrison, K. (2011). *Research Methods in Education* (7th ed.). Routledge.

Creswell, J. (2014). *Research design: Qualitative, qantitative, and mixed methods approaches* (4th ed.). Sage Publications.

Farrell, L., Bourgeois-Law, G., Regehr, G., & Ajjawi, R. (2015). Autoethnography: introducing "I" into medical education research. *Medical Education*, *49*(10), 974–982. https://doi.org/10.1111/medu.12761

Fetters, M. D., Curry, L., & Creswell, J. (2013). Achieving integration in mixed methods designs - Principles and practices. *Health Services Research*, *48*, 2134–2156.

Fraenkel, J. R., Wallen, N. E., & Hyun, H. H. (2015). *How to design and evaluate research in education* (9th editio). McGraw-Hill Education.

Glaser, G. M., & Strauss, A. L. (1967). *The discovery of grounded theory*. Aldine.

Johnson, R., & Onwuegbuzie, A. (2004). Mixed methods research: A research paradigm whose time has come. *Educational Researcher*, *33*, 14–26.

Kearney, G. P., Corman, M. K., Hart, N. D., Johnston, J. L., & Gormley, G. J. (2019). Why institutional ethnography? Why now? Institutional ethnography in health professions education. *Perspectives on Medical Education*, *8*(1), 17–24. https://doi.org/10.1007/s40037-019-0499-0

Kennedy, T., & Lingard, L. (2006). Making sense of grounded theory in medical education. *Medical Education*, *40*, 101–108.

Koshy, E., Koshy, V., & Waterman, H. (2011). *Action research in healthcare*. Sage Publications.

LaDonna, K. A., Taylor, T., & Lingard, L. (2018). Why Open-Ended Survey Questions Are Unlikely to Support Rigorous Qualitative Insights. *Academic Medicine*, *93*(3), 347–349. https://doi.org/10.1097/ACM.0000000000002088

Lincoln, Y. S., & Guba, E.. (1985). *Naturalistic inquiry*. Sage.

Lingard, L., & Kennedy, T. (2010). Qualitative research in medical education. In T Swanwick (Ed.), *Understanding Medical Education: Evidence, theory and practice* (pp. 371–384). Wiley Blackwell.

McNiff, J. (2013). *Action research: principles and practice* (3rd ed.). Routledge. https://doi.org/10.1177/0340035206070163

Meadows, K. (2003). So you want to do research? An introduction to quantitative methods. *British Journal of Community Nursing*, *8*, 519–526.

Neubauer, B., Witkop, C., & Varpio, L. (2019). How phenomenology can help us learn from the experiences of others. *Perspectives on Medical Education*, *8*, 90–97.

Norman, G., & Eva, K. W. (2014). Quantitative research methods in medical education. In Tim Swanwick (Ed.), *Understanding medical education: evidence, theory and practice* (2nd ed., pp. 349–369). John Wiley & Sons.

O'Brien, B. C., Harris, I. B., Beckman, T. J., Reed, D. A., & Cook, D. A. (2014). Standards for reporting qualitative research: a synthesis of recommendations. *Academic Medicine*, *89*(9), 1245–1251. https://doi.org/10.1097/ACM.0000000000000388

O'Cathain, A. (2015). Assessing the quality of mixed methods research: Toward a comprehensive framework. In *SAGE Handbook of Mixed Methods in Social & Behavioral Research* (pp. 531–556). https://doi.org/10.4135/9781506335193.n21

Onwuegbuzie, A., & Leech, N. (2005a). On becoming a pragmatic researcher: The importance of combining quantitative and qualitative research methodologies. *International Journal of Social Research Methodology*, *8*, 375–387.

Onwuegbuzie, A., & Leech, N. (2005b). Taking the "Q" out of research: Teaching research methodology courses without the divide between quantitative and qualitative paradigms. *Quality & Quantity*, *39*, 267–296.

Patton, M. (2002). *Qualitative research & evaluation methods*. Sage Publications.

Plano Clark, V., & Ivankova, N. (2016). *Mixed methods research: a guide to the field*. Sage.

Ravenek, M. J., & Rudman, D. L. (2013). Bridging conceptions of quality in moments of qualitative research. *International Journal of Qualitative Methods*, *12*, 436–456.

Reeves, S., Kuper, A., & Hodges, B. (2008). Qualitative research methodologies: Ethnography. *BMJ*, *337*, 1–7.

Reeves, S., Peller, J., Goldman, J., & Kitto, S. (2013). Ethnography in qualitative educational research: AMEE Guide No. 80. *Medical Teacher*, *35*(8), e1365-79. https://doi.org/10.3109/0142159X.2013.804977

Regehr, G. (2010). It's NOT rocket science: rethinking our metaphors for research in health professions education. *Medical Education*, *44*(1), 31–39. https://doi.org/10.1111/j.1365-2923.2009.03418.x

Richards, L., & Morse, J. (2013). *A user's guide to qualitative methods*. Sage Publications.

Smith, D. E. (2005). *Institutional ethnography: a sociology for people*. Altamira Press.

Tavakol, M., & Sandars, J. (2014). Quantitative and qualitative methods in medical education research: AMEE Guide No. 90: Part II. *Medical Teacher*, *36*, 838–848.

Teherani, A., Martimianakis, T., Stenfors-Hayes, T., Wadhwa, A., & Varpio, L. (2015). Choosing a Qualitative Research Approach. *Journal of Graduate Medical Education*, 7(4), 669–670. https://doi.org/10.4300/JGME-D-15-00414.1

Tracy, S. J. (2010). Qualitative quality: eight "big-tent" criteria for excellent qualitative research. *Qualitative Inquiry*, *16*(10), 837–851. https://doi.org/10.1177/1077800410383121

van Enk, A., & Regehr, G. (2017). HPE as a field: implications for the production of compelling knowledge. *Teaching and Learning in Medicine*, 30(3), 337–344. https://doi.org/10.1080/10401334.2017.1392864

Williamson, G. R. (2012). *Action Research in Nursing and Healthcare*. SAGE Publications Ltd. https://doi.org/10.4135/9781446289112

Yilmaz, K. (2013). Comparison of quantitative and qualitative research traditions: Epistemological, theoretical and methodological differences. *European Journal of Education*, *48*, 311–325.

Chapter 4

Ethical Issues in Health Professions' Education Research

N. Ananthakrishnan, Shanthi Ananthakrishnan

ABSTRACT

Ethical issues are important for judging the quality of research. Unfortunately, the importance of ethical conduct of research is not taken seriously in health professions education research (HPER) in comparison with rigorous guidelines practiced for clinical trials. There also exists considerable variability in dealing with the ethical issues among different countries. As a result, a young researcher is often confused about the standard practice which should be followed in HPER. This chapter highlights the perception change regarding HPER from, being considered non-harmful and a mere audit, to one which is now on par with social science research regarding strict regulatory guidelines. The inputs which led to this change have been highlighted. The principles and practices of bioethics viz., confidentiality, autonomy, informed consent, beneficence, non-malfeasance, inducements, influence of hierarchy, and conflict of interest have a slightly different perspective in HPER settings. These considerations will have implications for the procedures to be followed by the Institutional Review Boards and Ethical Committees (IRB and IEC), which have been highlighted in this chapter. Though the chapter is contextualized in the Indian scenario, it is possibly, applicable in other similar environments.

Key Words: medical education; ethics, ethical principles, health professions education research

ASSESS NEED

Medical Research is growing with great rapidity along with growth in medical knowledge due to various causes. It is estimated that the doubling time of medical knowledge in 1950 was 50 years; in 1980, 7 years; and in 2010, 3.5 years. In 2020 it is projected to be 0.2 years—just 73 days. (Densen, 2011)

Along with expanding medical knowledge, Health Professions' Education Research (HPER) is also growing. Yet there are still sceptics in the medical professional community who scoff when the term "Medical Education Research" is mentioned (Christner, 2020). There is lack of appreciation of the value of research into various aspects of medical education in our medical schools. This is unfortunately because Education Research does not fetch big grants or lead to great recognition in the health profession and remains a poor cousin in the research field (Todres, Stephenson and Jones, 2007). There is an even greater degree of unawareness regarding the ethical issues concerned with HPER. Teaching of ethics to medical students and postgraduates has been largely ignored till recently in India leaving young faculty researchers without a proper understanding of ethical issues involved in research. It is not so only in India; it is so in other countries as well (Ramana, Kandi and Boinpally, 2013).

HPER is what facilitates an understanding of what works or does not work as well, in the teaching/learning process and in the organisation of the curriculum and provides information enabling decisions regarding improving the quality of the outcome. An educational research based on planned, systematically obtained and analysed data is a stimulus for quality control and improvement. In the past, research in medical education was largely a process of auditing of existing teaching/learning or curricular practices, comparing them and drawing conclusions as to which one was more superior. Waiver of ethical approval was the norm then (Olle ten Cate, 2009). There are still countries where this situation exists. Olle ten Cate mentions that the Netherlands is among those countries which do not require ethical approval for medical education research (Olle ten Cate, 2009). However, this is not the situation in many other countries including India where a rigorous approval process is mandatory.

BRIEF

This chapter will deal with issues regarding:

- Possible ethical pitfalls in the conduction of research in health professions' education,
- Guidelines regulating this type of research
- Process for getting approval from the concerned Ethics Committee
- Taking care of concerns of students
- Understanding the principles of conflict of interest between the role as a teacher and that of a researcher.

CONTEXTUALIZE

Some of the incidents narrated below will highlight the issues which may arise in Health Professions' Education research (HPER).

i. A first MBBS student was asked to participate in an educational research by a teacher who wished to relate their learning styles to their performance in formative evaluation. Since the student was told that participation is voluntary, he declined to participate. Subsequently in the summative examination, the same teacher was the examiner. The student failed and attributed his failure to not participating in the teacher's research. His parents also lodged a complaint since the student was below the age of consent as per Indian law and their permission for participation was not taken as is required in Indian guidelines.

ii. A Ph.D proposal was submitted to the Ethics Committee for assessing the effect of Emotional Intelligence and Motivational Interview training to undergraduates to improve their interaction with patients. Half the batch was to be used as controls with no such training and the other half was the experimental group. The Ethics Committee declined to give consent since one half of the students was being deprived of the benefits of a process which has proved in other countries to contribute to improving communication with patients. The committee suggested that the experimental model may be modified to use historical controls or the students who are not given the opportunity of emotional intelligence and motivational training during the experimental phase, should be given this training after the experiment is over.

DESCRIBE

Introduction

Research in medical education is still largely based on observational studies and on undergraduate medical education. These two constitute 69% and 62% respectively of HPER (Todres, Stephenson and Jones, 2007). There are far fewer publications based on research on effects of continuing medical education or postgraduate training (Todres, Stephenson and Jones, 2007).

Previous studies were largely educational audits performed for quality control which were not always meant or suited for publication. Hence an atmosphere of laxity prevailed. Currently, more and more qualitative methods are used with planned and intrusive interventions in the educational process, some of which involve sensitive issues. As such, while in the past the process of approval of education research was practically non-existent and almost automatic as it was considered non-damaging, it is now subject to more rigid guidelines like other social sciences' research and is similar to that existing for Health research in general. It is, therefore, necessary for all researchers in the field of health professions research to be aware of the current guidelines and avoid the pitfalls which might result in refusal of permission by the concerned regulatory authority.

Existing Controversy

Olle ten Cate has mentioned three main factors in medical education research as stated below in justification of not having strict guidelines regulating educational research (Olle ten Cate, 2009).

1. *"Students determine the outcome of educational interventions far more than patients can determine the outcome of medical interventions."* The argument being that their participation is therefore, mandatory and should not be curbed.
2. *Potential harm resulting from education experiments does not compare with potential harm from medical experiments."* The implication here is hence research regulations need not be as strict. This hypothesis is, however, subject to dispute.
3. *"Why require ethical approval when methods are compared within cohorts but not historically or inter-institutionally?"* This opinion is obviously not unanimously approvable.

This is the reason that in the Netherlands no formal ethical approval is required for HPER. This premise has been disputed and the reasons why it is disputed will be discussed. The movement from mere audits to more and more social science research in education with sometimes intrusive questioning of personal details and inter-group comparisons without an opportunity of all to benefit by the intervention has led to this shift in perspective.

Hence the movement from laxity in permitting educational research to a great degree of strictness by applying the same ethical rules for education research as apply to general health research. ICMR in its guidelines on Ethical issues in social and behavioural science studies says that the risks of such research are non-measurable and dynamic in nature and therefore might be misconstrued as being in the category of no risk or minimum risk research when in fact they are not so (Indian Council of Medical Research, 2017). Hence special precautions need to be taken considering vulnerability, hierarchical pressure, confidentiality, principle of *"primum non nocere or above all no harm"* and voluntariness in obtaining informed consent. The Indian guidelines say that for social and behavioural science research in which some aspects of education research falls should conform to strict guidelines (Indian Council of Medical Research, 2017).

Changing Perspectives

Educational research has for a long time had the privilege of enjoying a special status amongst research activities being largely exempt from strict oversight (Howe and Moses, 1999). This attitude was welcomed by researchers in HPER since they felt that IRB members do not possess sufficient knowledge about research in education to be eligible to be regulators. In fact, there have been accusations of bias against the IRB regarding issues concerned with qualitative educational research (Murphy and Johannsen, 1990). To overcome this objection, the Code of Federal Regulations (CFR) of the USA, code 45 CFR 46, specifically mentions that IRBs should have representatives who represent a range of perspectives and interests including at least one member of the community who is not part of the organization and one member whose chief interests are non-scientific such as a lawyer, a layperson or a clergyman (Dougherty and Howe, 1990). These rules also apply to regulations enforced by the Indian Council of Medical Research in their guidelines on "Research on Human Participants" (Indian Council of Medical Research, 2017).

The only area exempt from requirements of 45 CFR 46 is *"Research conducted in established or commonly accepted educational settings involving normal educational practices such as (i) research on regular and special educational instructional strategies or (ii) research on the effectiveness of or the comparison among instructional techniques, curricular or classroom management methods."* (Howe and Moses, 1999). In the above circumstances also, the commission set up for prescribing rules for educational research laid down that even in areas exempt from strict regulation as stated above, there should be a process of administrative review in every case. This led to several universities prescribing more and more stringent rules to govern educational research for fear of litigation (Howe and Moses, 1999).

It has been suggested in this context that to make an appraisal of what constitutes "*a normal educational practice*" as defined above, there needs to be a board comprising of external members who are educationists (Dougherty and Howe, 1990).

Current Perspectives

Ethical issues in educational research may arise out of breach of prescribed well known ethical guidelines common with other health research or be specific to educational research only (Bassey and Owan, 2019). The common areas usually pertain to issues concerned with management and organisation of the research, data handling, plagiarism and issues concerned with publication ethics etc. which are all common to other types of research and other issues which are specific to education research (Bassey and Owan, 2019). The potential issues of concern are mentioned below.

1. **Research Management issues:**
    a. Grant issues
    b. Research supervision
    c. Data handling and management
    d. Confidentiality
    e. Fabrication and falsification of data
    f. Data analysis issues

2. **Publication Ethics issues:**
    a. Copyright infringement
    b. Plagiarism
    c. Citation and referencing issues
    d. Authorship and other publication ethics issues
    e. Conflict of interest
    f. Peer review issues

3. **Issues specific to education research**
    a. Data handling and confidentiality
    b. Discrimination issues both due to participation or non-participation, principle of beneficence and non-malfeasance.
    c. Vulnerability of subjects, principle of autonomy
    d. Age of the research subject
    e. Informed consent procedure
    f. Hierarchical organisation in an educational institution

This chapter will predominantly focus on issues specific to HPER since research management issues are common to all research and outside the scope of this chapter and the issues on publication ethics have been dealt with in a separate chapter.

Vulnerability and compromise of the principle of autonomy: The greatest concern in planning interventional research in education is due to a perception of vulnerability of the student population. This is a real issue since students largely constitute the subjects of educational research. It is considered that in the background of a very strict and overbearing hierarchical system in the medical colleges where the teachers have supreme authority, the ability or the independence of decision making of a medical student to withhold informed consent is seriously compromised. This is because there is a feeling, perhaps rightly so, that non-participation may result in adverse consequences in the summative examination process or academic career progression. ICMR in its National guidelines for Biomedical and Health Research involving Human Participants has classified students among individuals who have diminished autonomy due to dependency on being under a hierarchical system as a **vulnerable group** (Indian Council of Medical Research, 2017). As per guidelines laid down by ICMR, being research on a vulnerable population, all proposals for such review should come for a full board review of the concerned ethics committee. To avoid this concern of exploiting a vulnerable population, it may be advisable, where feasible, for a teacher to avoid research on his/her own current students under his/her hierarchical control.

Students should be treated as vulnerable and mandates to participate should be avoided. All educational research should preferably be part of the curricular process with provision for a cross over when comparing instructional methods. This is because innovation may be better or worse than the current practice and may be either harmful or beneficial to a selected few student only (Eva, 2007, 2009). One may also consider doing the research during extra-curricular hours using academic brake times. By carrying out research during spare time students are not inconvenienced and their interests are not adversely affected. However, they should have the freedom to either participate or not participate without fear of adverse consequences.

Beneficence and non-malfeasance: This specially applies to comparison of different teaching/learning methods during the curricular process between two groups of students, one of which is in the new intervention group and the other in the control group with the old methods. In this situation, if the new instructional strategy has been shown to be clearly and unequivocally superior to the old one in other studies, then having two groups of students one for the experimental group with the new interventional strategy and the other for the conventional intervention would be unethical unless those who missed out on the new instructional strategy during the conduct of the experiment are given an opportunity to learn by the new strategy after completion of the experiment. This objection would still apply even if "informed consent" has been obtained to be in the control group since this would be perceived to be due to hierarchical pressure. Hence in any such research involving comparison between two groups of students, there must be a cross over so that the benefit of the new intervention accrues to both groups for another topic of instruction.

Informed consent procedure: Informed consent for participation in the study must be obtained by an independent member of the research team who is not part of the hierarchy of educational control and who is not involved in the teaching/learning or assessment of the experimental subjects. Full information must be given on the purpose and consequences of the research, the benefits or potential harm which may accrue to all or some of the students and they should be explained, when in the control group, that they will also have an opportunity to experience the benefits of the new intervention for a future lesson. Opportunity and freedom to withhold consent must be provided, as also an opportunity to withdraw from the study at any time without assigning reasons without adverse academic consequences.

The informed consent process must educate the students about privacy, anonymity, equipoise, equitability, beneficence and non-maleficence etc. There is yet another issue regarding informed consent. In India, many of the students who are the subjects of research, including in health professions education institutions, are below the age of legal consent which is 18 years as per Indian guidelines. Hence serious consideration must be given to the need to get the legal guardians involved in the informed consent procedure. The procedure for obtaining informed consent for research for those below the legal age of consent is detailed in the ICMR guidelines (Indian Council of Medical Research, 2017). It has been suggested that the IRB should focus on the process of consent rather than the wording of the consent form (Silva and Sorrell, 1988)

For online questionnaires requiring anonymous feedback from students as part of research, the researcher must ensure that there is no way that the identity of the responder is revealed to the researcher and it remains anonymous. The students should not be asked to enter any identifiable data as part of filling up the questionnaire. They should not be asked to use their Universal ID No. or their mobile phone numbers for responding as these would be identifiable.

Process of obtaining approval from IRB or Institute Ethics Committee: The researcher should first determine whether the project qualifies as a research or a mere evaluation of existing practices. If it is an audit whose results are meant for local stakeholders to improve the curricular process without publication, it may not qualify as research. If, however, it is intended for publication and general dissemination, to add to the body of knowledge, it qualifies as research and requires ethical approval. The former may require only administrative approval, but the latter requires a formal application for approval to the IRB. If the IRB deems that the research is based on data already available which is being put to a secondary use for publication ensuring total anonymity, it may grant a waiver of approval after an expedited approval process. If, however, the committee feels that vulnerable population is involved it will go for a full board review.

IRB review process: All educational research which does not meet with the criteria of an in-house audit of practices must be submitted as a protocol to the IRB or the Institute Ethics Committee. Based on the protocol, the purpose of the research and the consideration of vulnerability issues, it is for the IEC to decide whether a formal waiver may be issued or whether it requires a full committee review and appraisal. The consideration is based on a case-by-case study and cannot be generalised. The IRB is likely to study in detail the age of the participants, issues of vulnerability, the informed consent process, intrusiveness of the data collection Proforma, post study usage of data and such other issues. The standards of approval are very similar to social science research although it may be less stringent than health research involving patients.

Use of secondary data: Often there is a perception amongst researchers that if data is already available it may be used for future research without any further approvals. This is an incorrect assumption. For example, there was a study in one institution to correlate the marks obtained in school leaving examination with academic progress after admission to a professional institute based on formative and summative examination scores. Although these scores were available with the academic section, it requires a second detailed proposal to the IEC describing the purpose of the study for fresh approval. Likewise use of previously obtained data, such as school leaving marks, for classifying students into those requiring additional curricular support, even with the justifiable intention of providing additional curricular support, still requires approval if the intention is to publish the research.

Confidentiality: Participant's identify must be protected while disseminating findings. The researcher must remember that inclusion criteria by themselves may serve as identifiers (Christakis, 1985, Forester and McWhorter, 2005). To avoid this, it is better to conduct a multidisciplinary or multisite research. This will also indirectly reduce the chances of being accused of exercising hierarchical pressure. If participants agree to have their identities revealed, this decision has to be made by the Ethics committee after verification of the consent process and permit it only if necessary for the study.

Data must be anonymized before it is provided for consultation by faculty. In the case of teachers involved with active teaching of the subject student participants, only independent research team members should be involved in collecting student information. There are two types of anonymization:

a. Anonymized data, irrevocably stripped of all identifiers and
b. De-identified data where the identifiers are replaced by a code kept by the independent member of the research team. This latter must be under strict control to be provided only where necessary on approval of the IRB.

Data must be protected against unauthorised access by measures such as:

a. Physical safeguards, data stored under lock and key
b. Administrative safeguards – enforcing organisational rules regarding privacy
c. Technical safeguards, encrypting, password protection etc.

Avoiding inducements: Participation in research should not fetch extra credits in the curricular process to the student participants. This would be considered an inducement which is unfair. This will also jeopardise participants right as per the Declaration of Helsinki (The World Medical Association, Declaration of Helsinki – Ethical Principles for Medical Research Involving Human Subjects, 2018) to withdraw at any time without assigning reason from the research. (Leentjens and Levenson, 2013)

Research By Medical Students as Part of the Curricular Needs

There are no specific guidelines on medical students pursuing short term educational research projects as part of their curriculum. In situations where the risk is less than minimal, as in situations where it involves mere analysis of data, already available in records in an anonymous manner, without any sensitive new issues being raised as part of the current research, auditing for quality control, etc. strict scrutiny may not be required. These may be submitted for exemption from review as per ICMR guidelines. In situations where comparison of instructional techniques is involved, particularly one whose superiority is obvious or has been noted in other studies, research is permitted only if all students have the benefit of the new intervention after the completion of the study and do not miss out on the advantages accrued to their fellow students.

As per ICMR protocol all studies involving vulnerable populations such as students must undergo a full committee review and is not subjected to a waiver without review. The general opinion about student research is that there cannot be any laxity regarding research done by the most inexperienced member of the research team such as students in comparison to those governing more experienced members (Dougherty and Hall, 1990)

SUMMARIZE

This chapter highlights the perception change regarding HPER from, being considered non-harmful and a mere audit to one which is now on par with social science research regarding strict regulatory guidelines. The inputs which led to this change have been highlighted. The following principles of bioethics which apply to HPER have been discussed in detail, viz.

i. Vulnerability and compromise of autonomy
ii. Principle of beneficence and non-malfeasance
iii. Question of inducements or hierarchical compulsion
iv. Informed consent procedure
v. Confidentiality
vi. Procedure for obtaining consent from the IRB or the IEC.
vii. Secondary usage of data collected for previous research
viii. Implications of students doing educational research

EVALUATE

It is hoped that after perusal of this chapter, the reader would be able to find answers to many questions, some of which are listed below pertaining to HPER.

1. Why has there been a change in perception regarding HPER from a belief that it was non-damaging to the subjects of research to the current practice of requiring strict regulation?
2. What measures need to be taken to protect the student population, who largely the subjects of research, in view of their vulnerability?
3. What are the principles and practices for obtaining informed consent from students for participation in HPER?
4. What types of HPER may be exempt from strict scrutiny by the IRB and be eligible for a waiver of approval?
5. What steps need to be taken to protect confidentiality in HPER?

ROAD AHEAD

This has been aptly summarised in a paper by Boileau et al in Medical Teacher in 2017 (Boileau, Petenaudeand St-Onge C, 2018). The tips modified from her paper are as follows:

1. Determine whether your project qualifies as a research or is a mere audit of existing practices.
2. Verify need for consent for secondary use of data obtained during normal academic process.
3. Ensure free and informed consent of subject participants.
4. Obtain consent through independent member of the research team.
5. Ensure confidentiality of participation.
6. Ensure data is anonymized before appraisal by faculty researchers.
7. Protect participants' identity.
8. Safeguard research data.
9. Treat student participants as being vulnerable.
10. Consider doing the research in extra-curricular time.
11. Avoid impression of positive or negative inducements.
12. Ask for a thorough review by the IRB or the concerned ethics committee to safeguard researcher and subjects.

REFERENCES

Bassey BA, Owan VJ (2019). *Ethical issues in Educational Research Management and Practice.* Retrieved on August 2021 from *https://papers.ssrn.com/sol3/papers.cfm?abstract_id=3516195*

Boileau E, Petenaude J, St-Onge C (2018). Twelve tips to avoid ethical pitfalls when recruiting students as subjects in medical education research. *Medical Teacher* 40:1, 20-25.

Christakis N (1985). Do Medical Student research subjects need special protection? *IRB*: 7:1.

Christner J (2020) *What is Medical Education Research?* Retrieved on August 2021 from *https://blogs.bcm.edu/2020/09/22/what-is-medical-education-research/*

Densen P (2011). Challenges and Opportunities Facing Medical Education. *Trans Am Clin Climatol Assoc*; 122: 48-58.

Dougherty K and Howe K (1990) Policy regarding educational research: *Report to the subcommittee on Educational Research of the Human Research Committee, unpublished manuscript, cited by Howe KR and Moses MS*

Eva KW (2007). The Yin and Yang of education research. *Medical Education* 41, 724-5.

Eva KW (2009). Research Ethics Requirement for Medical Education. *Medical Education*, 43: 194-95.

Forester JP, McWhorter DL (2010) Medical Students' perception medical education research and their role as participants. *Academic Medicine*, 80: 780-5.

Howe KR and Moses MS (1999). Ethics in Educational Research, *Review of Research in Education*;.24: 21-60.

Indian Council of Medical Research (2017). *National Ethical Guidelines for Biomedical and Health Research Involving Human Participants.* Retrieved on August 2021 from *https://main.icmr.nic.in/sites/default/files/guidelines/ICMR_Ethical_Guidelines_2017.pdf*

Leentjens AF, Levenson JL, (2013) Ethical issues concerning the recruitment of university students as research subjects. Journal of Psychosomatic Research, 75: 394-8.

Murphy M and Johannsen (1990) Ethical obligations and Federal regulations in ethnographic research and anthropological education. *Human Organisation*, 49, 127-134.

Olle ten Cate (2009) Why the ethics of medical education research differs from that of medical research. *Medical Education* 43, 608-10.

Ramana, Kandi and Boinpally PR (2013). Ethics in Medical Education, Practice, and Research: an insight. *Annals of Tropical Medicine and Public Health*, 6, 509-602.

Silva M and Sorrell J (1988). Enhancing comprehension of information for informed consent: A review of empirical research. *IRB: A review of Human Subjects Research*, 10, 1-5.

The World Medical Association, INC. (2018) *Declaration of Helsinki Ethical principles for Medical Research Involving Human Subjects.* Retrieved on August 2021 from *https://www.wma.net/policies-post/wma-declaration-of-helsinki-ethical-principles-for-medical-research-involving-human-subjects/*

Todres M, Stephenson A, Jones R (2007) Medical Education Research remains the poor relation. *BMJ* 335, 333-5.

Chapter 5

Sampling in Medical Education Research

Pushpanjali Krishnappa, Malu Mohan, Jyotsna

ABSTRACT

Samples are the key contributors of data for any type of research. Sampling is the process of drawing a representative sample from a population. It facilitates a robust research process within the constraints of available resources. However, there are certain considerations to ensure that the results generated are valid and credible. These include identifying and obtaining an appropriate sampling frame, defining specific inclusion criteria and adopting a sampling methodology appropriate to meet the objectives. The minimum sample size required is determined by several considerations. This chapter addresses sampling strategies for quantitative, qualitative and mixed-methods research employed in medical education.

Key Words: sampling, educational research, medical education, research methodology, sample size

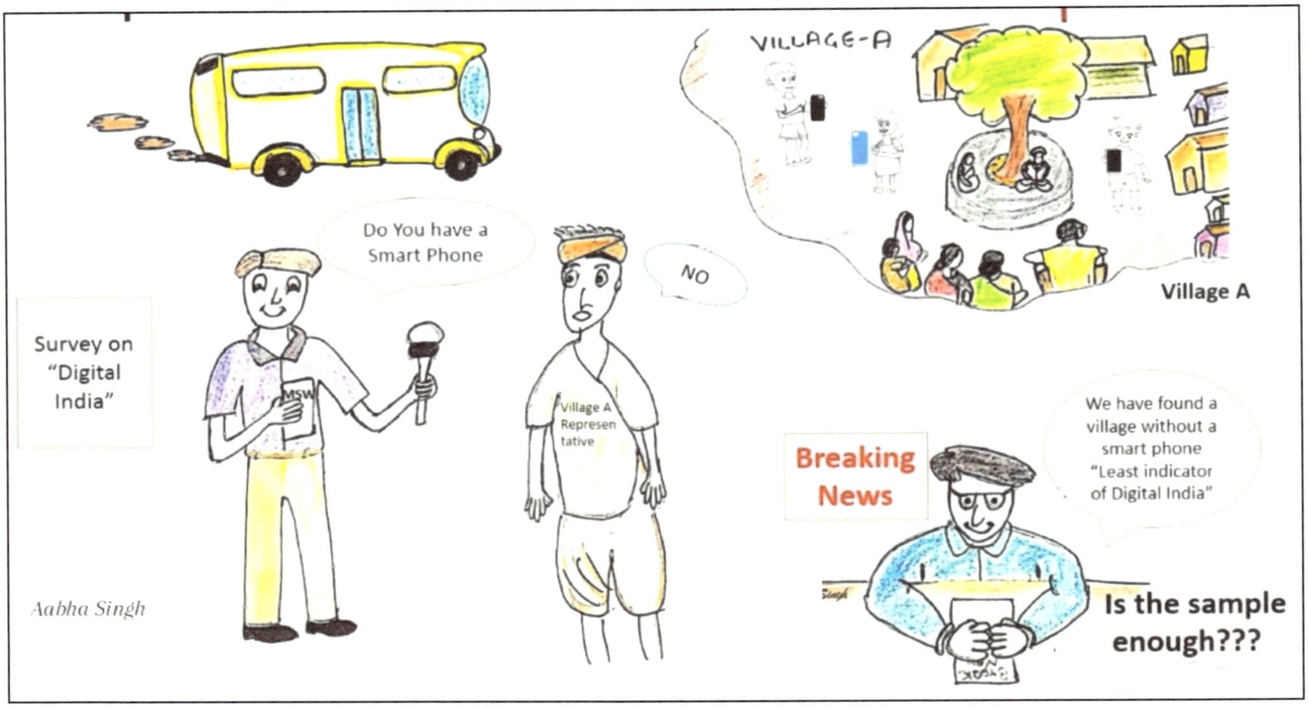

ASSESS NEED

Why Do We Need Sampling in Medical Educational Research?

The issue of sampling is crucial for researchers in general. It is not practical or feasible for researchers to study every individual from a population of interest. For instance, in an educational ecosystem under study, like a University, it is impossible to study the characteristics of interest of every student or teacher. When every individual from a target population is studied, it is called a **census**. However, more often than not, in research, we study a subsection of individuals from the target population, which saves time, money and man power. Such a subset of elements selected from a large population for the purpose of research is called a **sample**. The process of drawing a sample from a population is called **sampling.**

In medical educational research, depending upon the research questions explored, researchers may use quantitative methods, qualitative methods or a combination of both (mixed-methods). Quantitative research mostly aims to generate and test hypotheses explaining the occurrence of specific phenomena in any educational ecosystem so as to make generalizations about such occurrences. This often means that the samples drawn need to be reasonably representative of the target population. Qualitative research focuses on exploring certain phenomena, focusing on the perceptions and experiences of individuals. Qualitative researchers, hence, are interested in choosing a sample that will deepen their understanding of the phenomenon under study. Hence, their aim would be to ensure that there is as much diversity as possible in terms of the characteristics and experiences of those involved in the sample (Johnson & Christensen, 2014).

BRIEF

- Defining the population, target population and sample constitute integral steps in research
- Study samples are key contributors to the credibility of research
- Defining the sampling frame and inclusion criteria are the first steps
- Appropriate sampling methodology and adequate sample size are critical to ensure robustness of research

CONTEXTUALIZE

The leadership of a University requested the chairperson of a health professions education unit (HPEU), to submit a report on the challenges experienced by the teaching staff engaged in online teaching. This report had serious policy implications for decisions on investment in faculty development and infrastructure. So, it had to be based on valid research findings on the current infrastructure, perceptions and practices of teachers regarding online teaching and the challenges they faced. It was decided to conduct a survey to assess the knowledge, practice and attitudes (KAP) among the teachers regarding online teaching, using an existing tool, along with a qualitative exploration of their perceptions. A whole population approach was adopted for the survey including all the teaching faculty from all the five institutions functioning under the University.

The survey results showed favorable KAP scores among the participants, especially on items related to computer proficiency. However, more than half of the responses were from engineering staff, who, by virtue of their background, had better computer proficiency than others. The survey had included the responses of even those staff who had not conducted a single online teaching session until then. Thus, the research participants did not represent the actual composition of the staff engaged in online teaching, thereby affecting the validity of results.

What should have been the ideal approach to ensure valid results?

DESCRIBE

How to Select Your Samples in Quantitative Research?

In quantitative research, the researchers are interested in developing reasonably accurate generalizations about occurrences. The sample should therefore, resemble the population in all characteristics that are important to the research being conducted, except in total size. Such a sample is called a representative sample, while a sample that is systematically different from its population is called a biased sample (Johnson & Christensen, 2014; Creswell & Creswell, 2018) (Figure: 1).

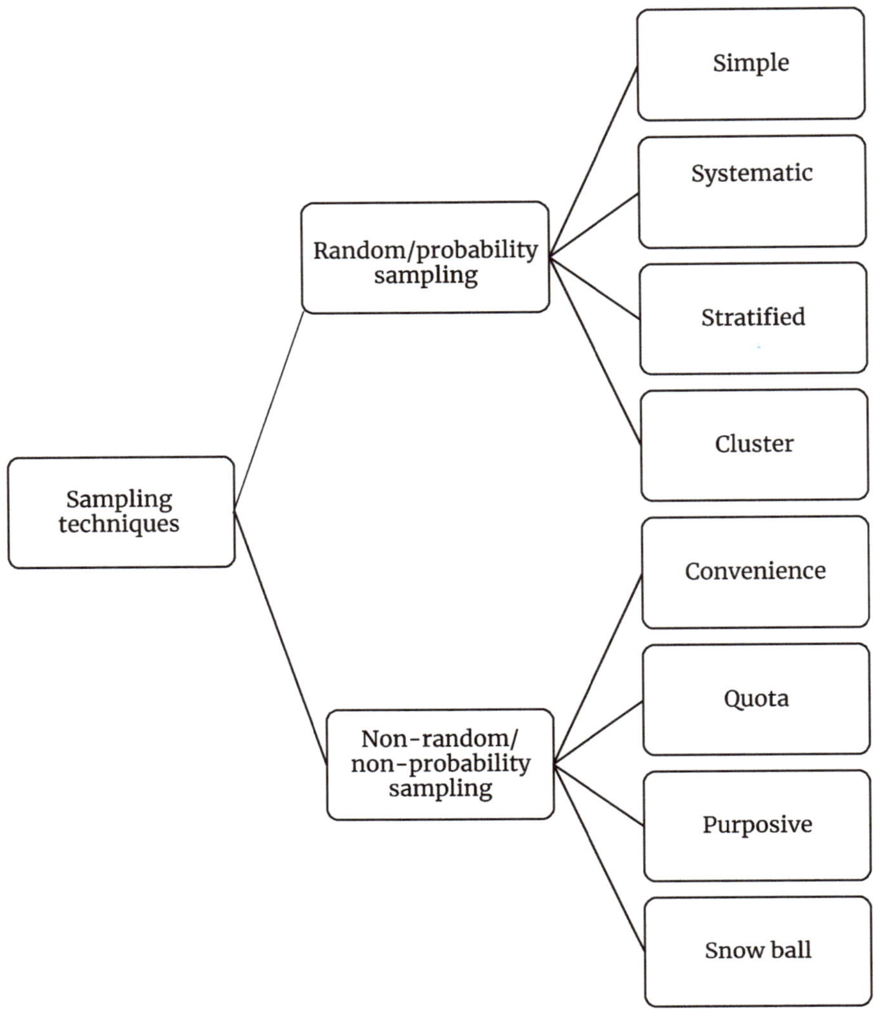

Figure 1: Sampling Techniques used in Quantitative Research

Broadly, there are two types of sampling methods used in quantitative research:

i. **Random/Probability sampling** – refers to sampling techniques which are based on the theory of probability. A key goal of studies which rely on probability sampling techniques, is to ensure generalizability of study results. This is achieved through the process of random selection. Random selection is the process of selecting people randomly from a population to ensure that the samples are representative (Table:1).

Table 1: Random/Probability Sampling Techniques

Types of Sampling	Description
Simple random	This is the most basic form of random sampling, where, every element in the population has an equal chance of being selected into the study. *If there are 1000 students attending a University and you need a sample of 100 students for a research study, then we randomly select 100 people using either a table of random numbers (a list of numbers that fall in random order) or random number generators (computer programs which generate random numbers).*

Types of Sampling	Description
Systematic	Here, a sampling interval (symbolized by k) is fixed and a starting point is selected between the first number in the sampling frame and k (including both). The sampling interval is the population size N, divided by the sample size, n (N/n). The randomly selected starting point will be the first element to be included into the sample from the sampling frame and then we will continue to select every k^{th} element in the frame. *If there are a 100 medical teaching faculty (N=100) in a University and the estimated sample size, n=20, then k, the sampling interval will be 5. Now we can randomly select a starting point between 1 and 5 using simple random sampling. If the random number thus selected is say, 4, then the 4th name in the sampling frame will be the starting point and from there every 5th person in the list will be selected into the sample, until the required sample size of 20 is reached. This is useful when we have a ready sampling frame.*
Stratified random	If the population is heterogeneous, then the sample should also represent the heterogeneity. In order to do that, the population is divided into mutually exclusive groups called strata and then from each of these strata, we draw a simple random sample or a systematic sample. The variable that forms the basis of strata is called the stratification variable (age, gender, class, caste, etc.) (Figure: 2).
Cluster random	Clusters are collective units with multiple elements like schools, colleges, universities, households and so on. In cluster sampling, instead of randomly selected individuals, we would be randomly selecting clusters. When the elements in a population are geographically spread out, choosing clusters will save resources. (Figure: 3).

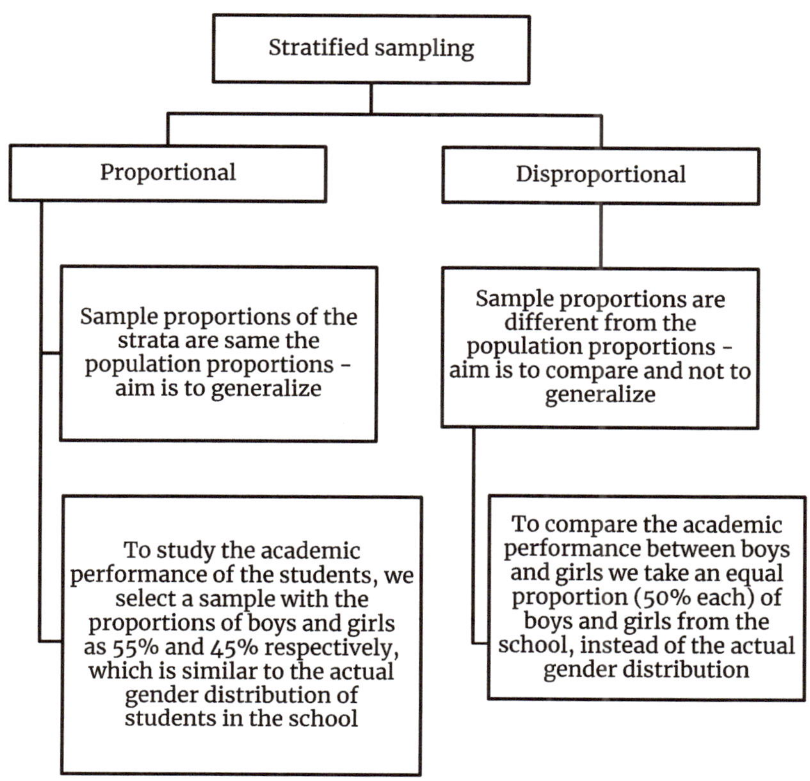

Figure 2: Types of Stratified Sampling

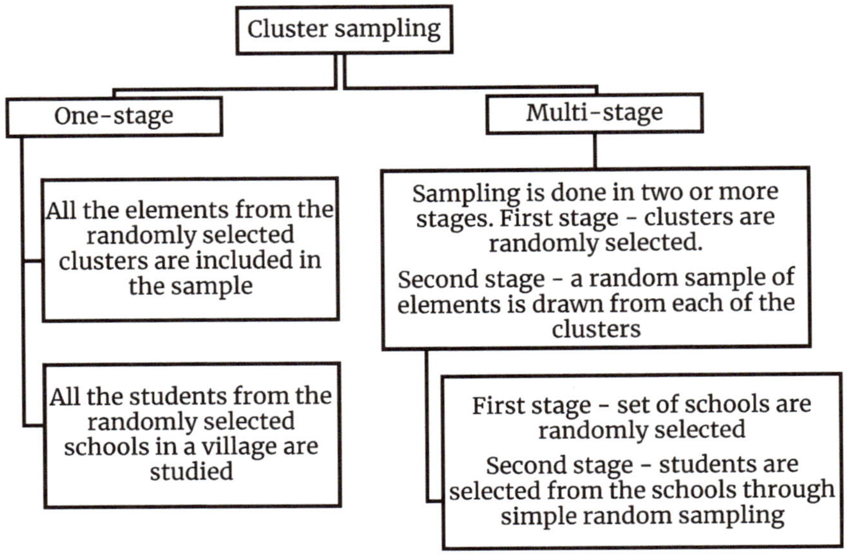

Figure 3: Types of Cluster Sampling

ii. **Non-random/Non-probability sampling** – refers to sampling techniques in which an element's probability of being selected into a sample is unknown. Since the probability of inclusion into the sample is unknown, it is very much possible that the samples drawn are systematically different from the population and thus are biased. Hence, non-probability samples are not ideal when generalizability of study findings is the goal of a research study (Table: 2).

Table 2: Non-random/Non-probability Sampling Techniques

Types of Sampling	Description
Convenience sampling	Here, researchers conveniently select those elements into the sample, based on their availability, willingness to volunteer or ease of recruitment. *For instance, we recruit the first 100 medical residents from a University, who expressed willingness and came forward to participate.*
Quota sampling	Here, the researcher identifies the major population sub-groups to be represented in the study, determines the required sample sizes or quotas for each of these sub-groups and then recruits the participants in each of these sub-groups through convenience sampling. *If the sample needed is 100, then keeping with the gender distribution in a medical college (60% males and 40% females), the researchers decide that there should be 60 male residents and 40 female residents in the study.*
Purposive sampling	This is also known as judgmental sampling. Here, the researcher defines the population of interest using specific characteristics and then locates individuals with those characteristics. *If a researcher identifies first time attendees of a boot camp as his/her population of interest, then he/she identifies them and approach only them.*
Snow ball sampling	This is particularly useful when the population of interest is hard to locate and when a sampling frame is not available. Here, each research participant is asked to identify and help locate other potential participants. *If a researcher explores why recent nursing graduates from a district chose alternate career options, then he/she could identify the first few candidates and then through them locate more nurses who are working in other fields.*

How to Select Your Samples in Qualitative Research?

Qualitative research involves in depth exploration of a phenomenon or focus of interest. Hence qualitative research sampling is predominantly **purposeful**. That is, we intentionally select individuals who will enrich our understanding of the phenomenon under study. Thus, it is essential to define the criteria or attributes that should be present in these individuals. The different types of qualitative sampling methods are provided in Table: 3. A combination of two or three sampling methods can also be used. The primary aim of sampling here, is to ensure that we choose individuals and sites which are "information rich". However, logical constraints, accessibility of potential participants and the cost of locating and enlisting participants for the study should also be accounted for (Creswell, 2012).

Table 3: Sampling Techniques in Qualitative Research

Types of Sampling	Description	Example
Comprehensive sampling	A technique where all relevant people/individuals/groups/settings are included in the sample. Although it assures representativeness, it is expensive and at times impractical.	*"A researcher wants to understand the factors which influence students' communication skills and chooses to explore the perceptions of all relevant stakeholders. All the students, staff and patients who have interacted with the students are included."*
Maximum variation sampling	A wide range of cases are purposively selected to provide a diverse, rich source of data reflecting the range of occurrence of the phenomenon in the population.	*"A researcher exploring the learning patterns amongst students chooses top, mediocre and below average performers in his/her sample to ensure maximum range".*
Homogenous sampling	The sample is small and homogenous. Few similar cases are selected for intensive study and in depth understanding of the research focus.	*"A researcher exploring the administrators' perceptions on quality assurance in education chooses a small sample of administrators and engages intensively with them".*
Extreme case sampling	The cases are selected from the extreme ends of a spectrum and compared.	*"A researcher explores the learning patterns of students by comparing consistently outstanding achievers and consistently extreme underperformers".*
Typical case sampling	An "average/typical case" that characterizes a phenomenon is defined through discussions within the research team.	*"A researcher exploring the educational environment in medical colleges defines the "average case" as any accredited institution which has been functioning in the state for a minimum decided period of time and studies only those institutions".*
Critical case sampling	This technique is adopted when the researcher wants to investigate, in depth, a previously identified or known case/phenomenon.	*"A previous study had identified the Dean as the educational leader for any health professional educational change and a researcher which aims to introduce changes in an institution, chooses to focus on the Dean and engage specifically with her on the initiative".*

(Contd...)

Types of Sampling	Description	Example
Negative case sampling	Here, the researcher purposefully selects cases which do not agree to/conform with and are contrary to his/her expectations of a phenomenon.	*"A researcher, who is theoretically aligned to the hypothesis that students have limited capacity to contribute to curriculum development, chooses to explore the students' inputs on it."*
Opportunistic sampling	This is exclusively adopted in qualitative research, where it might be impossible to identify all study participants at the start of the research. During the research process, the research focus might shift and opportunities to explore new research questions or aspects might arise.	*"As a researcher explores the students' perceptions on emotional health, he/she comes across a faculty team who has been extensively working to help students cope. So this team is included in the sample and their perceptions are explored."*
Mixed purposeful sampling	Here, more than one sampling strategy is adopted for data triangulation.	*"When a researcher includes critical case sampling, negative case sampling and extreme case sampling in his study to explore the learning patterns of students".*

How to Select Your Samples in Mixed-methods Research?

Mixed-methods research involves the use of both quantitative and qualitative research methods in a single study to explore and/or explain a research problem. Here, the sampling strategy is determined by the temporal relationship between quantitative and qualitative methods and the relationship between the two samples. These are in-turn determined by the research objectives and the research design (Johnson & Christensen, 2014; Creswell & Creswell, 2018) (Table: 4, Figure: 4).

Table 4: Sampling Strategies in Mixed Method Studies

Criterion for Classification	Types	Description	Example
Based on time orientation	Concurrent	If quantitative and qualitative samples are selected at the same time.	*"In a mixed-methods study to explore the practices and perceptions of teaching staff on online teaching, participants for the survey and the FGDs are selected at the same time."*
	Sequential	If the samples are selected one after the other.	*"First the participants of the survey are selected and then subsequently, after the survey is initiated or completed, the FGD participants are selected."*

Criterion for Classification	Types	Description	Example
Based on the relationship between qualitative and quantitative samples	Identical	Same samples are used in both qualitative and quantitative components.	*"A study exploring the practice preparedness among medical students uses the same sample for the survey and in-depth interviews."*
	Parallel	Different samples are drawn from the same population.	*"Different samples of medical students are selected for the survey and the interviews."*
	Nested	Participants selected for one phase represent a subset of those participants selected for another phase.	*"The participants for the interview are selected from amongst the highest and lowest scorers of practice preparedness from the survey."*
	Multilevel	Qualitative and quantitative sampling can be applied differentially for different levels/hierarchical situations of the population under study.	*"A case-control study is conducted comparing the learning patterns among high and low academic achievers among the medical residents in a University. In-depth interviews are conducted among a different sample of low achievers within the same target population to explore the specific challenges they face. Focus Group Discussions are separately conducted among the medium achievers to explore their perceptions and challenges."*

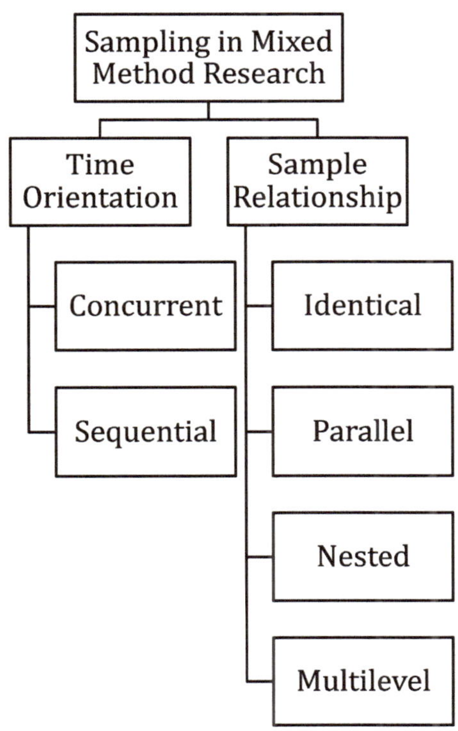

Figure 4: Sampling techniques in mixed-methods researc

How Do We Determine Sample Size for Quantitative Studies?

While selecting participants for any research study, an important consideration is the size of the sample. As a general rule, one can say that, the larger the sample, the better. This is because larger samples have potentially smaller sampling errors, bringing the sample statistics closer to the population parameters. However, selecting large samples may not always be feasible due to resource constraints. A common approach used to determine sample size in quantitative research studies, is to make an educated guess (x% of the population) as to what proportion of the population is required in the sample, considering the time and resources available. Previous research studies or pilot studies can assist in arriving at such an educated guess.

- One could also determine the sample size using appropriate formulas. In surveys and correlational research, we use the sampling error formula for sample size determination, which is based on the expected proportion of the sample with the desired characteristic, sampling error and a confidence interval. In the case of experimental design, we use power analysis, based on the desired power, level of significance and the effect size, which is the expected difference in the means between the control and experimental groups expressed in standard deviation units.
- A practical and rigorous approach is to systematically identify the required sample size based on appropriate sample size tables available in published texts, which are based on standard formulas. Fowler's (1988) table based on sampling error formula for surveys and correlational studies and Lipsey's (1990) table for experimental design based on power analysis are examples of such sample size determination tables.

How Do We Determine Sample Size for Qualitative Studies?

The primary thrust of sampling in qualitative research is on the quality of information rather than the number per se, since our goal is to assess the perceptions or experiences of the study participants to develop a deeper understanding of phenomena. However, this does not mean that sample size determination is not important in qualitative research, since inadequate sample sizes could affect the credibility of findings (Sandelowski, 1995; Vasilieiou et al., 2018). There are two common considerations in determining sample size:

i. **Data/theoretical saturation** – during the course of qualitative research, there will reach a point, when the analysis will show that no new information is emerging from the participants. This is the time to stop the study and size of the sample is not a consideration at this point.
For eg: If you are exploring the reasons for stress amongst students, then after conducting a round of focus group discussions or in-depth interviews, you will reach a certain point where no new information is emerging. Hence you stop conducting any more discussions and interviews after this.

ii. **Deep case oriented analysis** – this analysis involves deeper, nuanced analysis of the experiences and perceptions of fewer members requiring a smaller sample size.
For eg: You have been asked to analyse the curriculum from the stakeholders' point of view in your University. So your sample will include curriculum designers, course coordinators, teachers and students. Rather than a very large sample, here, you will have to go for an in-depth analysis of each of the stakeholder's views.

In general, when the population group is homogenous, a smaller sample size is required. When the population group is heterogeneous, a relatively larger sample size is required. Ideally, qualitative sample sizes should be large enough to allow a rich and textured understanding of the phenomenon under study, allowing data saturation, but small enough to allow a deep and nuanced case-oriented analysis (Sandelowski, 1995).

SUMMARIZE

Sampling is essential to ensure the robustness of any research process, so that valid and credible data are generated. However, the specific purpose of sampling varies according to the objectives of the research and the methods adopted to achieve them. Medical education research is predominantly focused on exploring and refining complex educational ecosystems. More often than not, the purpose of quantitative sampling methods employed here, is to generate samples which adequately represent these ecosystems so that the results can be generalized. The purpose of qualitative sampling is to ensure that the perceptions and experiences of the selected sub-group, such as students or mentors, enhance our understanding of the problem studied. Random/probability sampling methods are most suitable to generate representative samples, while non-random sampling methods are predominantly used for in-depth exploration of phenomena. A significant proportion of the current research in medical education employs mixed-methods, where the chosen sampling designs are determined by the relationship or time orientation between the quantitative and qualitative research components. The size of the study sample is an equally important consideration. The primary criterion for sample size determination in quantitative research is to ensure that the sample selected is large enough to minimize sampling error. In qualitative research, the sample size should be sufficient for a rich and nuanced analysis of the research problem.

EVALUATE

Revisit the questions we posed in the scenario (section 'Contextualize) and see if you can find the answers to these questions:

1. ***What was the type of research?***
2. ***What forms the population, the target population and the sample in this scenario?***
3. ***What is the appropriate sampling technique?***
4. ***How do we arrive at sample size for the chosen research method?***

- Since both quantitative (survey) and qualitative (FGD) methods were employed in the research, it is clearly a mixed-methods research.
- The staff from the five selected institutions within the University forms the whole population, while the target population will include only who are actively engaged in online teaching. A set of people drawn from this target population, adequately representing it forms the sample.
- The sampling technique for the survey should have been random, proportionally stratified from each of the five institutions. A criterion-based purposeful sampling, is most appropriate for the FGD and the selection criterion should have been the experience of conducting online sessions. If the researcher wants a more nuanced analysis, he/she could select a sub-set of survey participants who conducted the least and the most number of online sessions and interview them (maximum variation sampling and nested design).
- While data saturation should determine the number of FGDs to be conducted, an educated guess proportional to the target population size in each of the institutions would have been ideal for the survey.

ROAD AHEAD

Sampling forms important component of research. Medical education researchers need to be well versed with the sampling methods and techniques to get valid data. Selection of sample largely depends on the research objectives and the inclusion and exclusion criteria. The probability sampling methods sometimes refers to random number tables and computer-generated numbers.

More Resources to learn more about random allocation of subjects using computer generated random numbers.

- **https://levelup.gitconnected.com/how-do-computers-generate-random-numbers-a72be65877f6**
- **https://engineering.mit.edu/engage/ask-an-engineer/can-a-computer-generate-a-truly-random-number/**

There are many online courses on sampling and sampling methods in research. Few links are pasted below:

- http://nie.gov.in/niecer/niecer_page.htm
- https://onlinecourses.nptel.ac.in/noc19_ge24/preview

Your experience with sampling and sampling methods for the educational research at your institution

- What were your research objectives?
- What were your inclusion criteria?
- What was your research type?
- What method of sampling method and technique did you adopt? Do share your experience with the authors at the email addresses mentioned in the chapter.

REFERENCES

Creswell, J.W. (2012). *Educational research. Planning, conducting and evaluating quantitative and qualitative research.* Boston (Ma): Pearson Education INC.

Creswell, J.W., & Creswell, J.D. (2018). *Research design: qualitative, quantitative, and mixed methods approach.* Los Angeles: Sage.

Johnson, R.B, & Christensen, L. (2014). *Educational research. Quantitative, qualitative, and mixed approaches.* Los Angeles: Sage.

Sandelowski, M. (1995). Focus on qualitative methods: sample size in qualitative research. *Res Nurs Health.*, 18: 179- 183.

Vasilieiou, K., Barnett, J., Thorpe, S., Young, T. (2018). Characterizing and justifying sample size sufficiency in interview-based studies: systematic analysis of qualitative health research over a 15-year period. *BMC Med Res Methodol.* 18:148. https://doi.org/10.1186/s12874-018-0594-7

Chapter 6

Program Evaluation in Health Professions Education

Thomas V Chacko

ABSTRACT

With globalization of medicine and curricular shift towards outcome-based and transformative medical education, there is a need for capacity building of faculty and academic leaders in the field of Program Evaluation (PE) in health professions education. It is much sought after by educational program planners and accreditation bodies to ensure and assure that institutions are producing graduates who are competent health care providers. Market forces also drive the need for quality improvement in the educational programs so as to move towards excellence. This chapter gives an overview of the need, the theories and framework that guide the choice of model and process of program evaluation. It aims to bring awareness among the stakeholders of the systematic process that exists in conducting program evaluation. The "Road Ahead" section at the end of the chapter will help the readers get further guidance in conducting program evaluation in diverse settings and explore this field further.

Key Words: program evaluation, program theory, logic model, evaluation framework, quality improvement

ASSESS NEED

Medical Education in India, and in most parts of the world, is undergoing a transition to adopting competency based education focusing on graduate outcomes linked to health needs of society. This being a transition from traditional information-intensive teacher-centered paradigm to a student centered learning to acquire competencies, there is need to do PE more frequently and in a systematic manner.

Another major need for doing PE is the one forced by the COVID pandemic which has led to adoption of online and blended learning and it's benefits have led to it being accepted as the "new norm". The above statements is illustration of the need for the chapter. "Assess need" is also a critical first step in the process of Program Evaluation.

BRIEF

- Program Evaluation (PE) helps make defensible value judgments on the merits and fitness to purpose of a program;
- PE Theories, Models and Standards inform and guide the program evaluator on what to focus upon given the different contexts, circumstances and purpose defined by the stakeholders
- It uses robust research methods but the intent is not to prove but to improve the program;
- An evaluator needs to first understand the program before trying to evaluate it;
- Use of "Evaluation framework" helps the evaluator to conduct program evaluation in a systematic manner.

CONTEXTUALIZE

The following scenarios help to illustrate the need for PE stated in the changing context:

Scenario 1

Given the transition to the new CBME curriculum and with the medical schools gainfully adopting online learning, a number of questions arise in the minds of stakeholders:

- "Are the graduates of the Competency Based Curriculum job-ready to manage common ailments at the primary care level?";
- "Are the faculty competent to deliver Competency Based Curriculum and use assessment methods that are appropriate for performance testing?"
- "Are the educational inputs and processes being optimally delivered to ensure attainment of the stated outcomes? Is there scope for further improvement?";
- "Are all the routine ongoing teaching-learning activities needed to achieve the stated objectives and outcomes? Are some of them wastefully consuming precious resources?".

These questions would be the starting points for the program evaluator to design PE and communicate findings to the stakeholders for them to take corrective measures to improve it further.

Scenario 2

Your Academic Dean wants to know whether the new system of training that has been introduced is better than the traditional method that we all grew up learning in and teaching. She wants to make the institution "an Institution of Excellence". Which program evaluation model would you choose? How would you proceed? How will you identify the indicators of "success", "effectiveness" and "attainment of stated outcomes"? Is there a systematic framework or process to follow to accomplish this task? Are you equipped with competencies to carry out the task of program evaluation in a professional way as a "consultant" program evaluator?

DESCRIBE

What is Program Evaluation?

The word evaluate suggests a value judgment. Professionals who are entrusted to do this task engage in the process called program evaluation. During this process to determine value, quality, utility, fairness, effectiveness or significance of a program, evaluator uses inquiry and judgment methods that include determining and applying international program evaluation standards for judging quality, identifying key stakeholders, collecting, analyzing and communicating relevant information.

Program evaluation refers to the systematic collection of information about the activities, characteristics, and outcomes of programs, to reduce uncertainties, improve effectiveness, and make decisions. Program evaluation is intended to guide defensible judgments about the merit (technical value) and worth (social value) of programs (American Evaluation Association 2021) Hence program evaluation uses robust methods used in research so that the findings are defensible.

Educational Program Evaluation

Program evaluation in education has been described in different ways. Cook (2010) described it as "*Using information to judge value or worth of an educational program*". ACGME (2010) described it as "***Systematic collection and analysis** of information **related to** the design, implementation and outcomes of a program for the **purpose** of monitoring and improving the quality and effectiveness of a program*".

Why Program Evaluation?

1. **Program evaluation guides governance.** It helps the organizations to determine whether the program is worthy of adoption, continuation or expansion (value, quality, utility, fairness, effectiveness, or significance).
2. **Helps the institution to optimize inputs and processes.** This happens when inputs and processes are evaluated in relation to the program's intended outcomes.
3. **To improve the quality of medical education globally.** World Federation for Medical Education (WFME) has included having a system of program evaluation of educational programs and curricula as one of the global standards for ensuring quality in medical education.
4. **Helps in quality assurance for patient safety.** When the institution presents evidence of compliance to national/international program evaluation standards set by accreditation agencies, it serves the purpose of quality assurance for the society and country.
5. **Helps inform the institution, the regulators and the society about how the institution is executing its social responsibilities.** The curriculum that is implemented in an institution reflects the values and mission of the institution and describes the outcome attributes of the graduates of the program in line with its ethos for health care service.

Theories That Inform and Models That Guide Program Evaluation

Program evaluation theories inform and guide the program evaluator on what to focus on given the different contexts, circumstances and purpose the stakeholders would like to know more about the program in order to take decisions about the program (Anh 2018)

Table 1: Choosing a Model for Educational Program Evaluation: An Overview of Theories and Models

Purpose of Evaluation (Well suited for)	Evaluation Orientation & Proponents	Distinguishing Characteristics	Concerns/limitations	Situations where commonly used
Helps evaluators know "To what extent Program objectives are achieved?".	**Objectives oriented** Tyler's **Objective Model** (Goal-based Evaluation).	• Uses objective methods of data collection to compare measurable objectives (actual Vs intended).	• Only internal comparisons possible. • Doesn't provide feedback on processes for program improvement. • Cannot diagnose why a curriculum has failed.	• Curriculum development and Evaluation. • Define objectives for new curriculum linking it to needs of society. • Monitoring Participant's progression towards Course Outcomes.
Proactively provide Information needed for decision making and retroactively provide information for educational accountability for the actions, decisions taken.	**Management oriented** Stufflebeam's Context - Inputs - Process – Product (**CIPP**) Model for Evaluation.	• Systematic process allows rational decision making and evaluates at all stages of program development. • Ongoing efforts to identify and correct gaps in inputs and processes mainly "to improve & not to prove".	• If the whole model (all components of CIPP) are applied, it is expensive and time consuming. • Overvalues system efficiency and so caters mostly to top managers rather than users of system (users have less voice).	• Comprehensive framework for both Formative (improvement) and summative (effectiveness) evaluation. • Continuing Quality Improvement.
To inform consumers about education products so that they can make decision on which educational program to choose from.	**Consumer Oriented** Scriven's (Goal-free) Evaluation.	• Inform users/ consumers • Does product evaluation against benchmarked standards using a variety of methods including checklists, needs assessments, cost analysis, experimental and quasi experimental designs.	• Conceptually abstract and theoretical with lack of guidelines about how to conduct it and so limited to its use only by experts. • Chance that some most important effects may be missed and so should be used as supplement to Goal-based evaluation.	• Used by Standards and "Watchdog" agencies about the actual worth of the program to consumers independent of what is claimed (intended outcomes & effects) by program proponents.

Purpose of Evaluation (Well suited for)	Evaluation Orientation & Proponents	Distinguishing Characteristics	Concerns/limitations	Situations where commonly used
To provide professional judgment on quality of an Institution, program & its activities.	**Expertise Oriented** Flexner, Eisner's Connoisseurship & Criticism model, Accreditation Groups.	• Relies on individual's professional expert judgment, experience and human wisdom. • Use of consensus standards & site visits. • Qualitative rather than quantitative.	• Subjective opinion of the expert in the absence or narrowness of standards to assess the criteria.	• Self-study to identify gaps against standards for its improvement. • Accreditation Bodies for judging quality & areas of its improvement.
To respond to Stakeholder's need for information. Helps evaluators better understand the program and determine which issues and concerns are most important.	**Participant Oriented** Stakes Responsive Model.	• Orients more to program activities than intents. • Reflects multiple realities & interpretations based on the person's points of view, beliefs & interests. The role of Evaluator is to capture these opinions of people about the program. • Use of inductive reasoning and discovery.	• Since it is interactive and responsive to stakeholders need for information in an inductive and discovery way, it is time consuming, not easy to conduct; being responsive to information need of stakeholders, may fail to maintain focus to answer specific evaluation questions.	• Participants in and around the program use the findings to identify program scope, the activities, strengths and shortcomings of a program. • Evaluator finds out what is of value to the audiences (stakeholders).
To carry out Program Evaluation on Effectiveness of Professional Training programs.	**Training Effectiveness Oriented** Kirkpatrick's four levels hierarchy framework model.	• Training program effectiveness looks at four levels with three on the learner's. 1) Reaction/ satisfaction. 2) Learning (change in Knowledge/ Skill/Attitude) . 3) Behaviour (application of learning at work) and for the Institution sponsoring the training. 4) Results & Return on Investment/ Expectation.	• Evaluation becomes more expensive as we go up the levels. • Some feel it is not a Model (Kirkpatrick called it a "framework"). • Too simplistic for it to be used to evaluate higher education programs. Other models also need to be used to bring out the complexity of inputs and multifarious environments.	• To evaluate the effectiveness of educational programs. • Develop indicators for evaluation of the training program's success. • Impact of the training on the learner's learning.

What Next?

1. A Program Evaluator First Understands the Program Before Its Evaluation

An educational program is generally designed to help the learner achieve predetermined graduate outcomes to become competent to deliver on-the-job professional tasks. Teachers often implement curricular innovations to enhance the learning experiences for better learning outcomes. In the long-term, these are aimed at improving patient outcomes. To better understand the programs well as iteratively engage the stakeholders (to ensure their acceptance of the evaluation report), the tools known as LOGIC MODEL for the PROGRAM THEORY or THEORY OF CHANGE are commonly used. Whereas the Program Theory explains WHY a program is needed and expected to work, the Logic Model ILLUSTRATES a Program Theory. In developing the program theory, one starts with the problem or the needs that the program is expected to address. The program evaluator then elicits from the stakeholders in a series of "if-then" statements, the chain of outcomes that a particular activity or intervention leads to (Fig 1) (Woodrow & Oatley, 2013) (CDC 2021) Conversely, by following this program theory, if at the end of the outcomes chain the problem gets solved, it is a vindication that the program intervention was well designed.

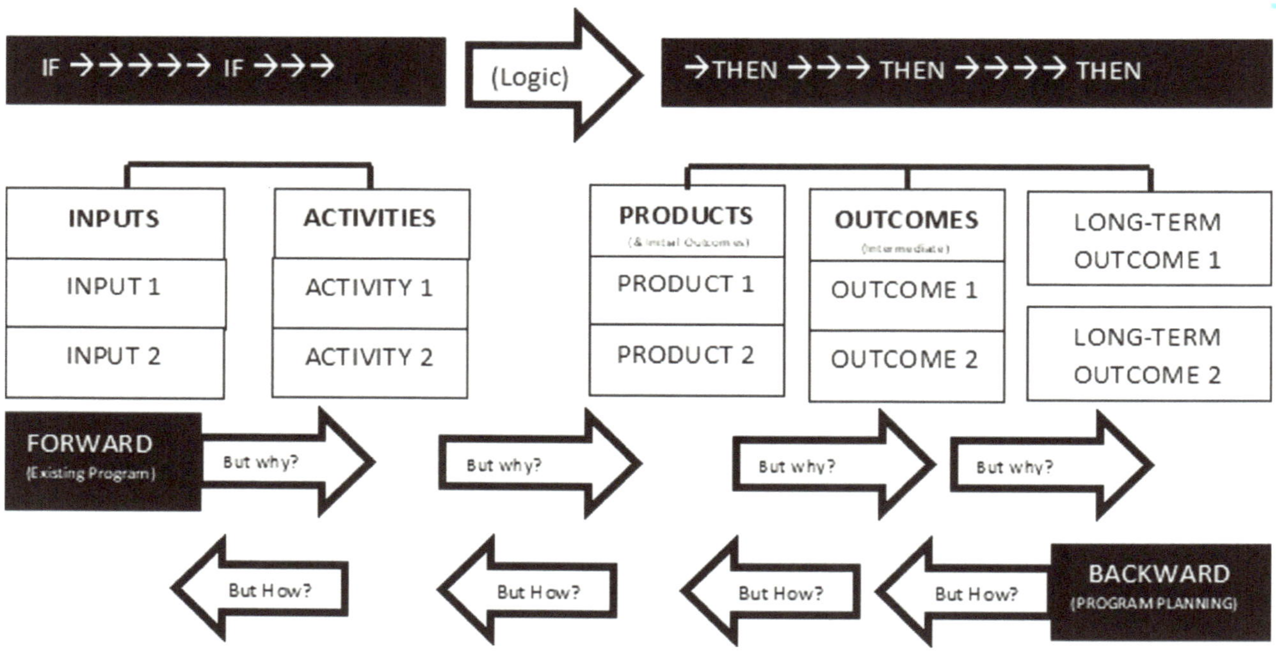

Figure 1: Logic Model Components and Thinking for Program Planning and Evaluation

When the program is already in existence, a **forward Logic Model** is constructed by the evaluator by eliciting the information starting from left to right (as in the figure 1) with further elicitation of its rationale (logic) by asking "**but why?**" question to better understand a program before moving to evaluate the program. When the Program is in planning stage, **a backward Logic Model** is constructed starting from the right (program outcomes) by asking the question "**but how?**" to elicit what activities are needed and for each activity what resources are required. If one's logic is sound, using this approach, a blueprint is ready that will ensure that the program activities **will** lead to the specified outcomes.

Uses of Logic Model and Program Theory in Program Evaluation

The Logic Model links the inputs (resources) and activities to program products(outputs) and outcomes (impact/goals) while communicating the logic (theory) behind the program's reason for existence. Benefits of doing this logical linking process, include:

1. **It helps identify the gaps and unmet needs** in the existing program
2. **It helps build a strong program design with focus on change and results rather than activities.** It helps identify the extraneous activities that do not contribute to the achievement of program objectives by identifying them and eliminating them. This way, the extra cost and resources can be avoided or better utilized.
3. **Helps in program monitoring and evaluation** by identifying the short-term, intermediate and long-term outcomes
4. **Helps initiate mid-course corrections** if needed through periodic review of resources-activities-outcomes.

2. Identifying Measurable Outcome Indicators for Program Evaluation

Whereas the outputs of a program are the direct products of program activities, outcomes are benefits or changes for individuals or population groups -in terms of behavior, knowledge, attitudes brought out during or after participating in a program. For the program evaluator to establish that the program is effective, outcome indicators should be identified. Indicators are specific, observable and measurable items of data that can be tracked to measure how well the program is achieving an outcome (Table 2). The outcome benefits may take time to manifest but we can measure changes in the beneficiaries over a period of time, from the time they undergo a program. **Initial outcomes** are the benefits to those who underwent the program experience immediately and can be measured in terms of changes in knowledge, attitude and behavior or skills. They are not the endpoints in themselves but are essential steps towards the desired program goals and so they are the indicators of participant's progress towards that final goal. **Intermediate outcomes** link initial program outcomes with the long-term outcomes those are expected for its participants. They are often participant's change in behavior that results in their change in knowledge, skills and attitudes. The **long-term outcomes** are the ultimate program outcomes for which the program is created.

Who and *what* changes as a result of the impact of the program helps identify the *indicators* of effectiveness of the program. The following outcomes evaluation matrix (Table 2) will help a program evaluator for mapping the evaluation questions and corresponding indicators.

Table 2: Outcomes Evaluation Matrix for Identifying Indicators and Evaluation Questions

Outcomes	Evaluation Questions	Indicators	Study Design	Data Source	Data Collection methods
Impact of the program on participants.	They reflect purpose, needs of stakeholders.	Specific, observable & measurable markers of success.	Appropriate to evaluation question.	Where from info' available?.	Detailed steps to collect for each indicator, source.
Short-term: change in knowledge, attitude, skill.	How well did the program work? Have the key short-term outcomes of the program been achieved?.	Percent increase in Post-Test Scores (K); improvement in performance scores (S); extent of change in perspective (A).	Descriptive study; Experimental & Quasi Experimental (Retro-Pre, Pre-post etc) as appropriate to the evaluation question.	Participants in program, Progress reports, Portfolios.	Assessments, Quiz; Retro-pre survey, Self-reports, document study.
Intermediate: Change in behaviour.	How well did the program lead to knowledge transfer on to the job?.	Percent trainees applying the new learning on the job.		Participants at workplace, Supervisors, Performance appraisals.	Observation of changes in practice of participant; exit interview/survey.
Long-Term: Change in status/ condition of participant or user of service provided by them.	Did the smoking cessation training program succeed in helping trainees' target group to stop smoking?.	Percent trainees fulfilling criteria for excellence in teaching. Improved learning by students taught by trainee.		Users of service delivered by Participants at their workplace.	Service beneficiaries exit interview/ survey. Institution's Quality Systems document study.

3. Types and Uses of Program Evaluation

There are several types of program evaluations but by building on the Logic Model that helps identify key activities and outcomes and the CDC's Program Evaluation Working group's types of PE (CDC 2021), the evaluations can be classified as:

Formative Evaluation

Undertaken before full implementation is completed or when a new program or activity is being developed or when an existing one is being modified. It helps test the logic used in planning the program and to identify the "fit" between the program activities and the program needs. It thus ensures that a program or program activity is feasible, appropriate, and acceptable thereby improving the likelihood of success of the program.

Process/Implementation Evaluation (and Program Monitoring)

Undertaken during the program implementation including in periodic cycles by reviewing the activities and output components identified in the program's logic model. It determines whether program activities have been implemented as intended and how well the program is working & is accessible and acceptable to the program users.

Outcome/Effectiveness Evaluation (and Objectives Based Evaluation)

Undertaken immediately after implementation by starting a review of the outcome components listed in the program's logic model. It measures program effects in the target population by assessing the progress in the outcomes or outcome objectives that the program is to achieve in terms of change in target group's behaviours.

Impact Evaluation

Undertaken after implementation – at least a year after the program was concluded to assesses program effectiveness in achieving its ultimate goals in the long term. It shows the degree to which the program meets its final goal.

4. Framework for Program Evaluation (Steps and Standards for Effective PE)

The PE framework includes steps in evaluation practice and standards for effective evaluation. The two are used together throughout the evaluation process for each step in an iterative way by applying the standards (utility, feasibility, propriety and accuracy) to ensure that the program evaluation is effective in achieving the purpose for which it is carried out (Carter, 2019)

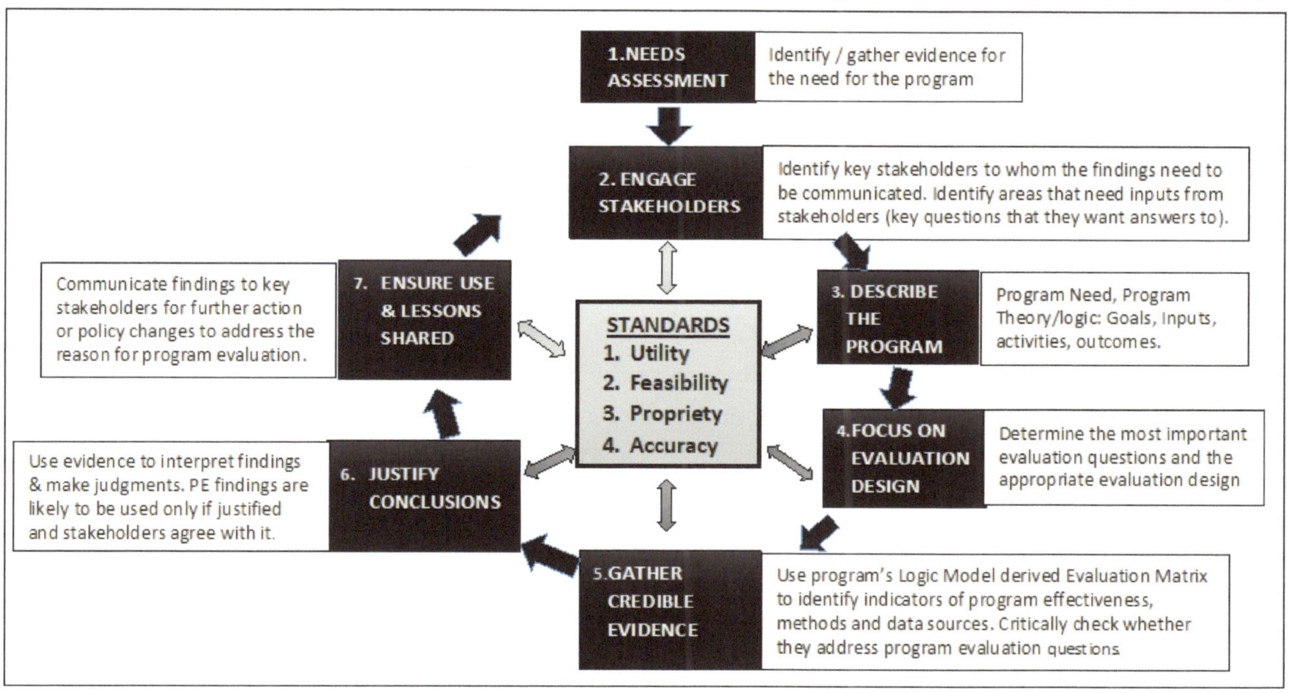

Figure 2: The Evaluation Framework (Steps in Conjunction with Evaluation Standards)
Source: Adapted and Built on CDC Working Group's Evaluation Framework (CDC, 1999)

International Standards for Program Evaluation

As shown in the program evaluation framework (Fig 2), educators with interest in educational program evaluation need to apply program evaluation standards at every step in their practice of program evaluation. This is to ensure credible and beneficial program evaluation for the stakeholders. For this purpose the Joint Committee on Standards for Educational Evaluation proposed a set of 30 Standards that are meant to help with assessing the quality of evaluation activities, determining whether a set of evaluative activities are well-designed and working to their potential. These 30 Standards are grouped into four sets – utility, feasibility, propriety, and accuracy and following these standards demonstrates the professionalism among program evaluators. (Mathison, 2013)

1. **Utility standards** ensure that an evaluation will serve the information needs of intended users in a timely manner. They include:
   - U1. **Attention to Stakeholders** so that their needs are addressed;
   - U2. **Evaluator Credibility**: the need to be trustworthy and competent to ensure PE reports are acceptable;
   - U3. **Information Selection and Scope** to address pertinent questions of the client;
   - U4. **Values Identification** to enable clarity in making value judgments;
   - U5. **Report Clarity** with essential information in an easy to understandable way;
   - U6. **Report Timeliness** including interim reports and distributed to intended users;
   - U7. **Evaluation Impact** evaluations need to be planned, conducted and reported to stakeholders to increase likelihood of evaluations being used.

2. **Feasibility standards** are intended to ensure that an evaluation will be realistic given the time, resources and expertise at hand, diplomatic, and frugal. They include:
   - F1. **Practical Procedures** to avoid disruptions and ensure needed information is collected;
   - F2. **Political Viability**: recommends keeping in mind the positions of different interest groups to ensure they cooperate;
   - F3. **Cost Effectiveness** by being efficient in producing only information of value.

3. **Propriety standards** are intended to ensure that an evaluation will be conducted legally, ethically, and with due regard for the welfare of those involved in the evaluation, as well as those affected by its results. They include:
   - P1. **Service Orientation** by designing it to serve the needs of all;
   - P2. **Formal Agreements** on what, how and by whom and when in writing so that all parties comply or can be renegotiated upon,
   - P3. **Rights of Human Subjects;**
   - P4. **Human Interactions** respecting human dignity;
   - P5. **Complete and Fair Assessment** to be fair in reporting both strengths and weaknesses so that strengths can be built on and problem areas addressed;
   - P6. **Disclosure of Findings** in full including the limitations to all stakeholders;
   - P7. **Conflict of Interest**: need for open disclosure;
   - P8. **Fiscal Responsibility**: need for fiscal prudence and be ethical so that expenditures are accounted for and appropriate.

4. **Accuracy standards** are intended to ensure a valid and reliable evaluation that will reveal and convey technically adequate information about the features that determine merit of the program being evaluated. They include:
   - A1. **Program Documentation**: clarity in description and documentation of program;
   - A2. **Context Analysis**: so that it's influences on the program can be identified;
   - A3. **Described Purpose and Procedures** in detail so that they can be monitored and assessed;

A4. **Defensible Information Sources** so that its adequacy can be assessed;

A5. **Valid Information** so that the interpretation arrived is valid for the intended use; A6) Reliable Information choose or develop procedures so that information obtained is sufficiently reliable for the intended use;

A7. **Systematic Information** that is collected, processed, and reported should be systematically reviewed, and any errors found should be corrected;

A8. **Analysis of Quantitative Information;**

A9. **Analysis of Qualitative Information** to be done appropriately and systematically for effectively answering evaluation questions;

A10. **Justified Conclusions** should explicit so that stakeholders can assess them;

A11. **Impartial Reporting** guarding against distortion and biases;

A12. **Meta-evaluation**: The evaluation itself should be formatively and summatively evaluated against these and other pertinent standards, so that its conduct is appropriately guided and, on completion, stakeholders can closely examine its strengths and weaknesses.

The evaluator can also use the 30 Standards as a checklist to guide conduct of program evaluation and while writing the evaluator's report.

Program Evaluation for Quality Assurance & Excellence

Program evaluation thus has many applications and one of the key reasons why a system of program evaluation (Fig. 3 below) should be in place in all educational institutions is for the purpose of patient safety through a quality assurance in the educational system that would ensure competent health care professionals.

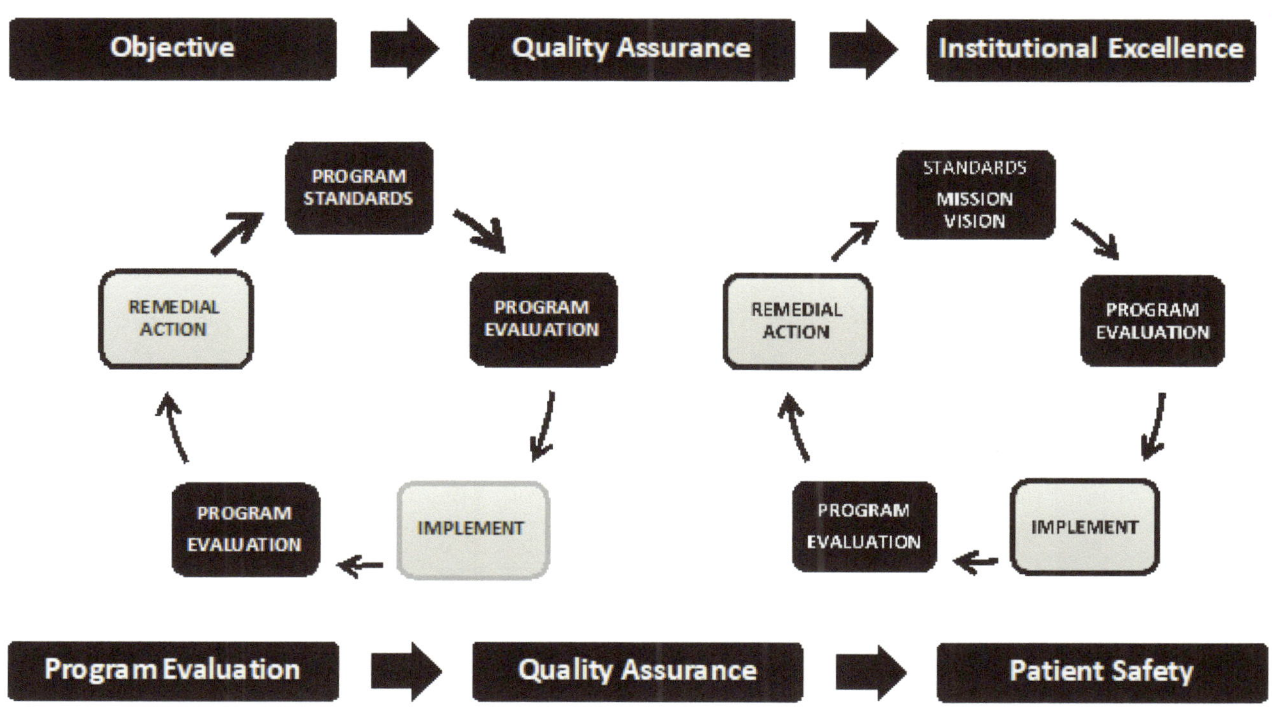

Figure 3: Role of Program Evaluation Ensuring Competent Health Care Professionals & Excellence

SUMMARIZE

Program evaluation also helps the institution achieve excellence through quality improvement facilitated by a systematic program evaluation (audit) process being in place:

- Program Evaluation helps make defensible value judgment on the merit and worth of a program.
- It uses robust research methods but the intent is not to prove but to improve the program.
- An evaluator needs to first understand the program before trying to evaluate it.
- Use of evaluation framework helps the evaluator to systematically conduct evaluation
- International evaluation standards help the evaluator to demonstrate professionalism in conducting and reporting program evaluation to the stakeholders for decision making

EVALUATE

What program evaluation approach would I pursue? If:

- I want to know whether the training course that I conducted is effective:
    - ______________________________
    - ______________________________
- I am hired to evaluate an ongoing training program to ensure health care providers are competent:
    - ______________________________
    - ______________________________
- I am tasked to be project officer for quality improvement and institutional excellence:
    - ______________________________
    - ______________________________
- I am asked to write a grant proposal for an educational program to reduce depression among college students in the state:
    - ______________________________
    - ______________________________
- I must conduct program evaluation of an educational institution aiming for being included in the top ten in the country and submit a report that will be used by stakeholders:
    - ______________________________
    - ______________________________

ROAD AHEAD

Resources to Further Guide PE

The chapter gives only an overview on program evaluation. To actually undertake a program evaluation, the following resources would come in handy as they provide the needed detail:

A. **Resources for planning**

1. **Center for Disease Control (CDC) Program Evaluation Web Resources.** Accessible from https://www.cdc.gov/eval/framework/index.htm. (Good resource for Program Evaluation Framework steps and Evaluation Standards, Logic Models, Indicators, Templates)
2. **United Way. A guide to Developing an Outcome Logic Model and Measurement Plan** accessible from https://www.yourunitedway.org/wp-content/uploads/2015/12/UWGRP-Guide-to-Outcomes-and-Logic-Models-6-8-15.pdf (Good resource for developing outcomes based Logic Models, your outcomes measurement plan with examples)

B. **Resources for implementation/Methods/Report writing**

1. **W K Kellogg Foundation's EVALUATION HANDBOOK** accessible from https://www.wkkf.org/~/media/62EF77BD5792454B807085B1AD044FE7.ashxLast accessed on 20th July 2021. (blueprinting Program Evaluation planning and its implementation and utilization)
2. **Evaluation Cookbook** (1998) Learning Technology Dissemination Initiative Heriot-Watt University Edinburgh. Accessible from http://www.icbl.hw.ac.uk/ltdi/cookbook/cookbook.pdf Last accessed on 20th July 2021. (for Practical tips and tools useful for Program Evaluation)
3. **CDC. Developing an Effective Evaluation report** accessible from https://www.cdc.gov/eval/materials/developing-an-effective-evaluation-report_tag508.pdf (for explaining the steps mentioned in Evaluation Framework and writing an effective evaluation report)

REFERENCES

Anh, V. T. K. (2018). Evaluation Models in Educational Program: Strengths and Weaknesses. *VNU Journal of Foreign Studies*, *34*(2). https://doi.org/10.25073/2525-2445/vnufs.4252

Carter, M. W. (2019). *In Support of Effective Interventions*. 43, 1–14. https://doi.org/10.1097/OLQ.0000000000000281.Program

CDC(2021), Step 2B logic models - centers for disease control and ... (n.d.). Retrieved March 28, 2022, from https://www.cdc.gov/oralhealth/funded_programs/pdf/logic_models.pdf

CDC (1999). Framework for program evaluation in public health. *MMWR. Recommendations and Reports : Morbidity and Mortality Weekly Report. Recommendations and Reports / Centers for Disease Control*, *48*(RR-11), 1–40. https://www.cdc.gov/mmwr/preview/mmwrhtml/rr4811a1.htm

Centers for Disease Control & Prevention (2016). *Program Performance and Evaluation Office (PPEO)*. 1–34. https://www.cdc.gov/eval/tools/logic_models/index.html

Cook, D. A. (2010). Twelve tips for evaluating educational programs. *Medical Teacher*, *32*(4), 296–301. https://doi.org/10.3109/01421590903480121

Frye, A. W., & Hemmer, P. A. (2012). Program evaluation models and related theories: AMEE Guide No. 67. *Medical Teacher*, *34*(5). https://doi.org/10.3109/0142159X.2012.668637

Goldie, J. (2006). AMEE Education Guide no. 29: Evaluating educational programmes. *Medical Teacher*, *28*(3), 210–224. https://doi.org/10.1080/01421590500271282

Mathison, S. (2013). The Program Evaluation Standards. *Encyclopedia of Evaluation*, *126*, 125–126. https://doi.org/10.4135/9781412950558.n446

Woodrow, P., & Oatley, N. (2013). Practical approaches to theories of change in conflict, security & justice programmes. *Collaborative Learning Projects*, *March*, 1–29. https://assets.publishing.service.gov.uk/government/uploads/system/uploads/attachment_data/file/304613/Practical-approaches-theories-change-conflict-security-justice-prog.pdf

Section II

Practice

Chapter 7

Identifying A Research Problem and Formulating A Research Question

Indika Karunathilake, Gominda Ponnamperuma

ABSTRACT

Identifying a research problem and formulating a research question are often considered the toughest part of a research. The reason for this is it is often considered that the research questionis the heart or the engine of a research. The process of developing a research question is fraught with constant traps and pitfalls. Avoiding these need a structured, methodical, and disciplined approach. The first step of such an approach is identifying a research problem which is of practical and theoretical value. Deriving a research question from the research problem is an iterative process of subjecting the research question to repeated scrutiny using three basic question forms: what, why, and how. These three question forms facilitate the critical review, refinement, and conversion of an initial broad and non-specific research question into a focused, specific, unambiguous, and researchable research question. This chapter explores the finer aspects of the art and science of identifying a research problem and converting it to a research question.

Key Words: hypothesis; health professions' education research, medical education

ASSESS NEED

Health professions teachers are trained well in research in their own disciplines. They know how to identify a research problem, wade through the literature around that problem, carve out a research question from it, and conduct a research that stretches the knowledge base in their discipline. Health professions teachers also encounter many educational situations that they do not know how best to tackle. Many do not consider the problems that these situations pose as fertile grounds for research. The reason for this is educational research considerably differs from most health professions research. The lens through which an educational problem should be viewed to make it the starting point of a successful research study requires training in educational research. Such training offers a way of thinking to the health professions teachers so that an educational issue at hand could be transformed into a researchable question. This chapter takes the reader through the steps of the thinking process of developing such a research question.

BRIEF

- Health professions education research demands a unique skill set, often distinct from the traditional discipline-based research that the health professionals have been trained in.
- Like in any other field, the research question is the make-or-break element of a research that determines its quality.
- Developing a good health professions education research question requires a sound knowledge in core theories of health professions education, an in-depth understanding of a way-of-thinking unique to educational research, and hands-on experience in developing research questions.
- Identifying a research problem that has both practical and theoretical relevance is the key to designing a research question.
- Constructing a good research question can be achieved by figuring out the answers to the three questions of what, why, and how, in an iterative process.

CONTEXTUALIZE

A physiology lecturer has been teaching online almost exclusively due to the on-going Covid-19 pandemic. He has been often wondering how effective what he does when compared with the traditional face-to-face teaching. However, he acknowledges that online learning also offers some fabulous facilities for the students to learn, un-learn and re-learn at their own pace, while interacting with a wide range of learning resources. He wonders whether offering the student both online and on site options so that the student can blend the two modes based on their own learning preferences would be the best option. This pushes him to look for an answer from the literature. He types in the words the search terms: "blended learning", "effectiveness" and "health professions education". The results show that almost all articles have found blended learning either more effective than or at least as effective as another type of learning (Liu et al., 2016). He languishes that although the evidence seems to be convincing it is certainly not beyond reasonable doubt. There may be instances that blended learning is only as effective as (and not exclusively more effective than) other modes of learning. He wonders why blended learning is only 'as effective as' other learning modes? It may be that in different study settings the circumstances, learning facilities, ratio of blending, and student preferences and preparedness are different (Berliner, 2002). Since the results seem to be contextual rather than universal, at least to an extent, he decides that the only way to find out whether blended learning is more effective than other modes of learning (online or onsite) is to conduct his own research.

So, he plans a research to find out the effectiveness of learning with different teaching and learning modes, i.e., blended, online, and onsite learning. His preliminary research question is: what is the effectiveness of blended learning when compared with online or onsite learning?

However, he realizes that this research question is rudimentary and unrefined yet. To refine it further, he asks himself a few more questions. "What exactly are the type of learning that I am investigating? Who are my study participants? Is it feasible to divide the participants into three groups to administer blended, online, and onsite learning?" Answers to these questions do not come to the lecturer effortlessly. He expands on the previous literature search with a view to learning from how other researchers have tackled similar research questions. What he learns from the literature along with his own thinking provides him with his updated research question: what is the effectiveness of blended learning when compared with online or onsite learning related to cardiovascular physiology among the first-year medical students?

This updated research question too is far from complete. The lecturer is still unclear about: "Who exactly are the three student groups? What am I measuring to find the effectiveness? Is it fair, and ethical to create these three groups? How can I measure learning in each of the three methods?" When answering these questions, the lecturer conducts an even more thorough literature search and tries to learn how other researchers have conducted similar research. Both through what he has learned from the literature and what he has figured out for himself through a structured, methodical thinking process he manages to devise the following complete research question: when blended, online and onsite learning modes are compared, what is more effective in assimilating knowledge on cardiovascular physiology, by the first-year medical students at Medical School X in 2021?

DESCRIBE

What is a research question?

A research question has a few critical features. First and foremost, it should be a question. However, it should not be just a question. It should be a question that is researchable. In the above scenario, one could argue that the research questions produced both initially and after the first revision are non-researchable questions. The initially produced question states: what is the effectiveness of blended learning when compared with online or onsite learning? This question is non-researchable because it does not specify what is meant by effectiveness. Effectiveness can be simply based on the participant (i.e., students, teachers) perceptions or it can be more objectively measured using a purpose-made assessment. The research question also does not state effectiveness on what. Is it effectiveness in relation to particular content area, e.g., cardiovascular physiology, anatomy of the locomotor system? Hence, no one knows how effectiveness should be measured in this research study. Even after the first revision, the research question still does not convey what effectiveness means although it is more specific about the content area, i.e., cardiovascular physiology. Similarly, the first two attempts do not exactly specify who the research participants are. With such research questions, almost anything is possible. By contrast, the final research question is researchable as it is specific to a level that will produce a comparable study no matter who conducts it.

The next crucial feature of a research question is that it should lead to a research. This, then poses the question: what is a research? There are a few cardinal features of a research (Thabane et al., 2009). An investigation, to be called a research, should be based on data, should produce results generalizable beyond the study, and most importantly, must lead to new knowledge or at least extend the existing knowledge. It is the latter feature that a research question is mostly responsible for. In the above scenario, for example, there seems to be considerable evidence that blended learning is more effective than online or onsite learning. In that case, what the researcher should ask themselves is that how can he justify conducting such a research. How the researcher has justified this study is by finding a gap in the existing evidence. That is a relative lack of evidence for the effectiveness of blended learning in a setting similar to the present study. This justification is further vindicated by the fact that all previous research has not unequivocally indicated that blended learning is more effective than the other modes of teaching and learning (Liu et al., 2016).

The other important features of a good research question are that it should be clearly worded without any ambiguity, it should be succinct, and it should be readily understandable or easily and uniformly interpreted.

Why a research question?

The research question forms the heart of a research (Lipowski, 2008). This means all other steps in a research are dependent on how good the research question is. To illustrate this, the above scenario could be extended to show how the research question is instrumental in determining the next steps of a research.

Once the research question is ready, the most important next step is to identify a broad research approach. There are three broad research approaches in health professions education research: quantitative, qualitative, and mixed methods. In the scenario above, given that the researcher considers investigating the effectiveness in terms of assimilation of knowledge, it is likely that the researcher considers assessment of knowledge to find the answer to the research question. Since knowledge is traditionally assessed by quantifying knowledge using scores or grades, this research question seems to point towards a quantitative approach.

That said, it is not impossible to find out what the students have learned using interviews, and then qualitatively compare the richness of the knowledge gained by the participants in the three different groups. If the researcher wants to adopt such an approach, however, it would be better if the research question is slightly modified: when blended, online and onsite learning modes are compared, what are the differences in the richness of knowledge on cardiovascular physiology, assimilated by the first-year medical students, at Medical School X in 2021? Thus, removing the term 'more effective' has given the research question a more qualitative outlook.

Similarly, the original research question can be used for mixed methods approach, if 'effectiveness' can be operationally defined to include both assessment (quantitative data) and student perception (qualitative data).

The foregoing illustrates how the research question determines the broad methodological approach that the researcher should adopt. Not only the methodological approach, but every step in the research process is also controlled and determined by the research question. For instance, in the above scenario, the next step would be to identify the specific research methods. Given the nature of the final research question in the scenario, if a quantitative approach is selected, then the researcher can adopt an experimental study design. Within an experimental study design, if a classical pre-post test comparison is used with the online group as the control, then the researcher should evaluate a few critical issues (Norman, 2003). For example, does the researcher has sufficient numbers in the study sample to form three groups; is random assigning of students ethical, given that the group that they are assigned to may not be their preferred learning mode; and how the researcher plans to control cross-contamination, given the tendency of students to use multiple learning modes at home? If the answers to any of these questions are less than satisfactory, researcher must either change the study design from an experimental to a quasi-experimental study or change the research to a qualitative study approach. In the case of the latter, the researcher may have to go back to the research question and modify it as discussed earlier within this section.

Study design apart, the data collection methods and tools, and the data analysis methods that the researcher uses should generate results capable of answering the research question. Finally, the conclusion of the study should accurately answer the research question (Mattick et al., 2018). All this shows how important the research question is in determining the course of a research.

Steps of developing a research question

As can be seen by the above discussion, developing a high-quality research question is the key to the success of a research. Given its importance, a carefully planned, structured approach is needed when developing a research question. There are two main steps in the journey towards a successful research question. First, an appropriate research problem should be identified (Gelling, 2009). Second, a systematic, methodical, and stepwise process should be followed to develop the research question from the thus identified research problem (Ringsted et al., 2011). These two steps are further explained below.

A good research problem must ideally have two components: practical relevance and theoretical relevance. Practical relevance means the results and conclusion of the research should improve on-ground practice. In the above scenario, for example, the researcher has a practical problem to solve and that is to find out what is the most effective mode of teaching and learning for cardiovascular physiology. Finding an evidence-based answer to this problem will improve the educational practice of not only the researcher but many others in similar settings. The latter is the generalizability of the conclusion that is expected from a research. Usually, it is the practical relevance that initiates a research project by a ground-level practitioner such as a teacher. However, if the research question is sound, it should also provide some theoretical relevance. This means the solution to the research question should also provide some useful information at least to extend the current theoretical understanding in the field of study (McGaghie et al., 2001). In the above scenario, theoretical relevance is not extensive as it is a practical problem that triggers the research. However, since educational theory or at least how the theory can be applied is contextual and content-specific (Eva, 2003), in contexts similar to the researcher's setting there seems to be a lack of evidence as to which teaching and learning mode is most effective. This is further supported by the current evidence that blended learning may either be more effective than or as effective as other modes of teaching and learning. So, even from the theoretical standpoint, the research that this researcher plans to conduct is justifiable as it will add to the knowledge base to further clarify this ambiguity in evidence and contribute to either tipping the balance toward or away from blended learning. This would be theoretical relevance of this study.

Once the practical and theoretical relevance have been established, the formal development of the research question should begin, adopting the systematic and structured process alluded to above. The key to this process is to consider the development of a research question as an iterative, as opposed to a one-off, process of testing the original research idea with a series of critical questions. These critical questions form the basic building blocks of constructing a research question. They can be summarized as what, why, and how. 'What' is to specify 'what is being researched?' 'Why' indicates 'the reasons or justifications for the research' and 'how' is to detail 'the methods of research'. The researcher must ask these questions iteratively in several rounds. The question developed in the first few rounds would be broad and non-specific (Ringsted et al., 2011). In each round, the research question would be narrowed down to a more specific and refined question. When answering the three questions in each round, the relevant literature should be consulted, and the possible research methods should be evaluated. This process must go on for at least three rounds before finalizing the research question.

In the above scenario, 'what' refers to 'the effectiveness of the three modes (blended, online and onsite learning) of teaching and learning'. Non-specific and broad question as it may be, the researcher could not have come up with this question, had he not referred to the existing literature to verify whether there is already convincing evidence to answer this question. The researcher decides to go ahead with the research once it is confirmed that there is a gap in the current evidence base. In the next round (i.e., first revision), the researcher further narrows down the initial part-formulated question to a more specific question, by adding 'the effectiveness of the three modes of teaching and learning related to cardiovascular physiology among first-year medical students'. This may have happened after further considering the practical relevance and after consulting the literature to identify a relative paucity of literature on teaching and learning of cardiovascular physiology. In the third (and in this case the final) round, the researcher further cones down the research question by further specifying and qualifying what is meant by 'effectiveness': 'the effectiveness of assimilating knowledge on cardiovascular physiology when the three modes of teaching and learning are compared among the first-year medical students at Medical School X in 2021'. It is clear from this example that it is not only the place, but the timing of research should also be indicated within the research question. The above illustration is only concerned with the question 'what'. The other two questions (i.e., why, and how) should also be addressed similarly when developing a complete research question. The possible questions that should go through a researcher's mind when formulating the research question for all three questions is summarized in Table 1.

Table 1: Summary of the steps of developing a research question, using a practical example

Round/ iteration	Question form	Exact question	Answer	Research question
Round 1	What	What is the broad area of my study?.	Effectiveness teaching and learning modes, i.e., blended, online, and onsite.	What is the effectiveness of blended learning when compared with online or onsite learning?.
	Why	Why should I study this area of research?.	Because there is ambiguity in the current evidence, and it is not known whether the existing evidence is applicable to the current study setting.	
	How	How should I study this concern?.	By comparing the three modes of learning.	

Round/ iteration	Question form	Exact question	Answer	Research question
Round 2	What	What exactly is the type of learning that I am investigating? Who are my participants?.	Cardiovascular physiology First-year medical students.	What is the effectiveness of blended learning when compared with online or onsite learning related to cardiovascular physiology among the first-year medical students?.
	Why	Why am I investigating knowledge from this particular content area?.	Because there is no evidence on the effectiveness of the three modes of learning related to this content area.	
	How	Can I divide the participants into three groups to administer blended, online, and onsite learning?.	Since an estimated 150 students will consent for this research, each group will have enough numbers to derive conclusion with sufficient power.	
Round 3	What	What exactly am I measuring to find the effectiveness?. Who are the three student groups?.	Knowledge assimilation and retention of cardiovascular physiology. First-year students voluntarily assigned to the three group from Medical School X during 2021.	When blended, online and onsite learning modes are compared what is more effective in assimilating knowledge on cardiovascular physiology by the first-year medical students at Medical School X in 2021?.
	Why	Can I still justify conducting this research, given that this is on assimilation of cardiovascular physiology?.	There is no literature in this area of study. Given the context-specificity of most literature and given that there is ambiguity in the existing literature, it is still justifiable.	
	How	How can I measure learning in terms of knowledge assimilation in each of the three methods?. Is it ethical to divide participants into three groups?.	Measuring knowledge will be through multiple choice questions administered before and after learning. Random sampling may be unethical. So, I need to consider the student preferences when allocating the students into the three groups and force them to follow a particular type of learning only.	

During every round, if the researcher identifies the answer to a particular question unsatisfactory, then the researcher will have to address it then and there, and then go through the previous round/s to find out whether the research question as a whole makes sense. Sometimes the researcher may have to start the process again from a previous round.

SUMMARIZE

Writing a fit-for-purpose research question is both challenging and enjoyable. The process starts by identifying a practically and theoretically relevant research problem. Converting the research problem into a research question is never finalised until it is put through a structured and rigorous thought process. This thought process comprises three question forms: what, why and how. Known as the basic building blocks of a research question, these three question forms should be used iteratively to test and refine the evolving research question. During each iteration or round, the research question should become more specific, focused and researchable. If the evolving research question is found wanting during a given round, amendments should be made and the process should be restarted from the initial rounds. The finalised research question should then be used to guide every step of the research process.

EVALUATE

This section is meant to encourage the readers to reflect and self-evaluate their learning at the end of the chapter. The following assignments may help in this process:

Identify a research problem that you have been thinking of. Read the literature to find out if your problems have already been answered in the literature. Try to convert your problem into a research question. When doing so, try to answer the three fundamental questions: what, why and how. Think about the research approaches, study designs, data, and participants you will need to answer the research question. Go through this process iteratively until you are satisfied with the final research question. If you are not satisfied, make the necessary changes and go back the previous iterations to check that the line of thinking has no gaps. Finalise the research question and use it effectively to determine the next steps in the course of the research.

ROAD AHEAD

Writing a sound research question is challenging both to the experienced and the novice researcher (Doody & Bailey, 2016). If a research question is found to be having a critical flaw during its implementation, it may be irrecoverable or too costly to rectify. Or else, the flaw may be such that the study may prove untenable. To avoid such pitfalls, it is always good practice to bounce the inalized research question on a colleague for critical review and feedback (Mattick et al., 2018). Novice researchers should refer to standards texts of educational research and seek the guidance of a supervisor when conceiving and constructing their research questions. The following web resources, though not specific to education, may also prove useful.

1. *https://www.monash.edu/rlo/research-writing-assignments/understanding-the-assignment/developing-research-questions*
2. *https://www.scribbr.com/research-process/research-questions/*
3. *https://www.guide2research.com/research/how-to-write-a-research-question*
4. *https://libguides.ucmerced.edu/think_like_a_researcher/questions_lesson*

REFERENCES

Berliner DC. (2002). Educational research: the hardest science of all. *Educ Res.*, 31:18–20.

Doody O, Bailey ME. (2016). Setting a research question, aim and objective. *Nurse Res.*, 23(4):19–23. DOI:10.7748/nr.23.4.19.s5

Eva KW. (2003). On the generality of specificity. *Med Educ.*, 37(7):587–588.

Gelling L. (2015). Stages in the research process. *Nurs Stand.*, 29(27): 44-49. DOI: 10.7748/ns.29.27.44.e8745

Lipowski EE. (2008). Developing great research questions. *Am J Health Syst Pharm.*, 65(17):1667-1670. DOI: 10.2146/ajhp070276

Liu Q, Peng W, Zhang F, Hu R, Li Y, Yan W. (2016). The Effectiveness of Blended Learning in Health Professions: Systematic Review and Meta-Analysis. *J Med Internet Res.*, 18(1):e2. DOI:10.2196/jmir.4807

Mattick K, Johnston J, de la Croix A. (2018). How to...write a good research question. *Clin Teach.*, 15(2):104-108. DOI: 10.1111/tct.12776

McGaghie WC, Bordage G, Shea JA. (2001). Problem statement, conceptual framework, and research question. *Acad Med.*, 76(9):923-924.

Norman G. (2003). RCT = results confounded and trivial: the perils of grand educational experiments. *Med Educ.*, 37:582–584.

Ringsted C, Hodges B, Scherpbier A. (2011). 'The research compass': An introduction to research in medical education: AMEE Guide No. 56. *Med Teach.*, 33(9):695-709, DOI: 10.3109/0142159X.2011.595436

Thabane L, Thomas T, Ye C, Paul J. (2009). Posing the research question: not so simple. *Can J Anaesth.*, 56(1):71-79. DOI: 10.1007/s12630-008-9007-4

Chapter 8

Review of Literature

Chinmay Shah, Sanjay Bedi

ABSTRACT

Review of related literature plays a very important role for any research, its role starts before even researches is started and continue till your research gets published. Seed of any research begins with review of literature available in different Data Base. In this chapter we are going to discuss regarding, format in which literature is available, need of literature search, ways of doing literature search, use of information technology for literature search, different strategies to be used for literature search, its role in creating research proposal, different database available for literature search. Once research is complete, the next part is writing its result and discussion, where again literature review plays important role. Once the search done, we also need to learn how to write it as per the need of article or thesis.

Key Words: review, information retrieval, pubmed, google scholar, literature search

ASSESS NEED

What topic should be finalized for my research project? What topic should I give to my UG students for ICMR Short term Studentship? What topic should I give to my PG Students? Which area should I choose for my Ph.D.? Which topic should be chosen so that publication will be considered in scholarly Journal?

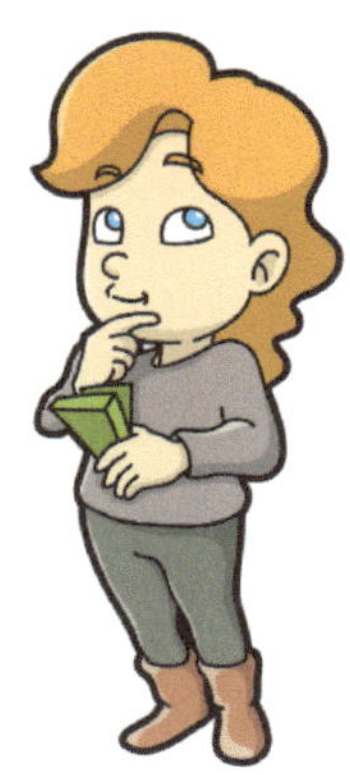

These are some of the questions which come to the mind of a research scholar when he starts thinking towards doing research. Once topic is finalized again questions come up like... How much people know about this topic?

What is already done in this area?

Which method has been used by previous researcher and succeeded?

What are the points which I should consider so that I will have minimum limitations?

What should I avoid? What is knowledge gap in topic under consideration?

Answer of all these questions lies in the review of existing literature.

Literature search will help us to ensure that work done by you is original and identifies a gap in the previous research. It will help in convincing the teacher that the student is choosing a particular topic after an effective literature review. It will help us to develop critical practices and to identify methodological approaches to be used in our own research.

It gives us idea to generate appropriate theory to support your work and explain why the results are similar/different from other researchers. Even as you put the finishing touches to your thesis you still need to be aware of any new research coming out in case it is raised during your thesis writing process.

Specifically, the review helps the researcher to articulate clear goals, show evidence of adequate preparation, select appropriate methods, communicate relevant results, and engage in reflective critique (Maggio, 2016).

Similarly, if you are a postgraduate student or research scholar or applying for grant, review of literature is an important part of project report/presentation. During presentation/publication of the research, literature search will help to finalize appropriate audience and Journal for sending the research for publication. It helps to demonstrate that our contribution is new and unique.

Once everything is finalized, you need to use appropriate method for managing references to cite them appropriately to give credit to original source.

BRIEF

- Why literature search
- Type of literature source
- How to do literature search for educational research
- What are different databases available
- Tips for conducting review of literature
- Writing review of literature

CONTEXTUALIZE

Let's start....take a pen and paper and write down title of your current project or projects you are intending to do in future. Now try to answer questions which are listed in previous section of the chapter. Take few minutes to do literature search as you have done till date and then proceed further to the next section of chapter.

For example: my research question is

Does flipped classroom improve student's retention of knowledge?

DESCRIBE

Before we go to details of literature search, let's in briefly look at the type and level of evidence in literature available (figure 1)[2]

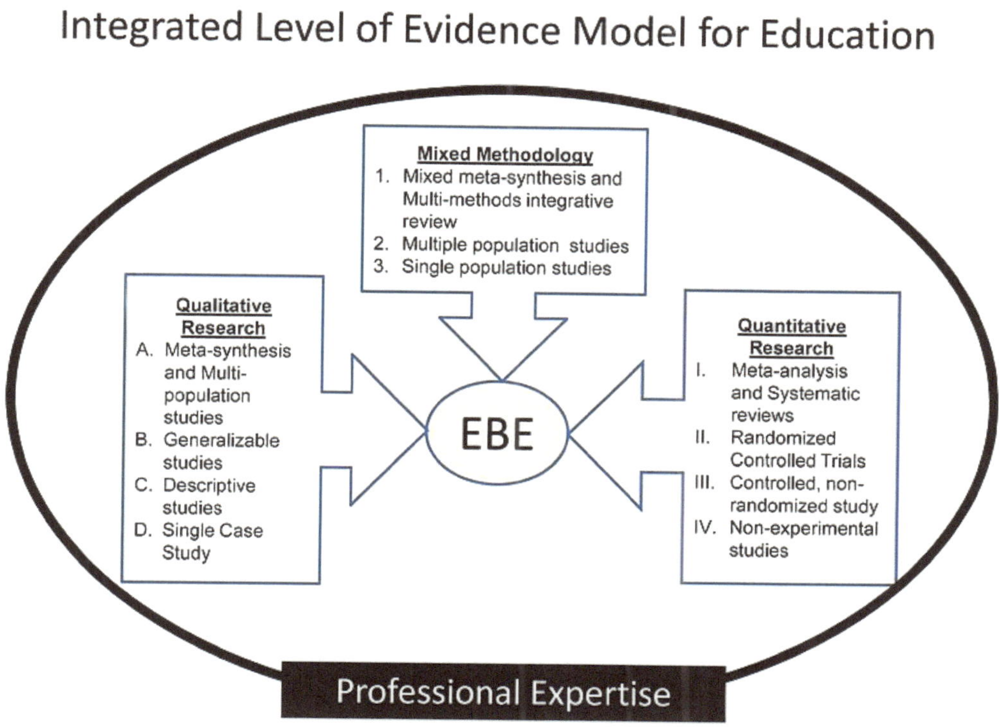

Figure 1: Different type and level of evidence in literature[2]

This will help us to decide what we want for our proposed project. Figure shows three type of research i.e qualitative, quantitative and mixed research. In all three the first type of research is having highest evidence value i.e in qualitative – multi synthesis and multi population studies have more evidence value than single case study.

As per the level of evidence we need to do the literature search in different databases. These databases can be in print or electronic form.

Type – I: Provide background/factual information: This type of information is available from text books, dictionaries, encyclopaedias resources like MIMS, CIMS, websites which are hosting collection of such resources, freebook4Doctors etc

Example of research question requiring type I database

- Basic/background information: What is flipped classroom?

Type – II: Current and past research: This information can be collected from printed or online Journals, Thesis & Dissertation, conference proceedings and abstracts, repositories, and bibliographic database etc, Sodhganga, Vidyanidhi, CTRI and WHO clinical registry can also provide us details of current and past research

Example of research question requiring type II database.

- What are the current tools which will help you to implement flipped classroom?

Type – III: Synthesis - analysis of research: This database will give us articles with highest level of evidence. These databases are the Cochrane Database of Systematic Reviews, DARE: Database of Abstract of Reviews of Evidence, Dynamed, BEME etc.

Example of research question requiring type III database.

- Use of flipped classroom V/s Traditional classroom in post Covid era.

So, once you frame your research question, you will know from which type of database you will get your required information, you will either go to the departmental or college library or will use information technology to search online database with the help of different search engines like Google, Yahoo, MSN search etc. Let's first see what are the steps involved in literature search.

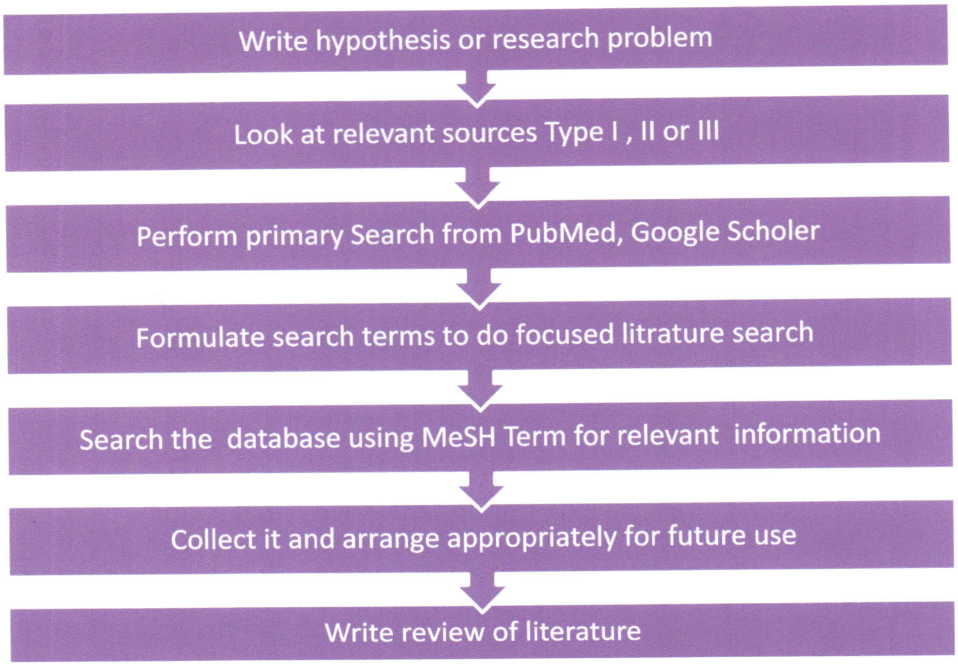

Figure 2: Steps involved in literature search

Let's Start with an example: My research question is: Does flipped classroom improve students' retention of knowledge?

Step 1: Search using human resources: discuss your topic with your colleagues, your guide, expert in the respective field and most importantly medical librarian.

This first step is very crucial as they may guide you further for next steps as well as expert/medical librarian may be aware of current status of area under research and they may help you to connect with stalwarts of respective field or with investigators doing similar research. They are also cognizant of strengths and limitations of different databases and search strategy.

Step 2: As per our habit we will search in Google, it may sometime give us more than 10,00,000 results and it will be difficult to go through these references and go through specific literature.

How to get desired results in Google?

1. Use explicit phrase: e.g., "Does flipped classroom improve student's retention of knowledge?"
2. Google has one specific section for scientific articles which is known as Google Scholar, try it – it reduces the result to 10% of simple Google search.
3. Use filter in Google scholar: we can filter search by

a. Duration

b. Relevance
c. Including or excluding Citations and patents

Once you search, you can also create alert so that if new article gets included in Google scholar, details will be sent to your mail. Google also has one more feature which help us to search based on image, which will help us not only in research but also in rare case report (image below)

Specific Search: As we all know, Google is a general search engine. When we want to use specifically for educational research we should focus on specific database. Box 1 below gives list of specific databases.

Box-1: List of Educational Data bases

- EBSCO
  - Academic Search Ultimate
  - British Education Index
  - Educational Administration Abstracts
  - Education Abstracts
  - Education Full Text.
  - ERIC
  - Education Research Complete
- Education Database (ProQuest)
- Education in Video (Alexander Street Press)
- Scopus
- Web of Science
- JSTOR
- The Best Evidence Medical Education (BEME)
- The Cochrane Library
- EMBASE (Excerpta Medica Database).
- PubMed Central
- PubMed
- Google Scholar

Academic Search Ultimate: *Academic Search Ultimate* includes rigorous creation of open access (OA) journals, which has resulted in a growing collection of 4,734 global OA journals. Once validated and certified for inclusion, these OA journals are treated with high-quality subject indexing and sophisticated, precise/accurate full text linking. (https://www.ebsco.com/products/research-databases/academic-search-ultimate)

British Education Index: covers all aspects of educational policy and administration, evaluation and assessment, technology and special educational needs. Indexing British education journals, theses and more, this resource is searchable by educational level and age group. (https://www.ebsco.com/products/research-databases/british-education-index)

Educational Administration Abstracts: is a database providing bibliographic records covering all areas of educational administration, including educational leadership, educational management and educational research. (https://www.ebsco.com/products/research-databases/educational-administration-abstracts)

Education Abstracts: is an education research database providing high-quality indexing and abstracts for hundreds of journals. Coverage spans all levels of education and includes adult education, multicultural education and teaching methods (https://www.ebsco.com/products/research-databases/education-abstracts).

Education Full Text: is a research database for students, professionals and policy makers. It includes full-text education journals that cover the essentials of education and related fields of study, including in-depth coverage of special education. (https://www.ebsco.com/products/research-databases/education-full-text)

ERIC (EBSCO): ERIC (Education Resources Information Center) is sponsored by the Institute of Education Sciences (US department of education). Included is educational research literature from journal articles, conference papers, reports, theses, book chapters and class programs (lesson plans and models). (https://www.ebsco.com/products/research-databases/eric)

Education Research Complete: *Education Research Complete* includes rigorous curation of open access (OA) journals, which has resulted in a growing collection of 303 global OA journals. Once validated and certified for inclusion, these OA journals are treated with high-quality subject indexing and sophisticated, precise/accurate full-text linking (https://www.ebsco.com/products/research-databases/education-research-complete)

Education Database (ProQuest): This easy-to-navigate educational database covers primary-, secondary-, and higher education. It also covers special- and adult education. It includes more than 1000 top educational publications (800 in full text). About 75% of the publications covered are scholarly journals. (https://proquest.libguides.com/)

Education in Video (Alexander Street Press): This is one of the first online collections of streaming videos, developed for training and developing teachers. Find videos with teaching demonstrations, lectures, documentaries, and primary-source footage of students and teachers in classroom environments. (https://alexanderstreet.com/marc/education-video-volume-i)

Scopus: It is one of the two big commercial, bibliographic databases that cover scholarly literature from almost any discipline. Besides providing research articles, Scopus also offers academic journal rankings, author profiles, and an *h-index calculator*. (https://www.scopus.com/home.uri)

Web of Science: it is also known as Web of Knowledge, is the second big bibliographic database. Usually, academic institutions provide either access to Web of Science or Scopus on their campus network for free. (https://clarivate.com/webofsciencegroup/solutions/web-of-science/)

JSTOR: Provides full-text access to the archives of core scholarly journals in the arts, humanities, social sciences, and sciences. Also include full text e-books and open access research articles. (https://www.jstor.org/)

Best Evidence Medical Education (BEME): This Collaboration (Harden et al., 1999) is an international group of individuals, universities and professional organisations committed to the development of evidence informed education in the medical and health professions. (*https://www.bemecollaboration.org/Home/*)

Cochrane Library: it is best known for its systematic reviews. There are 53 review groups around the world that ensure that the published reviews are of high-quality and evidence based. Articles are updated over time to reflect new research. (*https://www.cochranelibrary.com/*)

EMBASE (Excerpta Medica Database): It is a proprietary research database that also includes in its corpus PubMed. It can also be accessed by other database providers such as Ovid. (*https://www.embase.com/*)

PubMed Central: is the free fulltext/open access branch of PubMed. Full text for all indexed papers is readily available at PMC to read and download. You might also want to check out its sister site Europe PMC. (*https://www.ncbi.nlm.nih.gov/pmc/*)

PubMed: It is the number one resource for anyone looking for literature in medicine or biological sciences. PubMed stores abstracts and bibliographic details of more than 30 million papers and provides full text links to the publisher sites or links to the free PDF on PubMed Central (PMC) (*https://www.ncbi.nlm.nih.gov*)

Google Scholar: Google Scholar provides a simple way to broadly search for scholarly literature. From one place, you can search across many disciplines and sources: articles, theses, books, abstracts and court opinions, from academic publishers, professional societies, online repositories, universities and other web sites. Google Scholar helps you find relevant work across the world of scholarly research. (https://scholar.google.com/)

Out of all of the above databases most commonly used databases are PubMed and Eric Database. Below are few tips which you can use when doing literature search

1. **Avoid using stop words (Table below)**

	Stop words
A	a, about, again, all, almost, also, although, always, among, an, and, another, any, are, as, at.
B	be, because, been, before, being, between, both, but, by.
C	can, could.
D	did, do, does, done, due, during.
E	each, either, enough, especially, etc.
F	for, found, from, further.
H	had, has, have, having, here, how, however.
I	i, if, in, into, is, it, its, itself.
J	just.
K	kg, km.
M	made, mainly, make, may, mg, might, ml, mm, most, mostly, must.
N	nearly, neither, no, nor.
O	obtained, of, often, on, our, overall.
P	perhaps, pmid.
Q	quite.
R	rather, really, regarding.
S	seem, seen, several, should, show, showed, shown, shows, significantly, since, so, some, such.
T	than, that, the, their, theirs, them, then, there, therefore, these, they, this, those, through, thus, to.
U	Upon.
V	various, very.
W	was, we, were, what, when, which, while, with, within, without, would.

2. **Use field search (Table below)**

Field Search	
If you will search as	You will find your search term in the
Flipped classroom	All area except Full Text
Flipped classroom [Ti]	Title
Flipped classroom [tiab]	Title + Abstract
Flipped classroom [Jour]	Journal Title
Flipped classroom [Au]	Author
Flipped classroom [AD]	Author's Address
Flipped classroom [MeSH]	List of Mesh Term
1364 [Page]	Page Number
2019 [pdat]	Date/Year

3. **Let's see how to use Boolean operators/Connector mean AND, OR, & NOT**
Always use in **UPPER CASE,** Where **AND** narrows, **OR** broadens, **NOT** excludes the search terms. Using the Boolean operator AND between search terms returns only records that contain all of the search terms

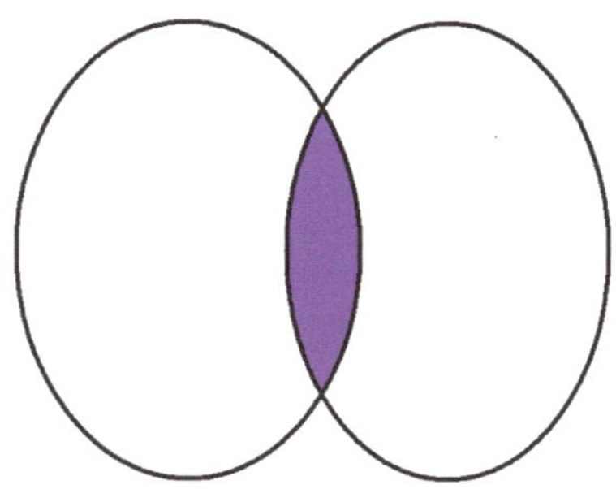

Figure 3: Flipped Classroom AND Student Retention

Using the Boolean operator OR between search terms returns all records that contain all of the search terms

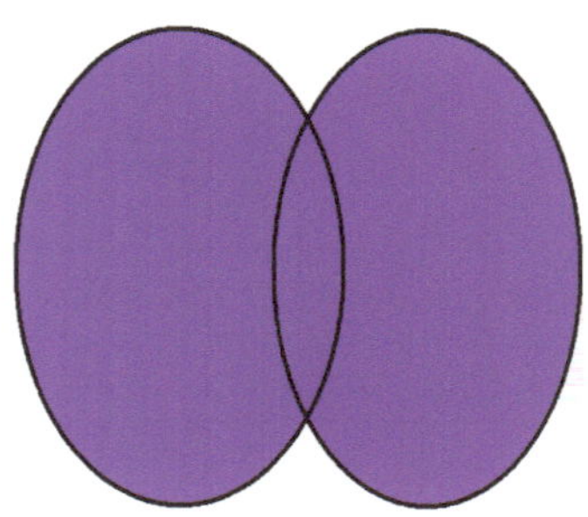

Figure 4: Flipped Classroom OR Student Retention

Using the Boolean operator NOT between search terms returns only records that contain the first search term and not the second.

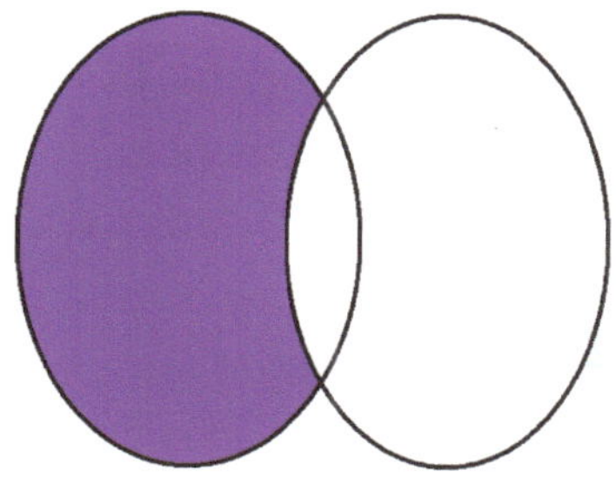

Figure 5: Flipped Classroom NOT Student Retention

As seen in Google, in PubMed also there are multiple filters like text availability, article attribute, article type, publication date, age, species, language, sex, subject, Journal category (Image Below). Detail explanation regarding how to use these filters are available on: **https://pubmed.ncbi.nlm.nih.gov/help/**

4. **Use MeSH term: One more method of refining search is use of MeSH terms: MeSH:**(Medical Subject Headings) Search topic is converted to MeSH. This method is useful in a way that it will give us all related terms which are used throut world for particular subject/intervention/disease
5. **Filter:** Refine your search using filters age group, language (English or other language), text availability (only abstract or full text), no. of years (5 or 10), etc

Once you finish your search you can save citations temporarily using the Clipboard, save citations indefinitely using My NCBI Collections, save citations as a text file and also create alert to remain updated for future additions of new articles.

There are more advance options available for PubMed search along with downloadable search strategies, which is used during writing article for meta-analysis as well as systemic review. Details regarding this can be found in further reading section.

In today's era of technology, multiple mobile app are also available for literature search like PubMed Mobile, PLOS one, Pubget, Pubmed etc.

Next Step...

Once you finish review of related literature you can classify it in to three broad categories which will help you in writing ROL as well as support you in explaining your results.

a. Literature having consensus and near consensus
b. Literature with disagreement or debate
c. Helped us to find gap analysis

Last category will help you to finalise your research question.

Writing review of literature

Once we get answer to your question under research, we will go for presentation, publication or thesis submission in case of research scholar perusing masters or Ph D. During presentation or publication we need to mention review of related literature as per the guidelines of university or Journal. Broadly it can be divided in to introduction, body and conclusion.

There are two ways we can write review of literature

1. Concept centric, where concepts are discussed in chronological order and
2. Author centric, where research of the authors is discussed in chronological order.

You can decide the way in which you would like to describe, based on your research question with goal to satisfy scholars regarding accumulated evidence on the topic.

You need to focus on tone and tense of your presentation when writing review of literature as it will inform readers regarding value and context of their view. You should also mention what you should know over and above what is already known to give a direction for future researcher. (Reference)

There are two places where we need to write review of literature with difference i. systemic review and meta-analysis.

When we write, meta-analysis, we need to average the results of the selected studies to get an overall index of the outcome or relationship. Commonly one gets confused between systemic review and review of literature, so let's see the difference first before knowing how to write review of literature. (Table 1.) (Lynn Kysh, 2020)

Table 1: Difference between systemic and literature review

	Systematic Review	Literature Review
Definition	High-level overview of primary research on a focused question that identifies, selects, synthesizes, and appraises all high quality research evidence relevant to that question.	Qualitatively summarizes evidence on a topic using informal or subjective methods to collect and interpret studies.
Goals	Answers a focused clinical question Eliminate bias.	Provide summary or overview of topic.
Question	Clearly defined and answerable clinical question. Recommend using PICO as a guide.	Can be a general topic or a specific question.
Components	Pre-specified eligibility criteria. Systematic search strategy. Assessment of the validity of findings. Interpretation and presentation of results . Reference list.	Introduction . Methods. Discussion. Conclusion. Reference list.
Number of Authors	Three or more.	One or more.
Timeline	Months to years. Average eighteen months .	Weeks to months.
Requirement	Thorough knowledge of topic. Perform searches of all relevant databases Statistical analysis resources (for meta-analysis).	Understanding of topic Perform searches of one or more databases.
Value	Connects practicing clinicians to high quality evidence. Supports evidence-based practice.	Provides summary of literature on the topic.

SUMMARIZE

Literature search is an integral part of any research/project, keep in mind following Principles during literature search:

1. Word Search: Contains your search terms anywhere
2. Field Search: Contains your search terms in fields you select
3. Combining terms using Boolean operators i.e. AND, OR, NO
4. MeSH Search: Contains your search terms in list of Mesh terms (in PubMed)
5. Use appropriate data base to search
6. Write literature search as per the need and context of question under research

EVALUATE

Now as you have gone through the chapter, please do following exercise with research question:

Does flipped classroom improve student's retention of knowledge?

1. Search in Google, you received.........................results
2. Search in Google with "question", you received.............results
3. Search in Google Scholar, you received......................results
4. Search in PubMed/Eric Database without filter, you received.............results
5. Search in PubMed/Eric Database with different filters, you received.............results
6. Write your ROL as you will write the research paper for the question under study

ROAD AHEAD

Please visit following link for going through detail:

1. Tutorial For PubMed Search
   https://learn.nlm.nih.gov/documentation/training-packets/T0042010P/
2. Tutorial For Eric Search
   https://paperpile.com/g/eric-research-database/
3. How to use the Cochrane Library
   https://www.cochranelibrary.com/help/how-to-use
4. Guide to advanced search in Google Scholar
   https://www.youtube.com/watch?v=FJH6MfuZs7s

REFERENCES

Level of Evidence Model for Education retrieved from https://commons.wikimedia.org/wiki/File:Level_of_Evidence_Model_for_Education.jpg (last accessed on 1st September 2021)

Maggio, L. A., Sewell, J. L., & Artino, A. R., Jr (2016). The Literature Review: A Foundation for High-Quality Medical Education Research. Journal of graduate medical education, 8(3), 297–303. https://doi.org/10.4300/JGME-D-16-00175.1

What's in a name? The difference between a Systematic Review and a Literature Review, and why it matters by Lynn Kysh, MLIS, University of Southern California - Norris Medical Library retrieved from https://guides.libraries.psu.edu/c.php?g=319063&p=5222056 (last accessed on 1st September 2021)

Chapter 9

Health Profession Education Research Methods and Tools

Mona Hmoud Al-Sheikh

ABSTRACT

In contrast with research in biomedical science, Health profession education research (HPER) addresses different types of research questions. The question may involve comparing the efficacy of two teaching or assessment methods, assessing an educational practice, or exploring a new method. This leads the need for a wide range of methods classified under quantitative, qualitative, and mixed methods. This chapter gives an overview of methods and gives an overview of toolbox for the researchers to address their research questions in an effective manner. Most popularly used quantitative methods are experimental/quasi-experimental, testing, observation, correlational studies and surveys; the tools used are questionnaires, tests, checklists, rating scales, observation schedules; Most popularly used qualitative approaches/methods are grounded theories, ethnography, phenomenology, action research and case studies. Focus Group Discussion (FGD), in-depth interviews, document analysis, narratives, and even social media. The methods used should be aligned with the research question and they should be evidence based

Key Words: educational research; research tools; qualitative research; quantitative research; research methods, critical appraisal.

ASSESS NEED

Health profession education research (HPER) is a rapidly growing field that is born out of an effective application of scientific research methods to answer questions faced by health professions educators in their diverse settings. It also helps in exploring new teaching/assessment methods, new curriculum designs, and evaluation. Once a problem is identified the next question is how one can go about to resolve the research question. The use of the appropriate method and tool for measurement or description becomes a matter of vital importance.

HPER can be quantitative, qualitative or mixed; quantitative studies test hypotheses and typically address questions what works, while qualitative studies are more exploratory and allow for probing into quantitative results to find out the reason behind them to generate hypothesis and answer the question of whether, how and why something works (Wolf, 2004; Wyse et.al., 2017). Quantitative studies can be descriptive (epidemiologic), measurement (psychometric, correlational) or interventional (experimental) while qualitative can be descriptive or exploratory. Each of these approaches to educational research is useful on its own and is even more productive when used as complementary (Bordage, 2007; Lingard and Kennedy, 2010).

There is a toolbox for each category of HPER and quality indicators. Tests (pre/post), surveys, checklists, rating scales, are quantitative tools, as they deal with measurement (numbers) using statistics while focus groups, personal interviews, Delphi technique are qualitative tools for capturing data in words.

While books in education give pure educational examples, this chapter will use examples from the HPER world to illustrate each of the highlighted issues.

BRIEF

- Health profession education research (HPER) is unique in its application of a) Quantitative approach which deal with numbers (quantification) b) Qualitative approach which deals words/expressions (qualification) and c) Mixed Methods Research combining quantitative and qualitative methods
- Most popularly used quantitative methods are experimental/quasi-experimental, testing, observation, correlational studies, and surveys
- The tools used under quantitative approach are questionnaires (offline and online); pretest/posttest, checklists, rating scales, observation schedules etc.
- Most popularly used qualitative approaches/methods are grounded theories, ethnography, phenomenology, action research and case studies
- Qualitative research being explorative, uses a variety of tools and techniques, Focus Group Discussion (FGD), in-depth interviews, document analysis, narratives, and even social media.
- The methods used should be aligned with the research question and should be evidence- based

CONTEXTUALIZE

Scenario 1

YOU are the Head of Medical Education Department in a medical school that has adopted a Parallel Integrated Problem-Based Learning (PBL) Program in addition to the traditional curriculum. The Dean of the medical school has requested you to compare the educational environment in the two programs from students' perspective and to prepare a report for the Ministry of Education.

*The research question was: **WHAT** is the students' perception of the PBL and traditional educational environment for medicine?*

In order to answer this question you need to chose a tool You can chose DREEM (Roff et al., 1997; Roff, 2005) as a tool to measure students' perceptions of the educational environment. The DREEM is a validated fifty-item questionnaire, each of five- point Likert scale. It measures students' perceptions of five subscales namely Learning, Teachers, Academic Self, Social, and Atmosphere. The method you selected was ***Quantitative*** *research design and the tool was* ***DREEM****. Suppose the results are in favor of the PBL curriculum.*

But the Dean asks you ***WHY*** *the PBL curriculum is perceived superior to traditional by students?*

Now you need to select ***Qualitative*** *research design to answer that question. So, you select a stratified sample of students from PBL and another one from traditional program and you use the* ***Focus Group*** *tool.*

The scenario reveals that the choice of the method or tool depends upon the research question besides other factors such as feasibility in terms of time and cost.

DESCRIBE

Quantitative methods

Most popularly used quantitative methods are experimental/quasi-experimental, testing, observation, correlational studies and surveys.

Experimental/quasi-experimental

Experimental Design "The experimental method is the only method of research that can truly test hypotheses concerning cause-and-effect relationships. It represents the most valid approach to the solution of educational problems, both practical and theoretical, and to the advancement of education as a science" (Leppink, 2019).

It requires complete randomization of the groups involved and double blinding of subjects and observers. This is not always feasible in educational research. For example, if you are interested in finding out if adding a "Simulation Component" to training nursing students on Leopold maneuver (used to palpate the gravid uterus systematically). Your experimental design should include two groups one receives theoretic instruction, then goes immediately to practice on patients in the wards. And the other group takes after theory a simulation session on mannequins before practicing on real pregnant ladies. Then you compare the performance levels of the two groups at the end of training. Complete randomization of students and controlling all other factors like the instructor, time of instruction, academic level of participating students in each group are characteristics of a true *Experimental Design*. Experimental Design leads to powerful evidence of cause and effect relationship, but it is not always feasible as these students are usually allocated in groups from the beginning of the academic year. So, you resort to *Quasi Experimental Design* which allows you to keep students in their respective groups and still perform the study. So, the difference between the two methods is summarized as follows:

- In a true experiment, subjects are randomly assigned to either the experimental or the control group, whereas there is no randomization in a quasi-experiment. This makes experimental design more internally valid.
- In a quasi-experiment, both groups differ not only in terms of the intervention like teaching method or mode of instruction they receive, but also in other factors, like the instructor, timing of instruction, baseline academic level of subjects. Additional statistical methods are needed in a quasi-experiment to cancel the effect of any confounding variable.

- Because complete randomization is lacking in quasi-experiments, there may be several competing hypotheses to explain the difference in the outcome of the two groups.

It is generally hard and most of the times not feasible to maintain internal and external validity in social science research (Cook, & Beckman, 2010).

The Tools under Quantitative methods

The tools used under quantitative approach are questionnaires (offline and online); pretest/posttest, checklists, rating scales, observation schedules etc.

Testing

Tests are commonly used in quantitative research to measure attitudes, personality, self-perceptions, aptitude, and performance of research participants. They can include single or multiple item formats which aligns with the purpose of the measurement.

Survey or questionnaire

A self-report data-collection tool that allows research participants to express their information about the thoughts, feelings, attitudes, beliefs, values, or perceptions about a particular research objectivities a list of statements designed by the researcher to measure degree of agreement of a sample of respondents to these items. Statements should be stating facts or opinions and should not be in question format. The subjects are requested to respond by either Yes/No or by selecting their level of agreement on a 3-point to 9-point Likert scale. Surveys are good to measure perceptions of subjects of specific items and should undergo validity and reliability measurement. Surveys can cover a wide selection of topics from learning preferences and styles to satisfaction measures (Saxon et.al., 2003). They are particularly useful for determining perceptions and attitudes of a large sample towards a particular issue at a particular time. Surveys are criticized for relying on personal judgement which is not always accurate (Bargh and Chartrand, 1999; Gordon, 1991; Walsh, 2013).

It is preferable to have an even number of levels of agreement and to exclude neutral from the choices. Surveys can be used for screening purposes to find people with specific characteristics to include them in the qualitative in-depth study (Paladine et. al., 2018). Response rate should be reported as the percentage of responses received over the total surveys sent and should not be less than 60 percent. Lower response rates are associated with low reliability scores. Informed consent, confidentiality and anonymity are important ethical considerations of surveys (Israel and Hay, 2006; Roberts and Allen, 2015). There are fifteen principles for using questionnaires in educational research (Christensen & Johnson, 2019). Questionnaires can be used as a qualitative tool when the questions are open-ended. In the example of the educational environment measurement, following the fifty-item, five-point Likert scale questionnaire, students were given three open-ended questions that said; a. mention the best course/activity you had in the college so far, mention the worst course/activity in your college so far, c. why do you think it was so? Answers to these simple three questions shed light into the students' experiences and overall perception of their undergraduate experience.

Checklists, rating scales, observation schedules

Checklists: they are lists of performance categories that candidates are evaluated for by a check if available. The major weakness of checklists is that they are dichotomous and only informs if the candidate did or did not do a certain behavior. A rating scale on the other hand gives levels of performance for each behavior category and is much more indicative of skill acquirement or mastery of a certain procedure. For example, during the OSPE examination of second year medical students, the instructor evaluates students on their skill in measurement of heart rate using recordings of pulse rate on a physiograph. If the observer uses a checklist, the findings are reduced to mere recording of whether the student chose the correct transducer, attached it to the physiograph, performed the recording, and calculated the heart rate. It misses information of how many trials and errors the student did in order to obtain the required record. It ignores completely how skillful the student was in fixing the transducer to the machine and to the finger of the subject, and so on. There were incidents when a student was very confident in choosing the proper transducer, fixing it to the physiograph and elegantly getting the record or calculation as opposed to another who clumsily tries two or three wrong transducers before reaching the correct one, tries to fix it in the wrong direction to the physiograph and uses force to do that, drops the transducer to the floor and picks it up after almost breaking it, and hesitantly obtain the ECG record and calculation. Both candidates will get the same score if the tool is a checklist. Using rating scale, the observer has more space to reflect on the difference in the level of performance between the two candidates. Checklists can be enhanced by a global rating at the end of three to seven levels to record the subjective evaluation by the observer of the candidate's performance.

Observation: Is defined as watching a behavioral pattern. It is a standard process to obtain reliable research data. It involves standardization of the observer, observe, and the context as in the location of the observation, timing and duration. The results of observations are usually in the forms of counts of the frequency of a certain behavior was attempted or a score that evaluates that behavior. Observations differ from questionnaires as the former records behavior while the second captures attitude. Observations are time and money consuming. Subjects can behave differently when they know they are observed. They can be made in a simulated environment like OSCE/OSPE or in the natural world like Workplace Based Assessment or mini-CEX. Blind observation in a natural world is more reliable.

The Pre-Posttest

This is the most commonly used quantitative experimental tool. The purpose of this tool is to measure the cognitive growth after an intervention. It is loaded with confounding variables as it is very difficult to assume that the change in the learners' knowledge or skill is solely due to the intervention. To avoid this dilemma, the use of two-groups randomized controlled trials erupted (Campbell and Stanley, 1963; Hatch, Duarte, and De Gregorio, 2018). The issues of dilution or spread of intervention from one group to the other and blinding should be addressed (Suter, 2012). This is what distinguishes educational research from clinical and scientific research where the subjects are under direct control of the researcher. Tests can measure performance in knowledge, clinical reasoning, intelligence, personality, or empathy. Achievement tests are designed by teachers to measure learning over a period while aptitude tests measure the ability to learn or schemata formation. Diagnostic tests are designed if a student is.

Qualitative methods

Most popularly used qualitative approaches/methods are grounded theories, ethnography, phenomenology, action research and case studies.

Grounded theory

A qualitative approach to generating and developing a theory from the narrative data that the researcher collects. It uses an inductive approach for generating theories or explanations. It is the study of a concept and not the description of a problem (Glaser, 2010).

Ethnography

Ethnography is a type of qualitative research that collects observations, interviews, and narrative data to describe an educational phenomenon. It is a research tool where the firsthand reflections of a participant on his experiences about a certain phenomenon in education as related to cultural settings (Reeves, Peller, Goldman, and Kitto, 2013).

Phenomenology

Is a methodological endeavor performed by professional educators? In this tool, the researcher personally experiences the phenomena under investigation, and later reflects deeply on that experience (Vallack, 2015). The relation between phenomenology and educational research is the characterization of educational situations and in the logic of educational practices (Saevi, 2014). In phenomenology, the researcher first documents an experience of the research in question, then progresses through five phases of the methodology to reach an answer to the research question. It is a useful tool to portray knowledge about first-person events, or the lived experiences of students in certain educational contexts (Stolz, 2020).

Action research

The researcher here plays an active role in changing the outcome of the research question. He seeks transformative change through the simultaneous process of taking action and doing research, which are linked together by critical reflection. In other words, action research is a form of problem-based investigation by educationists into their teaching, thus it is a process. It combines the concepts of human nature in action science and cooperative inquiry to obtain actual change in behavior as a result of corrective actions (Efron and Ravid, 2019).

Case studies

Robert E. Stake (1995) defines case study as "the study of the particularity and complexity of a single case, coming to understand its activity within important circumstances". It gives a holistic view of the context of an experience in education. The rich details that accompany case studies makes it a useful tool for educational research (Merriam, 1998). Case studies are useful as a preliminary research that provides data about the scope of data collection and sets the stage for future more comprehensive research.

Data collection and analysis in case studies is time consuming and there is high risk of researcher's bias. Lack of generalizability and extrapolation power of the evidence is another weakness ((Johnson & Onwuegbuzie, 2004).

The Tools under Qualitative Methods

Qualitative research being explorative, uses a variety of tools and techniques, Focus Group Discussion (FGD), in-depth interviews, document analysis, narratives, and even social media.

Focus group discussion

Focus Group Discussion (FGD) is an effective method of investigating a research question that addresses what people think about a particular phenomenon, why they think so, expressed in their own words and gestures. For some researchers any discussion in which the participants are actively engaged and attentive in group interaction becomes an FGD (Kitzinger and Barbour, 1999).

Focus groups are normally of four to twelve candidates and the researcher acts as a facilitator to guide a relevant discussion to the research question. The group is carefully selected to have common features for example: students of the same level, gender, or learning strategy. They are particularly useful to probe for answers why a particular measurement was found, or to propose solutions to a problem (Wilson, 1997; Nel, Romm, and Tlale, 2015).

It is a dynamic interactive data collection method that can explore into attitudes, underlying assumptions or causes of certain behaviors. Focus groups are semi-structured and are recorded and coded for analysis of responses). They are criticized for being not suitable for private matters. Another disadvantage is that an influential candidate can change the opinion of the whole group (Barbour, 2005; Brown, 1999).

Interview

One of the most important tool in qualitative research is the qualitative interview. It can be categorized into unstructured, semi-structured and structured (Crabtree, & Miller, 1999; DiCicco-Bloom, & Crabtree, 2006). The most important part in interviews is to identify the "Key informants" considering their knowledge, role or willingness (Poggie, 1972). In unstructured interviews, the researchers ask questions as they emerge to explore the meaning of a certain behaviour or observation. Semi-structured in-depth interviews are the most widely used tool for qualitative medical education research and can be either with a single person or with a group (Brown and Danaher, 2019). Typically, an interview takes half an hour to several hours and is face-to-face but telephone and email interviews (Glogowska, Young, and Lockyer2011, James, 2016) have also been used. Individual interviews allow for probing into private issues while group interviews give a wider perspective. The responses of each interviewee are recorded in addition to the group dynamics and interpersonal interaction (Johnson, 2002). The analysis of interview data has been described elsewhere in this book. It can be supported by photos or videos of the interviewees.

Observation notes

Researchers opt for these records or field notes to study how students perform or act in certain situations rather than what they think or say they do (Hammersley and Atkinson, 1995). Field notes are structured to include the content, context, and audience, and may include audio recording of spontaneous conversations. Observations are criticized for being influenced by the presence of the observer. This can be minimized by obscuring the purpose and research objective from candidates, and by ensuring passivity of the observer. It is a useful tool for common events but not for rare incidences. Lupton (2016) describes the use of social media in qualitative research (Lupton, 2016).

There is increasing interest in the use of blogs (Wilson, Kenny, and Dickson-Swift, 2015) and social media like *Facebook* (de Jong, 2015), *Twitter* (Hingle et.al., 2013), *Telegram* (Iqbal et.al., 2020), and *WhatsApp* (Klein et.al., 2018).

Document Analysis, Narratives, and Social Media

Narrative enquiry is a research tool that collects qualitative descriptions to reach a conclusion about the research question. It is a reliable tool to measure performance and has been used to evaluate neurology residents (Kelly et. al., 2020). Narrative enquiry used to detect professional identity roles (Katsarou, & Tsafos, 2016). In the latter study, deconstructing the narrations provided by participants helped recognize their professional identities, their views and assumptions and thus provided them with rich feedback. Confidentiality of participants is a concern in this type of research.

The combined use of visual narratives has been used to study and record behavior of preschool children in day care (Ridgway & Quiñones, 2016).

One should realize that the selection of methods and tool largely depend upon the research question. For example, if the research question involves how students perceive integrity and professional behavior or how they would behave in an ethical dilemma, then interview would be the most suitable tool. Alternatively, if the research topic is about medical errors and how students perceive malpractice, then focus group is a better tool as similar experiences of other students help candidates crystallize their thoughts. If the research question is about residents' reaction to criticism of their diagnosis and management in the morning report then observation notes of morning reports will be the best data collection tool.

Mixed methods can enrich the findings of either one alone and can accomplish a methodologically rigorous study design and lead to rich and comprehensive findings.

SUMMARIZE

The table below gives a summary tools and methods for Educational Research.

Research tool Name	Qualita-tive	Quantita-tive	General-izability	Time Consum-ing	Money Consum-ing	Reliabil-ity	Re-searcher Role	Re-searcher bias
Testing		Yes	Yes			Yes	Passive	No
Questionnaire		Yes	Yes			Yes	Passive	No

Research tool Name	Qualita-tive	Quantita-tive	General-izability	Time Consum-ing	Money Consum-ing	Reliabil-ity	Re-searcher Role	Re-searcher bias
Checklist	Yes	Yes	Yes			Yes	Passive	No
Rating scale		Yes	Yes			Yes	Active	Yes
Observation notes			Yes			Yes	Passive	
Pre/post test	Yes	Yes	Yes			Yes	Passive	
Focus group	Yes		Yes			Yes	Active	
Interview	Yes		No	Yes	Yes	No	Active	Yes
Narrative enquiry	Yes		No	Yes	Yes	No	Active	
Grounded theory	Yes		Yes	Yes	Yes	Yes	Active	
Ethnography	Yes		No	Yes	No	No	Passive	Yes
Phenomenol-ogy	Yes		No	Yes		No	Active	Yes
Action research	Yes		No	Yes		No	Active	Yes
Case studies	Yes		No			No	Passive	Yes

EVALUATE

YOU are the Vice-Dean of Academic Affairs at an established medical school. Graduates of medical schools in your country set for a Medical Licensure Exam (MLE) as soon as they graduate in order to be allowed to practice or enroll for postgraduate training. The Dean requested you to evaluate student performance in the MLE over the years.

The research question was: **WHAT** is the trend of students' performance in MLE?

If it has declined **WHY** the students' performance in MLE has declined over the years?

And to prepare an improvement plan WHICH method(s) will you suggest?

ROAD AHEAD

Research in health professionals education requires several successive steps, from formulating the correct research question to deciding the method for dissemination of the results. Each step has its own importance One of the key steps is choosing the correct method for the research Each approach has advantages and disadvantages and should be chosen according to the question being asked and the specific goal of the study. The road ahead should aim at well-conducted education research using the appropriate methods and tools that allow progression towards the important goal of using evidence-based education in our teaching institutions.

Identifying priorities for research efforts,selecting the appropriate tools and methods for the same and engaging a range of stakeholders in research priority setting exercises has been posited as an effective triad leading to the road towards reducing researcher bias and increasing social accountability

REFERENCES

Barbour RS and Barbour RS (2005) Making sense of focus groups. Medical Education. 39: 742 – 50

Bargh JA and Chartrand TL (1999) The unbearable automaticity of being. American Psychologist. 54: 462 – 79.

Bordage G (2007) Moving the field forward: going beyond quantitative - qualitative. Academic Medicine. 82: S126 – 8.

Brown, A. & Danaher, P.A. (2019), "CHE Principles: facilitating authentic and dialogical semi-structured interviews in educational research", International journal of research & method in education, vol. 42, no. 1, pp. 76-90.

Brown J (1999) Focus group interviews. In: Crabtree B and Miller W (eds) Doing Qualitative Research, pp. 109 – 24. Sage Publications, Thousand Oaks, CA.

Campbell DT and Stanley JC (1963) Experimental and Quasi - experimental Designs for Research on Teaching. Rand McNally, Chicago, IL.

Christensen, L. & Johnson, R.B. (2019), Educational Research: Quantitative, Qualitative, and Mixed Approaches, Sage Publications.

Conle, C. (2000), "Narrative Inquiry: Research tool and medium for professional development", European journal of teacher education, vol. 23, no. 1, pp. 49-63.

Cook DA, Beckman TJ. Current concepts in validity and reliability for psychometric instruments: Theory and application. Am J Med. (2006); 119:166. e7–166.16. 6 Deeks J, Dinnes J, D'Amico R, Sowden A, Sakarovitch C. Evaluating non-randomised intervention studies. Health Technol Assess. 2003; 7:186.

Cook, D.A. & Beckman, T.J. (2010), "Reflections on experimental research in medical education", Advances in health sciences education: theory and practice, vol. 15, no. 3, pp. 455-464.

Crabtree B, Miller W. *Doing Qualitative Research.* 2nd edn. Thousand Oaks, California: Sage (1999); 18– 20.

de Jong, Peter G. M (2015), "Theme for 2015: Integration", Medical science educator, vol. 25, no. 4, pp. 479-479.

DiCicco-Bloom, B. & Crabtree, B.F. (2006), "The qualitative research interview", Medical education, vol. 40, no. 4, pp. 314-321.

Efron, S.E. & Ravid, R. (2019), Action Research in Education, Second Edition: A Practical Guide, Guilford Publications, New York.

Glaser, B.G. (2010), "Naturalist Inquiry and Grounded Theory",

Glogowska, M., Young, P. & Lockyer, L. (2011), "Propriety, process and purpose: considerations of the use of the telephone interview method in an educational research study", Higher education, vol. 62, no. 1, pp. 17-26.

Gordon MJ (1991) A review of the validity and accuracy of self - assessments in health professions training. Academic Medicine. 66: 762 – 9.

Hammersley M and Atkinson P (1995) Ethnography: principles in practice. Routledge, London.

Hatch, T., Duarte, D. & Lisa K. De Gregorio (2018), "Pre- and Post-Tests and Assessments" in Corwin, Thousand Oaks, pp. 169.

Hingle, M., Yoon, D., Fowler, J., Kobourov, S., Schneider, M.L., Falk, D. & Burd, R. (2013), "Collection and visualization of dietary behavior and reasons for eating using Twitter", Journal of medical Internet research, vol. 15, no. 6, pp. e125-e125.

Iqbal, M., Alradhi, H., Alhumaidi, A., Alshaikh, K., AlObaid, A., Alhashim, M. & AlSheikh, M. (2020), "Telegram as a Tool to Supplement Online Medical Education During COVID-19 Crisis", Acta informatica medica, vol. 28, no. 2, pp. 94-97.

Johnson J. In-depth interviewing. In: J Gubrium, J Holstein, eds. *Handbook of Qualitative Research*. Thousand Oaks, California: Sage (2002); 103– 19

Johnson, R. B., & Onwuegbuzie, A. J. (2004). Mixed methods research: A research paradigm whose time has come. Educational Researcher, 33(7), 14-26.

Katsarou, E. & Tsafos, V. (2016), "Recognising participants' professional identities through analysis of narratives in educational Action Research/Reconociendo las identidades profesionales de los participantes a traves del analisis de narrativas en la investigacion-accion educativa", International journal of action research, vol. 12, no. 3, pp. 248.

Kelly, M.S., Mooney, C.J., Rosati, J.F., Braun, M.K. & Thompson Stone, R. (2020), "Education Research: The Narrative Evaluation Quality Instrument: Development of a tool to assess the assessor", Neurology, vol. 94, no. 2, pp. 91.

Kitzinger J, Barbour RS. Introduction: the challenge and promise of focus groups. In: Barbour RS, KitzingerJ, eds. Developing Focus Group Research: Politics, Theory and Practice. London: Sage 1999:1–20.

Klein, A.Z., Junior, José Carlos da Silva Freitas, Mattiello da Silva, Juliana Vitória Vieira Mattiello, Barbosa, J.L.V. & Baldasso, L. (2018), "The Educational Affordances of Mobile Instant Messaging (MIM): Results of Whatsapp® Used in Higher Education", International journal of distance education technologies, vol. 16, no. 2, pp. 51-64.

Lingard, L. & Kennedy, T.J. (2010), "Qualitative Research Methods in Medical Education" in, ed. T. Swanwick, Wiley-Blackwell, Oxford, UK, pp. 323-335.

Leppink, J. (2019), Statistical Methods for Experimental Research in Education and Psychology, Springer International Publishing AG, Cham.

Lupton, D. (2016), "The use and value of digital media for information about pregnancy and early motherhood: a focus group study", BMC pregnancy and childbirth, vol. 16, no. 1, pp. 171-171.

Merriam, S. (1998). Qualitative research and case study applications in education. San Francisco, CA: Jossey-Bass.

Nel, N.M., Romm, N.R.A. & Tlale, L.D.N. (2015), "Reflections on focus group sessions regarding inclusive education: reconsidering focus group research possibilities", Australian educational researcher, vol. 42, no. 1, pp. 35-53.

Poggie J. Toward quality control in key informant interview data. *Human Organization* 1972; **31**: 23– 32.

Reeves, S., Peller, J., Goldman, J. & Kitto, S. (2013), "Ethnography in qualitative educational research: AMEE Guide No. 80", Medical teacher, vol. 35, no. 8, pp. e1365-e1379.

Ridgway, A., Li, L. & Quiñones, G. (2016), "Visual narrative methodology in educational research with babies: triadic play in babies' room", Video journal of education and pedagogy, vol. 1, no. 1, pp. 1-18.

Roff, S., McAleer, S., Harden, R.M., Al-Qahtani, M., Ahmed, A.U., Deza, H., Groenen, G. & Primparyon, P. (1997), "Development and validation of the Dundee Ready Education Environment Measure (DREEM)", Medical teacher, vol. 19, no. 4, pp. 295-299.

Roff, S. (2005), "The Dundee Ready Educational Environment Measure (DREEM)-a generic instrument for measuring students' perceptions of undergraduate health professions curricula", Medical teacher, vol. 27, no. 4, pp. 322-325.

Saevi, T. (2014), Phenomenology in Educational Research, Oxford University Press.

Saxon, D., Garratt, D., Gilroy, P. & Cairns, C. (2003), "Collecting Data in the Information Age: Exploring Web-Based Survey Methods in Educational Research", Research in education (Manchester), vol. 69, no. 1, pp. 51-66.

Seidel J, Kjolseth R, Seymour E. The Ethnograph: a user›s guide. Littleton, Connecticut: Qualis Research Associates 1988.

Spindler, G. & Hammond, L. (2006), Innovations in Educational Ethnography: Theories, Methods, and Results, Psychology Press, Mahwah.

Stolz, S.A. (2020), "Phenomenology and phenomenography in educational research: A critique", Educational philosophy and theory, vol. 52, no. 10, pp. 1077-1096.

Suter, W. (2012), "Research Bias and Control" in, 2nd edn, SAGE Publications, Inc, Thousand Oaks, pp. 186.

Vallack, J. (2015), "Alchemy for inquiry: a methodology of applied phenomenology in educational research", Australian Association for Research in Education,

Walsh, K. (2013), "Medical students as human subjects in educational research - the importance of responder bias", Medical education online, vol. 18, no. 1, pp. 20757-20757.

Wilson, E., Kenny, A. & Dickson-Swift, V. (2015), "Using Blogs as a Qualitative Health Research Tool: A Scoping Review", International journal of qualitative methods, vol. 14, no. 5, pp. 160940691561804.

Wilson, V. (1997), "Focus Groups: a useful qualitative method for educational research?", British educational research journal, vol. 23, no. 2, pp. 209-224.

Wolf, F.M. (2004), "Methodological quality, evidence, and Research in Medical Education (RIME)", *Academic medicine,* vol. 79, no. 10 Suppl, pp. S68-S69.

Wyse, D., Selwyn, N., Smith, E. & Suter, L. (2017), "The Role of Theory in Quantitative Data Analysis" in SAGE Publications Ltd, 55 City Road, pp. 699.

Wyse, D. & Torgerson, C. (2017), "Experimental trials and 'what works?' in education: The case of grammar for writing", British educational research journal, vol. 43, no. 6, pp. 1019-1047.

Chapter 10

All About Questionnaires

Pathiyil Ravi Shankar, Ian G Wilson

ABSTRACT

Questionnaires are among the cost effective and most efficient means to obtain information from large number of respondents, widely used in educational research. Efficient use of time and resources, anonymity of respondents, use of standardized questions and a high participation rate are advantages. Adapting an existing questionnaire may be easier than constructing an entirely new instrument. Both open-ended and close-ended questions can be used. Validity and reliability are two important issues to be considered.

Qualitative and quantitative are the two basic types of questionnaires. Online questionnaires are becoming increasingly common. Questionnaires can be administered face-to-face, using a telephone, through mail or online. A Likert scale is often used to measure attitudes. Pilot testing is important before a questionnaire is administered. Validating a questionnaire is a complex and time-consuming process. Recruiting subjects and analysing responses could be challenging. This chapter also highlights attributes of a good questionnaire.

Key Words: Attitude, Research, educational; Research, qualitative; Research, quantitative; Students; Surveys and questionnaires

ASSESS NEED

Why are questionnaires commonly used in educational research?

Questionnaires are probably the most widely used instrument in educational research.

A questionnaire is a research instrument consisting of a set of questions or other type of prompts aiming to collect information from respondent(s) (QuestionPro, 2021).

Both quantitative and qualitative information can be collected using a questionnaire. Questionnaires are widely used in research. They are the cost effective and most efficient way to obtain information from a large number of respondents (Munn and Drever, 1990). Responses can be quantified and subject to statistical analysis. Questionnaires can be administered to respondents in different ways. They can be completed by a data collector while interviewing the participants. The most common method, however, is for the respondents to complete the questionnaires by themselves. The investigators may be contacted in case of any queries or difficulties. You should certainly know about online questionnaires, which are becoming increasingly common.

The main advantages of using a questionnaire in medical educational research are efficient use of time, respondent anonymity, use of standardized questions and the possibility of a high return rate (Munn and Drever, 1990).

Designing a questionnaire, obtaining feedback from the respondents about the questions, and pilot testing the instrument are time-consuming steps.

Several questionnaires have been developed with a few notable examples being *Dundee Ready Educational Environment Measure (DREEM), Jefferson Scale of Physician Empathy (JSPE), Communication Skills Attitude Scale (CSAS), Self-directed Learner Readiness Scale (SDLRS)* among others.

For most educational research purposes, it may be easier and efficient to adapt an already designed questionnaire. However, one must be careful while adapting the questionnaires used in western countries to the Asian and Indian context.

The authors have extensively used questionnaires to carry out research studies in several areas including student attitudes or perception toward transferable skills, complementary and alternative medicine, the doctor-patient relationship, care seeking behavior for childhood illness, integrative medicine, psychological morbidity, sources of stress and coping strategies.

BRIEF

- Questionnaires are commonly used in medical educational research
- They are more efficient to gather information from large groups, with high response rate, maintaining respondent anonymity.
- The questionnaire data can be analysed using quantitative and qualitative methods.
- Various issues should be carefully considered while planning and administering a questionnaire.
- Online questionnaires are becoming increasingly common in COVID era
- A good questionnaire fulfills several important characteristics.

CONTEXTUALIZE

Scenario 1

You are a medical educator at a medical school which was started three years ago. The Dean of the medical school has requested you to study the educational environment at the school in terms of different parameters like faculty, students, and students' self-perception. The perception of the educational environment among different cohorts of students and according to gender and other demographic characteristics is to be compared. A detailed information from subgroups of students who have lower perception scores is also needed. How will you go about this task?

One of the instruments to study student perception regarding the educational environment is the DREEM questionnaire developed in the Western context (Roff et al., 1997). This questionnaire has been used and validated in several settings (Roff, 2005). The scores can be compared among different groups and sub-groups of students.

Scenario 2

You are the Dean of Clinical Sciences at an established medical school. Students are selected from among the best talent in the country. You have been concerned by anecdotal reports of decline in empathy among medical students as they progress through the undergraduate medical course and especially by suggestions that the maximum decline may be taking place during the third year when students enter clinical training. How can you obtain a fair measure of attitude and empathy of students, which can help to answer your queries?

The Jefferson Scale of Physician Empathy (JSPE) was developed by Hojat et al. to measure empathy among physicians, health care professionals and students (Hojat et al., 2002). Several studies have been conducted using the instrument globally and also in India (Biswas et al., 2018; Shashikumar et al., 2014). A student version of the instrument has also been developed and used in several studies. Different cohorts can be studied in a cross-sectional manner and a particular cohort can also be followed longitudinally.

These two examples highlight how a variety of parameters can be measured or studied in medical education using appropriate questionnaires. In these two instances we used previously developed and validated instruments.

DESCRIBE

Issues relating to questionnaires

A questionnaire is perhaps the most used instrument in educational research. A distinction is made between open-ended and close-ended questions. An open-ended question requires the respondents to provide their answer while in a close-ended question the respondent picks the correct one among a choice of options (Singh, 2017).

Two important issues regarding a questionnaire are *validity* and *reliability*. We will now examine what these terms mean. The validity of a questionnaire is related to whether it measures what it is supposed to measure. There are two measures of validity- internal and external (Singh & Masuku, 2012). Good internal validity means lack of error in the measurements and the possibility of drawing inferences from the data. External validity refers to the applicability of the findings of the study to the population from which the sample was selected. Different constructs of validity have been discussed in the literature. See Table 1.

Table 1: Types of Validity and what do they mean?

Types of Validity	Criteria
Face validity	Does the questionnaire look like it will measure what it is intended to measure?.
Content validity	The extent to which the content matter experts agree on the content.
Construct validity	The ability to measure the concept adequately.
Predictive validity	The extent to which the questionnaire findings can predict results in future.
Concurrent validity	The extent to which the results are supported by using other tests.

The reliability of a questionnaire is also important. During test-retest reliability the same questionnaire is administered at different intervals to the same respondents obtaining similar results. Inter-rater reliability is another aspect and examines whether two individuals using the questionnaire score items similarly (Singh, 2017). Internal consistency examines the correlation between different items in the questionnaire. Cronbach's alpha is widely used as a measure of internal consistency. A value greater than 0.7 is regarded as internally consistent.

Among important issues to be addressed before the start of the study are:

- Identifying the target population
- The types of questions which will be used
- Whether the respondents can interpret the questions correctly
- Writing of individual questions avoiding pitfalls in construction, language
- The sequence and organization of questionnaire
- The process of validation and
- Pilot testing

We usually start with more general questions and then go onto more specific and sensitive questions. Demographic information is now often asked at the end of the questionnaire. If demographic questions are asked first, they may be seen as intrusive. If they are asked at the end respondents may be committed to the questionnaire and are more likely to respond.

Types of questionnaires

Questionnaires are divided into two basic types – qualitative and quantitative ('Questionnaire', 2020). Qualitative questionnaires also called unstructured or exploratory questionnaires are used to collect qualitative data which is not numerical in nature. An example can be collecting free-text comments about a particular class or session. They are usually used in the initial stages when not much is known about a topic.

Quantitative questionnaires are also known as formal structured questionnaires. These are used to collect numerical data which can be counted. The data can be subject to statistical analysis. We often use a Likert scale evaluating a respondent's agreement with a statement to convert perceptions and attitudes to numerical values which can be analysed statistically. These are usually used when we have more information about the subject or topic we are studying. Many questionnaires use a mixture of quantitative and qualitative elements within a standard questionnaire and use of free-text comments.

There are also computer, inhouse, telephone and mail questionnaires depending on how we administer the questionnaire. During the ongoing pandemic computer or online questionnaires are widely used to collect data. Google forms (*https://www.google.com/forms/about/*), Microsoft forms (*https://www.office.com/forms/about*) and SurveyMonkey (*www.surveymonkey.com*) are some freely available resources to create and administer questionnaires online. There are different online sources to obtain information on how to use these forms. The data collected can be directly downloaded in different formats.

Telephone interviews can be conducted in a short time, but respondents may be reluctant to answer certain questions over the phone. During an inhouse survey the interviewer visits persons in their homes or workplaces. If a good rapport is established this can be a good method of collecting data but it can be expensive, laborious and respondents often may not be comfortable having the interviewer at their homes or workplaces. Questionnaires can be sent through mail often with a prepaid return envelope allowing respondents to answer at their leisure. However, it can be expensive, and response rates can be low.

Various types of questions can be used in a questionnaire. These can be open-ended, and close-ended (multiple choice, dichotomous, scaled and pictorial) ('Questionnaire', 2020; 'Questionnaires', n.d.). Open-ended questions allow respondents to answer according to their choice without imposing any restrictions on their answers. Among close-ended options, multiple choice questions are commonly used and ask the respondent to select a choice from several options (usually four or five). Dichotomous questions provide respondents with a set of two responses (usually Yes/No, Agree/Disagree or True/False).

Use of scales

Scaled questions are used to judge the degree of the respondent's feeling about something. Likert scales, rating scales and semantic differential scales are different types.

A Likert scale measures attitudes directly and is usually a five or seven point scale allowing the respondent to express how much they agree or disagree with a particular statement (Likert Scale Definition, Examples and Analysis | Simply Psychology, n.d.). A semantic differential scale asks respondents to rate an entity within the frames of a multipoint rating option (Semantic Differential Scale, Example, and Question Types | QuestionPro, n.d.). The two ends of the scale have opposite choices. Pictorial questions substitute pictures instead of text and usually has a higher response rate.

The process of developing and validating a new questionnaire

As mentioned previously constructing a questionnaire is a complex process requiring significant statistical expertise. The first step is to determine what you want to measure using the questionnaire. Questionnaires are ideal for determining the prevalence of events or opinions in communities. They can also be used to determine the occurrence of certain illnesses. They work well in screening for illnesses such as depression or anxiety, or similar conditions. They can measure latent variables such as quality of life. It is obvious that the structure of questionnaires will vary significantly.

Table 2: Writing of individual questions avoiding pitfalls in construction, language

Type of question	Example	Issue
Double question	Do you think medical students should have more lectures or experience more clinical work?.	Many respondents would like to answer YES to both options.
Push polling	Elite medical schools produce better doctors than other schools.	There is a strong suggestion which may direct respondents to a specific answer.

Validation and Pilot Testing

Once the questions are framed and compiled, a pilot test should be run to determine the readability of the questions and the pilot can also be used to conduct the validation of the questionnaire. This is a vital step in the process of finalising the questionnaire. The validation process determines if the questions are capable of measuring what we want it to measure, and if it can measure it reliably. It is only when we can demonstrate that the questionnaire is valid and reliable that we should use it for research.

It is because of the complexity of the validation process that many researchers seek to use questionnaires that have been validated in prior research. This must be undertaken with caution. Just because a questionnaire has been validated with one community does not mean it is valid in other contexts. The questionnaire needs to be revalidated. However, using an established questionnaire means that you do not have to go through the process of writing the questions.

As a minimum the questionnaire should be subject to a pilot test. Many quote Cronbach's alpha based on the research findings and assume that this will validate the instrument. Cronbach's alpha is important for reliability, but it does not confirm validity. A pilot test will enable you to determine the acceptability of the language for the subjects of the study. It will also enable you to explore the validity of the questionnaire.

Validating a questionnaire is a complex process. It covers face validity where context experts examine the questions to determine their ability to measure what they are designed to measure. It also determines that subjects read and understand the questions in the way they were designed. Validation also measures reliability, as this is a basic requirement of a valid instrument.

The scores are also examined in detail to determine their structure and relationship to other measures and the ability to predict scores in other areas. Having developed and validated the questionnaire it is now possible to conduct the research.

Determining and recruiting subjects

The first step is to determine who are the subjects. Developing a sampling frame through determining the selection criteria for the subjects ensures the subjects have a degree of commonality. Decisions then need to be made about how subjects are recruited. Options include Telephone recruitment with interview by a researcher, posters, advertisements in newspapers or magazines, online through websites. Recruiting students can be through lectures and during other sessions. Recruiting students directly requires ethics committee approval. It is likely that you sit in a position of authority over the students and the methods used will need to ensure this does not affect the recruitment.

Sampling Frame for Questionnaire studies

The sampling frame is determined by the criteria used to select or reject respondents. Often a convenience sample is obtained. The sample should be representative of the population being studied. Issues of sampling have been addressed in detail in other sections of the book. Random sampling, systematic sampling, stratified sampling, and snowball sampling can all be used. Snowball sampling is often used for sensitive topics where it may be difficult to recruit participants.

Compliance issue and Tips for enhancing compliance

Questionnaires are self-report instruments, and this limitation must be taken into consideration in analysing the results. The questions must be in a sequence that helps the respondent understand what is being considered. Easier questions should come first so that the respondent feels more comfortable responding. Compensating respondents for their time can be considered. The amount offered should not serve as an inducement to participate.

Analysing the responses

Having recruited the research subjects, it is necessary to organise the data into a form that enables it to be managed and analysed. Questionnaires completed on-line can be easily converted to a spreadsheet to enable analysis. Paper questionnaires need to be entered manually, although it is possible to design them so that they can be scanned. If they are to be entered manually it is possible to design the questionnaire to help the data entry person, ensure the data is entered correctly. If ensuring the quality of the entered data is critical then double entry with comparison of the data sets will ensure the final data quality.

Having created the data spread sheet analysis can occur. The researcher may want to enlist the support of a statistician if they do not have sufficient skills themselves. If the use of a statistician is planned it may be best to enlist their aid during the development of the questionnaire. Box 1 lists the characteristics of a good questionnaire.

Box 1: Characteristics of a good questionnaire (Parajuli, 2004)	
Characteristics of a good questionnaire (Parajuli, 2004)	Professional looking. Title is informative and clear direction on completing the questionnaire are provided.
	Short and easy to read.
	Purpose of the study is explained and the reasons why respondents should participate are provided.
	Unambiguous and terminology used is easily understood by the respondents.
	Questions grouped logically. Arranged according to themes. Easy questions are asked first, and demography is asked at the end.
	Branching is clearly shown. If some questions do not have to be answered by some respondents indicate it clearly.
	Capitalized, italics or font types can be used to deliver instructions.
	Provides alternative but does not use double-barrelled questions.
	Questions are worded neutrally and do not lead the respondents to answer in a particular manner.
	Asked both close and open-ended questions. Most questionnaires ask for open comments towards the end.
	Title should be concise, reflect the contents and be easily understood.
	A cover letter is attached with the questionnaire explaining details about the questionnaire and mention about confidentiality of responses.
	The questionnaire should end by thanking the respondents for their participation.

SUMMARIZE

This chapter has demonstrated the use of and the complexity of devising high quality questionnaires.

- Questions need to be aligned with the purpose of study, research questions, and the target audience
- High quality questionnaires need to undergo a thorough validation process.
- Using an existing questionnaire requires revalidation for the subjects in the new research.
- While questionnaires in quantitative approach help in describing and explaining the situation, the questionnaires in qualitative approach can provide exploratory data. Questionnaires can be combined with other methods
- Qualitative questionnaires can be devised to collect information that will provide more exploratory data.

EVALUATE

- Imagine that you have to conduct a questionnaire-based study to assess the attitude of health professions students toward interprofessional learning.
- First carry out a literature review to determine if there is an already existing questionnaire which can be used.
- If a questionnaire needs to be developed de novo, undertake a literature review to determine the questions that will be required.
- Does the questionnaire meet the characteristics of a good questionnaire mentioned in table 1?
- Does the questionnaire require modification for use in your context?
- How will you pre-test the questionnaire?
- Will the questionnaire be administered in English? If not, the issue of translation should be considered?
- How will you go about obtaining ethical approval or exemption for your research?
- Will you administer the questionnaire using paper forms or use an online form? How will you motivate students to participate?
- When will you close the survey?
- How will the data be analysed?
- How will you maintain anonymity of the respondents?
- How will you communicate the findings of the study among internal stakeholders?
- How will the findings be communicated externally?
- Kindly think through these steps for the two scenarios and instruments we had described in the Contextualize section of the chapter. These steps are important when you are doing a study using DREEM or JSPE or any other questionnaire and will improve the logistics, the method of the study and the quality of the data obtained.

Figure 1 highlights the important steps in developing and using a questionnaire

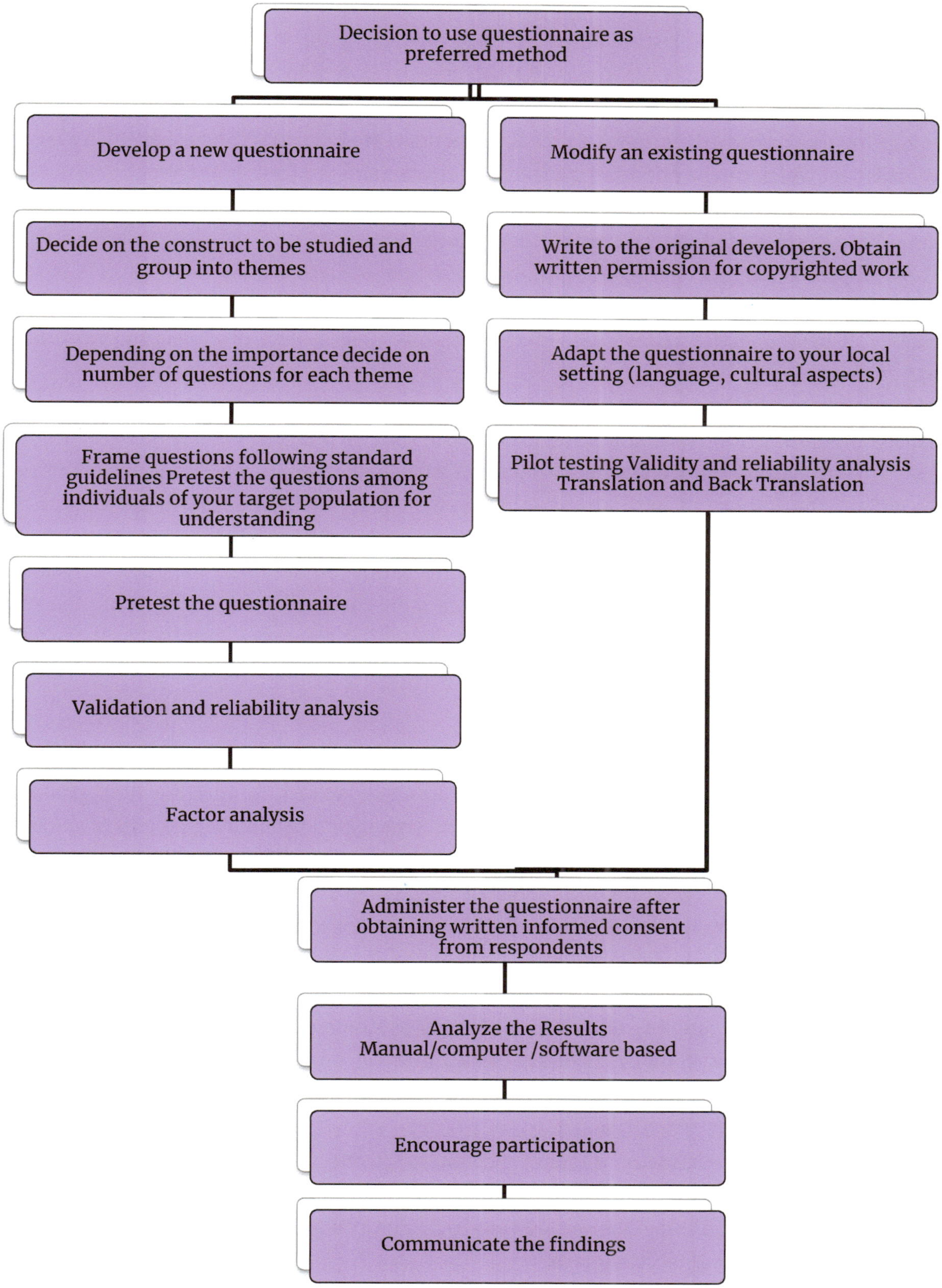

Figure 1: Developing and using a questionnaire in educational research

ROAD AHEAD

- Increasing use of online questionnaires
  Due to the ongoing coronavirus disease (COVID) pandemic and increasing use of online learning in health professions schools, online questionnaires will become increasingly common. They are easier to administer, and no printing and physical distribution are required. The data are also available as a spreadsheet which can be imported into statistical programs for further analysis.
- Resources to learn more about online questionnaires
  https://www.ncbi.nlm.nih.gov/pmc/articles/PMC5506389/
  https://www.snapsurveys.com/blog/10-tips-administering-online-surveys/
- Your feedback about questionnaires
  Have you used questionnaires? As a part of research? As a part of collecting information for accreditation purposes?
  Did you use a prevalidated questionnaire? How did you adapt it to your situation? Have you developed a questionnaire? Do you have statistical expertise in your institution? What challenges did you face? How did you address those challenges? Have you published research studies using questionnaires? Do write to the authors about these issues at the email addresses mentioned in the chapter.
- Can the process of questionnaire administration and analysis be automated?
  Will it be possible to use artificial intelligence to carry out the different tasks associated with questionnaire administration? These range from validation, pilot testing, preparation of online questionnaire, administering the questionnaire, analysing responses, reminding those who have not yet completed the survey, analysing the results, and generating a report.

REFERENCES

Biswas, B., Haldar, A., Dasgupta, A., Mallick, N., & Karmakar, A. (2018). An Epidemiological Study on Empathy and its Correlates: A Cross-sectional Assessment among Medical Students of a Government Medical College of India. Indian Journal of Psychological Medicine, 40(4), 364–369. https://doi.org/10.4103/IJPSYM.IJPSYM_109_18

Hojat, M., Gonnella, J. S., Mangione, S., Nasca, T. J., Veloski, J. J., Erdmann, J. B., Callahan, C. A., & Magee, M. (2002). Empathy in medical students as related to academic performance, clinical competence and gender. Medical Education, 36(6), 522–527. https://doi.org/10.1046/j.1365-2923.2002.01234.x

Likert Scale Definition, Examples and Analysis | Simply Psychology. (n.d.). Retrieved 3 May 2021, from https://www.simplypsychology.org/likert-scale.html

Munn, P and DreVer E.1990. *Using Questionnaires in Small-Scale Research. A Teachers' Guide.* Available from: *https://eric.ed.gov/?id=ED326488*

Parajuli, B.K. (2004). Questionnaire: a tool of primary data collection. Himalayan Journal of Sociology and anthropology 51-63. Available from: https://www.nepjol.info/index.php/HJSA/issue/view/123

Questionnaire: Types, Definition, Examples & How to Design Your Own. (2020, July 8). KyLeads. https://www.kyleads.com/blog/questionnaire/

Questionnaires. (n.d.). Research-Methodology. Retrieved 3 May 2021, from https://research-methodology.net/research-methods/survey-method/questionnaires-2/

QuestionPro. (2021). *The ultimate guide to great questionnaires.* Available from: *https://www.questionpro.com/blog/what-is-a-questionnaire/*

Roff, S. (2005). The Dundee Ready Educational Environment Measure (DREEM)—A generic instrument for measuring students' perceptions of undergraduate health professions curricula. Medical Teacher, 27(4), 322–325. https://doi.org/10.1080/01421590500151054

Roff, S., McAleer, S., Harden, R. M., Al-Qahtani, M., Ahmed, A. U., Deza, H., Groenen, G., & Primparyon, P. (1997). Development and validation of the Dundee Ready Education Environment Measure (DREEM). Medical Teacher, 19(4), 295–299. https://doi.org/10.3109/01421599709034208

Semantic differential scale, example, and question types | QuestionPro. (n.d.). Retrieved 3 May 2021, from https://www.questionpro.com/semantic-differential-scale.html

Shashikumar, R., Chaudhary, R., Ryali, V. S. S. R., Bhat, P. S., Srivastava, K., Prakash, J., & Basannar, D. (2014). Cross sectional assessment of empathy among undergraduates from a medical college. Medical Journal, Armed Forces India, 70(2), 179–185. https://doi.org/10.1016/j.mjafi.2014.02.005

Singh, A., & Masuku, M. (2012). Understanding and applications of test characteristics and basics inferential statistics in hypothesis testing. European Journal of Applied Sciences, 4(2), 90–97.

Singh, A. S. (2017). Common procedures for development, validity and reliability of a questionnaire. International Journal of Economics, Commerce and Management, V(5), 12.

Chapter 11

Consensus Group Methods: Delphi and Nominal Group Technique (NGT)

Medha A. Joshi, Nirmala Rege

ABSTRACT

Medical educators strive to use the latest findings from scientifically grounded research when making decisions regarding the health professions education. Empirical evidence from educational research, however, is often limited or contradictory. When faced with conditions of uncertainty or incomplete evidence, consensus group methods are widely used to synthesize expert opinions and enhance decision making. Two such methods *viz.* Delphi and Nominal Group Technique (NGT) which are commonly used for this purpose, are described in this chapter. These can be used in medical education research to determine components of a new or revised curriculum, develop items for assessment tools, define competencies, and develop educational resources. The readers will be familiarized with nuances of the process to conduct them and to maintain the quality as well as their advantages and limitations. The variants of these methods are also highlighted.

Key Words: consensus group methods, Delphi, nominal group technique (NGT), decision making, RAND appropriateness method, hybrid Delphi/NGT method, e-Delphi, policy Delphi

ASSESS NEED

In our personal as well as professional life, we come across occasions wherein we have to make selection of few from the available items, may they be resources, criteria, policy guidelines, or existing possibilities. for the benefits of others associated directly or indirectly with these items. Moreover, this selection needs approval from the group. We cannot make quick decisions based on what majority in the group wish but have to ensure that the decision is appropriate. This decision making becomes more crucial when the evidence supporting selection are not too strong or the group has varied and at times contradictory opinions. For this we need to discuss, take into consideration each other's opinion, critically look at all the pros and cons so that a consensus is reached among the group for the selection.

Processes to develop and measure consensus systematically are termed as consensus group methods (Murphy et al., 1998). As stated earlier, these methods are mainly useful when empirical evidence is insufficient or lacking or contradictory. In such situations it is expected that an accurate and reliable information can be best obtained by consulting a panel of experts and accepting their consensus (Humphrey-Murto, Varpio, Wood, et al., 2017). Consensus group methods are particularly applicable in medical education research as these methods can get inputs from the profession's collective knowledge and experience. In this chapter, we provide an overview of the two commonly used consensus group methods, which are well structured *viz.* the Delphi method and the nominal group technique (NGT).

BRIEF

- Delphi and NGT are a systematic means to measure and develop consensus on a topic.
- Suitable when empirical evidence is insufficient, inconsistent, or not present.
- The Delphi method involves a number of rounds. Participants never meet or interact directly.
- Advantage of Delphi is that it is possible to include a large number of experts spread around the world; the major limitation being it takes long time.
- NGT is a face-to-face interactive method and the number of participants are limited. It involves minimal discussion among the participants.
- Advantage of NGT is possibility of clarification and debate but the consensus is obtained from only a small number of participants, which is a limitation.
- A hybrid of these two methods (Hybrid Delphi) may be the solution to add benefits of both, yet minimize the limitations.

CONTEXTUALIZE

Please go through scenario-1 carefully. While reading the rest of the chapter, ask yourself why Delphi method has been chosen over the NGT by the chairman of the committee.

Scenario-1: The healthcare system in India is challenged with the shortage of skilled and competent workforce. Medical Education, which earlier focused largely on acquisition of knowledge was expected to produce competent and skilled medical practitioner. To meet the expectations of the stakeholders, the medical education has adopted competency based medical education (CBME). This paradigm shift in medical education has forced other healthcare education systems to relook at their curricula. Physiotherapy is one such highly skill -oriented healthcare system that is looking to bring about a change in their curriculum to introduce the competency-based education paradigm. Many developed countries already are offering CBE in physiotherapy, The Indian Association of Physiotherapists are planning to define competencies more suitable in the Indian context for a graduate physiotherapist.

The Association president has decided to form a small committee to finalize the competencies. The chairman of the committee thinks it would be highly relevant if inputs from the subject experts from India and other countries where CBE is in place are involved in defining the competencies. She has decided to adopt Delphi method.

DESCRIBE

Origination of Delphi and NGT

Olaf Helmer and Norman Dalkey from the RAND Corporation used Delphi method in 1950 for the first time (Rowe & Wright, 2011). They named it as Delphi, which is an ancient city in Greece. A priestess at a temple of Apollo at Delphi was famous for her prophecies. The Delphi method similarly helps to forecast the outcome of future scenarios, predict the likelihood of an event, tendencies and development, evaluate and make a decision about a particular topic or issue by collecting opinions/decisions from a group of experts (Belton et al., 2019; Gaba, 2007; Gary & Heiko, 2015; Rowe & Wright, 2011). The generation of new information and insights that shed some light on what might be in the future makes Delphi as an explorative tool (Steinert, 2009).

Similar to Delphi, NGT too obtains the opinions of experts on a given topic and brings about a group consensus, but unlike the Delphi technique, the key feature of NGT is structured, face-to-face meetings. NGT was developed in the 1960s as a procedure to facilitate effective group decision-making in social psychological research such as studies of program design in the NASA aerospace field, industrial engineering problems of social service, and environmental studies by program planners, and has since been employed in a wide range of fields including education and health. Authors that developed this technique, such as Van de Ven and Delbecq regarded NGT as a problem-solving method, based on the development of a consensual depiction of the problem (Delbecq & Van de Ven, 1971).

NGT provides a systematic procedure for obtaining relevant and reliable qualitative information from a group of experts. The collaborative nature of NGT increases the stakeholders' ownership of the ensuing outcomes and therefore increases the likelihood of acceptance and implementation of policies as this approach is democratic and transparent (Vella et al., 2000). The group is called a 'nominal group' because even though the participants form a group, interaction among the group members is nominal and they mostly work individually from the beginning till the end of the session (Boddy, 2012).

Purpose of Delphi and NGT

Both the methods have been extensively used in health education as well as health sciences. Some of the examples are as follows:

1. **Education and educational research** (Foth et al., 2016; Green, 2014; Humphrey-Murto, Varpio, Gonsalves, et al., 2017; Humphrey-Murto, et al., 2017).
    a. **Developing or reforming curriculum** including deciding educational goals and objectives; defining, developing, and assessing competencies; Identifying components of various phases (e.g. clerkship or internship); deciding assessment criteria and developing assessment tools; and educational resources
    b. **Futuristic planning** regarding advocacy of the institution, forecasting educational outcomes and exploring and describing any issues related to educational elements
    c. **For developmental research** pertaining to education, generating right research questions and refining them and clarifying or validating findings collected from various qualitative data collection methods

2. **Health care** (Belton et al., 2019; Boulkedid et al., 2011; McMillan et al., 2016; Niederberger & Spranger, 2020):
   a. In health care sciences both the techniques have been used to:
      - Evaluate healthcare quality; develop/select healthcare quality indicators, prescribing indicators, prognostic criteria for disease.
      - Formulate clinical guidelines or standards, recommend action and prioritize measures.
      - Determine cost-effectiveness or cost-benefit analysis of health care.

   b. Delphi method is also used for predicting trends in clinical practice/health care technology or forecasting future of various specialties or disciplines.

Steps/Process

Delphi Method

The four key elements of this method include

1. Anonymous responses,
2. Iteration,
3. Provision of all responses in form of summary to all group members, and
4. Statistical aggregation of individuals' response (Belton et al., 2019).

It is also known as estimate-talk-estimate technique (ETE). Multiple rounds of traditional Delphi minimize group bias.

Before initiation of first round: This period is termed as 'Exploration' stage.

- The researcher/s serves as a group facilitator with a neutral position. He/she defines the research question, the objective of the study and decides the rationale for selection of the Delphi as a method of data collection.
- He/she selects a group of experts based on the topic under consideration. They can be internal or external to the organization and may be from one field or with diverse background (heterogenous) depending on the problem.
- The researcher should do a pilot survey with the developed questionnaire by administering it to a subset of selected experts. This allows him/her to get an idea about the possible range of viewpoints expected. At this juncture, some open-ended questions can be included to get some ideas/issues that might have been missed by the researchers.

During rounds

- ***Round 1 of Delphi:*** After confirmation of participants, each member of the group is sent a questionnaire with instructions. The type of questions varies based on the topic of Delphi, a space is provided to enter personal opinion, experience, or previous research of experts as a supportive rationale for the response. Usually, 2-8 weeks period is given for responding.
- ***Summary report 1:*** The questionnaires are returned to the researcher who collates the comments and prepares a summary report, which has statistics of the group response (e.g. median and interquartile range for Likert scale measures). Sometimes reasons for the responses are given. However, the experts' identities remain unknown to the group members. A copy of the summary report is sent to each expert. to encourage them to state their opinions freely.

The researcher prepares a second questionnaire, which is based on the analyzed responses obtained in the first round. The changes are made in questions by identifying any similarities between answers. Irrelevant content is eliminated.

- ***Round 2 of Delphi:*** provides an opportunity to the group members to comment further. Their opinions may remain the same as in previous round or may change after going through the summary report of the first round when they get to know others' viewpoints.
- ***Summary report 2:*** Responses to the second questionnaire are analyzed and a second summary report of answers is prepared.
- ***Subsequent rounds of Delphi:*** The same sequence of events is followed in the subsequent rounds *viz.* compilation of responses and preparation of summary report, modification of questionnaires, and administration to experts to get their opinions. The questionnaire rounds can be repeated as many times as necessary to achieve a general sense of consensus.

Termination of Delphi

Usually, 2-3 rounds are sufficient to get stable responses and reach general agreement (consensus) (Belton et al., 2019; Heiko, 2012). The researcher decides if another round is necessary.

It should be noted that at the end of these rounds experts' opinions may remain stable but opposing each other (Rowe & Wright, 2001) or they may not be stable at all (Landeta & Barrutia, 2011). There may be a continuous dissensus or disagreement (De Loë et al., 2016; Rowe & Wright, 2001). In that case researcher should prevent having another round (Belton et al., 2019) as it will not provide any outcome.

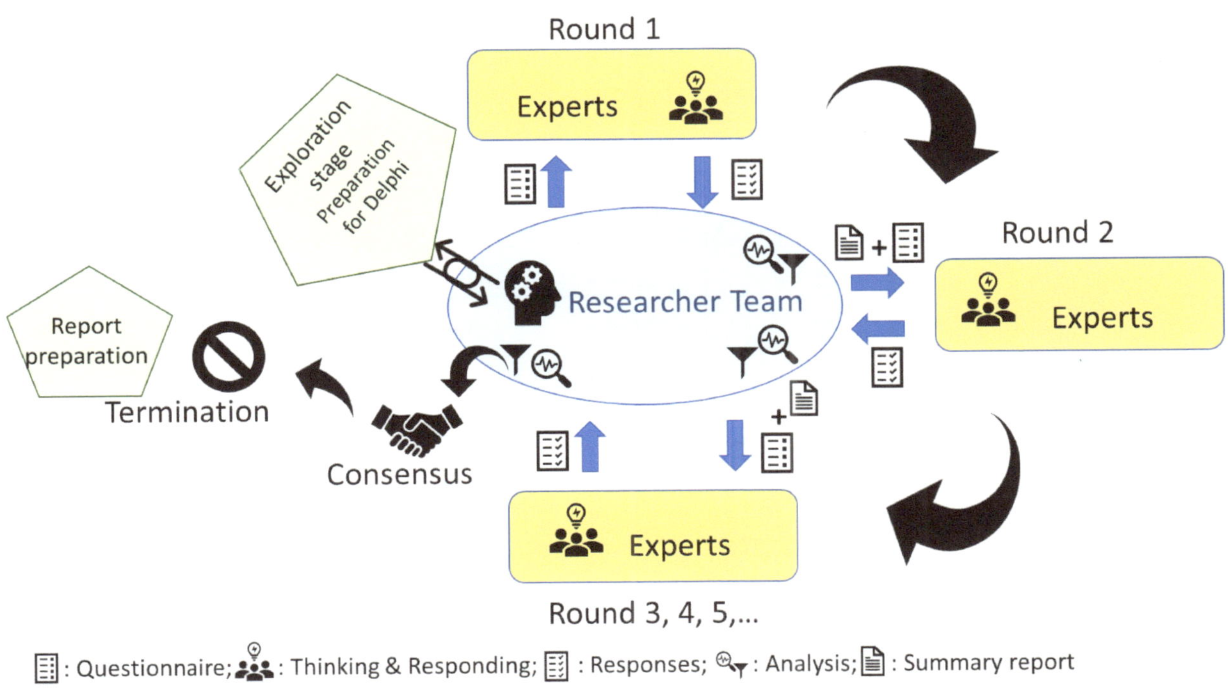

Figure 1: Delphi process

Nominal Group Technique (NGT)

Much of the success of a NG session depends upon the ability of the facilitator to remain neutral, non-judgmental and ensure that every participant contributes to the idea generation.

Step 1: *Opening the session* This is done by the facilitator by expressing the purpose of organizing the NG session, by stating the issue/question for which many ideas are expected to be generated by the group.

Step 2: *Generating the ideas*: Each participant in the group silently and independently generates as many ideas as possible in a short time (generally 5-10 mins; Abdullah & Islam, 2011) and writes them down on the paper provided. The ideas are to be written in short phases or statements.

Step 3: *Round Robin recording of ideas:* At the end of step 2, each group member is asked to tell their ideas in a round robin fashion. Facilitator starts from one end and asks each participant to tell one best idea out of all the ideas written down by her/him. These ideas are written down verbatim on a flip chart that is visible to all. Then the facilitator starts the second round of writing one idea from each participant. This goes on till all the ideas have been recorded on the flip chart in a serial order.

Step 4: *Discussing ideas*: Each recorded idea is discussed for clarification. This helps to offer the idea generator's logic behind an idea. Facilitator makes sure that there is no ambiguity on any idea in the minds of the participants.

Step 5: *Voting to prioritize the ideas*: In the next step, participants individually vote privately to prioritize the ideas based on their perception of top five ideas. Each of the top five ideas are written on five voting cards. The most significant idea is to be assigned a rating of five and the least among these five ideas will be rated one After all the participants finish the task of rating, the voting cards are collected and votes are written against the ideas on the flip chart or board. A sample is shown in Table 1. When all the votes are collated, the top five ideas can be easily listed based on these votes.

Step 6: *Final list of ideas:* based on the prioritized ideas a final list is generated, discussed and approved by the participants.

Table 1: Sample Voting Table

Serial No. of the idea	Idea	Vote	Total
1	Idea 1	4,5.2	11
2	Idea 2	1,2,4	7
3	Idea 3	3	3
4	Idea 4	3,4,1	8
5	Idea 5	5,5,4	14
6	Idea 6	4	4
45	Idea 45	4,5,5,2,5	21

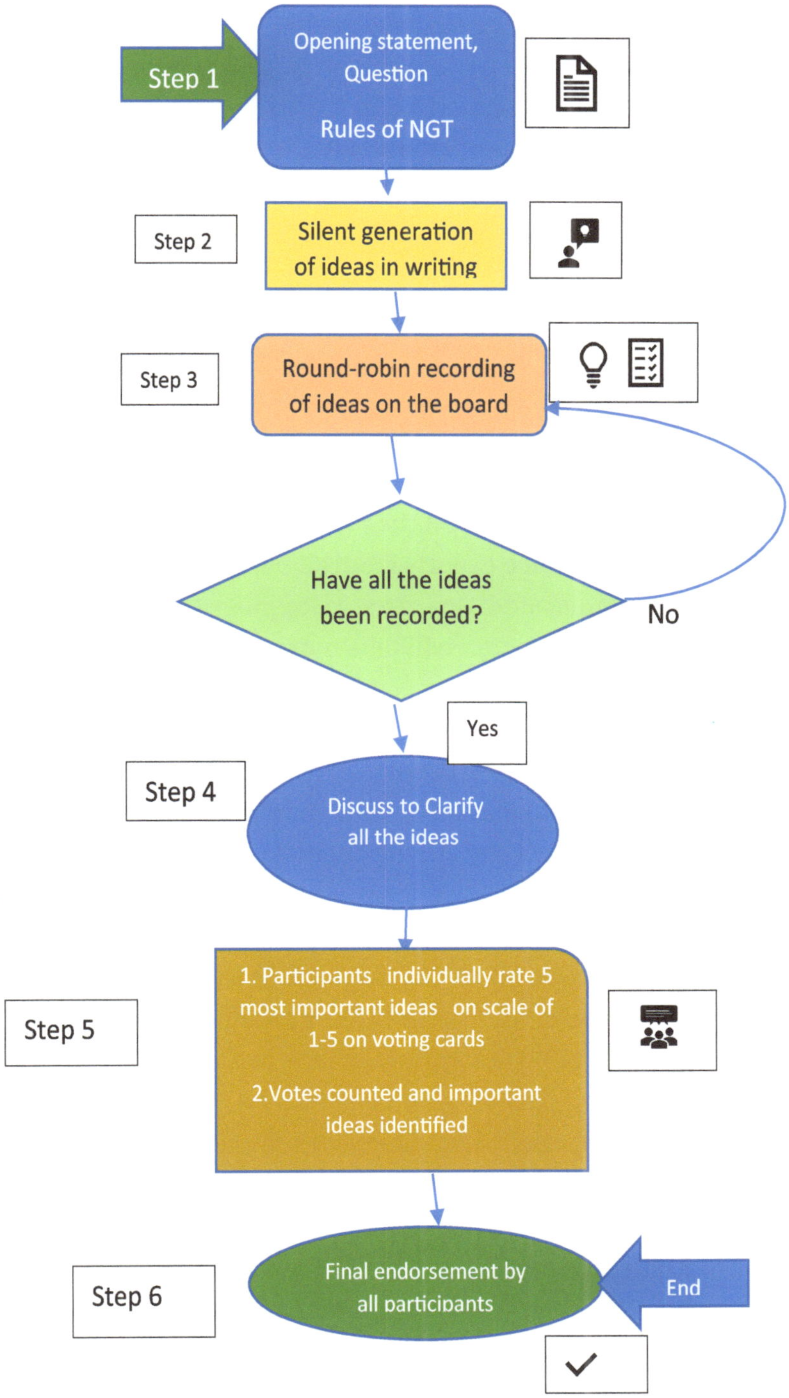

Figure 2: NGT process

Practical Tips to Gain Optimum Output from Both Methods

1. **Careful planning and efficient organization:** Whether it is Delphi or NGT, planning the time lines in advance and managing them is crucial. Right from planning to termination, all the steps are time consuming. In addition, experts should be given adequate time to respond.

2. **Selection of experts**: Experts need to be knowledgeable about the topic under consideration and hence the sample selected is purposive or convenient. Academic profile of the individual (including publications in the concerned topic), expertise in the professional field, membership of relevant organizations/institutions, interest in participation in the study can serve as the criteria. Sometimes in addition to "experts", stakeholders who are associated with the topic are also included. Heterogenous group, wherein the expert differ with respect to sector (academics, public, industry), demographics, geographical areas, is recommended as the opinions of this group will be more varied and therefore wider perspectives on the chosen topic gets covered (Spickermann et al., 2014) and they can visualize an issue from different angles (Abdullah & Islam, 2011). This increases accuracy of predictions and decisions (Devaney & Henchion, 2018; Hasson et al., 2000).
3. **Number of experts:** Usually 5–20 experts are considered for Delphi (Rowe & Wright, 2001) and seven to ten for NGT (Horton, 1980); however the literature shows that the number for the Delphi method varies from > 10 to > 1000. It also depends on the topic e.g., if one wants to decide about technology foresight, it may be required to include experts from all over the nation and in that case the number of experts may run into few thousands. One must remember that more the experts, more will be opinions and summary report preparation will take more time unless automated methods are used. Experts' task demands also increase in the subsequent rounds as they have to go through larger number of responses.
4. ***Confidentiality of data*** should be protected (Toma & Picioreanu, 2016; Trevelyan & Robinson, 2015). Responses in Delphi and ideas in NGT should be kept anonymous. Responses or ideas are important, not the generator of the same. Hence keep all responses/ideas including the voting nameless.
5. **Specific for Delphi**
   - ***Delphi questionnaire*** plays a crucial role in achieving response rate. The structure of questionnaire depends on the number and type of questions, which in turn depend on the research problem. If it is too focused then 10-15 questions are enough but for problems with wider scope and limited prior research, the number of topics and questions can increase (Belton et al., 2019; Toma & Picioreanu, 2016). However, general rule is not to have too lengthy questionnaire. Ideally, it should be answered in 30 min. These questions should be clear, unambiguous, in neutral language and arranged in logical sequence. For pilot round the questions are open ended but for subsequent rounds they are more structured and have responses either quantitative or qualitative. Quantitative responses can be rank- ordered (Likert scale), categorical or numerical; generally Likert scale with either 5, 7, or 9 responses is preferred, with 7 responses is favoured. The responses should bear descriptive anchors than having mere numbers, which will provide clarity and reduce incorrect responding. In addition, some space should be provided for experts to write their rationale for the opted responses or additional comments/questions (McMillan et al., 2016).
   - ***Questionnaire administration:*** Earlier the questionnaire was sent by post to the experts (the classic paper and pencil administration), but now-a-days the questionnaire is administrated using internet (email or online platforms) (McMillan et al., 2016).
   - ***Questionnaire analysis:*** While providing summary report, rationale for selection of a response is provided. Care should be taken to remove any indicator towards the majority opinion so that the experts will think only of rationale while reconsidering their choice and will be refrained from making a decision based on the majority opinion.

The important elements of analysis are 1. Stability of response and 2. Consensus measurement. The criteria for the same must be decided in the protocol prior to the start of the study (Chalmers & Armour, 2019). Stable response is defined as "the consistency of responses between successive rounds of a study" (Dajani et al., 1979), which can be considered as 15% change or lower in any two rounds. Standards for consensus however, are not rigorously established (Heiko, 2012). Researchers have used subjective criteria and descriptive statistics. Depending on the variable used, measures of central tendency (mode, median, and mean) and dispersion (interquartile range, coefficient of variance) are selected as a measure of consensus. Inferential statistics is used to quantify its degree (measure of association). Another consensus measure reported in the literature is the "Average Percent of Majority Opinions" (APMO) Cut off Rate. The consensus concept and strengths and weaknesses of different types of its measures has been described in the literature by Heiko Von der Gracht A (2012). Qualitative data analysis is presented using Ishikawa diagram (Fishbone diagram), mind mapping or other comparable tools (Steinert, 2009). Please note that both consensus and dissent-oriented analyses should be done to understand the generated data and draw meaningful conclusions. Such analysis can provide valuable trends.

- ***Dealing with participant attrition:*** Some dropout is expected as the rounds proceed. Hence the researcher should consider this possibility while deciding the number of experts in the panel (Hsu & Sandford, 2007). If there is a too low response rate as the rounds proceed, then this attrition leads to overestimation of the degree of consensus in the final results (Sinha et al., 2011). It may make a heterogenous group into homogenous one. At the final round each stakeholder group will not be adequately represented introducing response bias. 70% - 80% response rate is necessary at each round to maintain credibility of Delphi (Chalmers & Armour, 2019; Hasson et al., 2000; Mullen, 2003; Williamson et al., 2017). Hence the researchers need to keep the participants engaged throughout by using motivational techniques. These may include use of incentives (financial or social), direct personal communication (phone calls, text messages, e-mails) during rounds and by ensuring in the beginning that the experts understand purpose and relevance of Delphi using a questionnaire. However, these techniques have a flip side too. Incentives may be not be considered as ethical means. Maintaining person touch increases work burden of the researchers and question of undermining anonymity (which is a key element of Delphi) creeps in. It may happen that though experts understand the purpose and relevance in the beginning, during the rounds, they may face some uncertainties in the feedback and stop seeing the relevance. People with minority opinions are more likely to drop out, so attrition as rounds progress can lead to overestimation of the degree of consensus in the final results (Belton et al., 2019; Hsu & Sandford, 2007).

6. **Specific for NGT**
    - ***Infrastructure:*** A room with preferably a U-shaped table with a marker board or a flip chart at the open end of the U table. Marker pens, paper and pens for each participant, index cards for voting (five cards per participant).
    - ***A trained and experienced facilitator*** who will clarify the participant's role and importance of their contribution, along with the objectives of the session. The facilitator has to maintain the time, record the ideas verbatim, direct the discussion for clarification of the ideas and record the votes to generate the final prioritized list of ideas or solutions. The facilitator should be neutral and ensure that each participant's ideas are recorded without any bias.

- ***Do not criticize any idea:*** The main objective of NGT is to obtain a large number of ideas. As the ideas are being presented by each participant in step 3, a few may sound out of context or ridiculous. No one should object to, or laugh at it, this will prevent free flow of ideas from rest of the participants. This out of the box idea may lead to contribution of better ideas.
- ***No idea is bad unless it is voted out:*** Participants should not evaluate others' ideas. One can express their preference during voting. If an idea is not good, it is likely to get no/least votes and will be automatically voted out.
- ***Generate as many ideas as possible*** in step 1. As stated by Abdulla & Islam (2011) "*The larger the number of ideas produced, the greater is the probability of achieving an effective solution for an issue*".
- ***"hitchhiking" of ideas*** should be considered if two ideas can be combined or modified to generate a new, better idea (Dunham, 1998).

Advantages and Limitations Of Consensus Methods

It is well reported by Norman P. Uhl (1983) that:

> "*Decision making is often difficult and frustrating in the academic world. This is particularly true if a decision requires the approval and cooperation of a collective group such as the faculty, department heads, deans, and so forth...Unfortunately, agreement usually is hindered by great divergences of opinion, strong allegiances, and the varying vested interests that frequently characterize these groups.*" *(Uhl, 1983)*

This problem is overcome to the most extent by consensus methods as discussed above. They make use of 'collective knowledge' of professionals, which is considered as tacit knowledge. They have advantages over both, focus group and survey. The researchers require short period of training, though with experience the quality of process improves. These methods are participant- controlled methods and success depends on the quality of participants. However, a dominant participant cannot influence the result as anonymity of decisions is maintained. The results are available relatively soon but are not biased by "quick" decisions. Relatively less organizing ability is required than for a survey. A single series of consensus groups may achieve the same what a several pilots of survey achieve for sharpening the questions to be included in exploratory surveys that cover topics new to the researcher (List, 2001) Relatively low cost is required for using the technique and analyzing the results.

However, it may happen that the participants vote for what is perceived as majority. They may get a pressurized feeling to agree. It may also happen when they are not very knowledgeable about the topic or do not feel strongly about it to put forth their opinion. It may be an influence of culture wherein social cohesion is regarded highly than individual opinion e.g., some Asian countries. Nevertheless, there are ways to alleviate these problems (List, 2001).

These methods are also criticized for lacunae in the scientific rigor in conducting and reporting. The weaknesses in methodology can be attributed to questionnaire framing; the selection criteria used for participants; a priori definitions of number of rounds, level of anonymity, participant attrition and consensus and the feedback given after the round (Boulkedid et al., 2011; Foth et al., 2016; Sinha et al., 2011). Moreover, there are lot of variations introduced in the methodology by individual researchers so there is a poor standardization (Foth et al., 2016; Niederberger & Spranger, 2020). Practical guidance for using and reporting Delphi procedures has been provided in a systematic review by Boulkedid, et al, 2011.

For the advantages and limitations of individual methods please refer to (Foth et al., 2016; Green, 2014; Humphrey-Murto, Varpio, Gonsalves, et al., 2017; Humphrey-Murto, et al., 2017; Murphy et al., 1998).

Choice between Delphi and NGT

Though the intent and goals are similar, each approach has its supporters and critics. The choice between these two techniques depends on various factors viz. the research question, the perception of consensus required, the associated feasibility and availability of time (McMillan et al., 2016) as listed in Table -2.

Table 2: Factors governing choice between Delphi and NGT (Gallagher et al., 1993; Heiko, 2012; McMillan et al., 2016)

Factors	Delphi	NGT
Purpose	Conducted for addressing high-stakes or significant issues which require a thorough examination of options, time to research and respond and leveraging of expertise e.g. developing guidelines or policies, wherein wider and more reflective responses are needed from larger number of experts.	Conducted for small- to-medium sized decisions which require some group discussion e.g. problem identification, solution generation, exploring views of consumers and stakeholders. As idea generation is integral to NGT, for exploring ideas in relation to a problem or question and arrive at less consequential decisions. It also provides support to allow identification of personal problems and self-disclosure.
Problem	Can be done with wide range of problems, e.g. government planning, institutional, business and industry predictions, volunteer group decisions.	Needs a small group and better for more narrow problems e.g. curriculum implementation strategies of the institution.
Investigator's training and responsibility	Can be undertaken with short training but responsibilities are far greater- more procedural work involved in gathering, evaluating, and repeating the rounds.	Need a trained, experienced investigator to carry out technique in disciplined manner, to allow representation of all ideas and to reach a decision accepted by all the participants but responsibilities are less demanding.
Participant experts	When opinion of multiple stakeholders who are geographically dispersed is required.	When limited experts are required.
Flexibility	More flexible as based on responses to questionnaires, which are accessible to participants regardless of geographical location, time etc.	Less flexible and needs face-to-face meeting, which limits participant numbers and sites as it is difficult to find suitable time to all if widely dispersed.
Logistics	No requirements for travel/space, meeting scheduling.	Need to schedule meetings, arrange for travel of participants, space and infrastructure for meeting.
Ease of ad-ministration	Yes	No

Factors	Delphi	NGT
Time taken for results	It involves multiple rounds weeks apart (based on predefined criteria) so weeks or months to get results.	Single session so prompt results, which can then be refined through additional meetings as necessary.
Participant anonymity	Required.	Not required.
Motivation of experts	Experts need to be highly motivated throughout and so the investigator has to engage them.	Medium motivation of experts is alright to complete the process.
Perception of consensus	Analysis of data is more complex. Analysis of both, stability and level of agreement as descriptive and inferential statistics. Measurement of dissent should also be presented such as scatter plots, Subgroup analyses, or impact analyses, which provides understanding of data in toto.	Analysis of data is relatively easy. Mainly the descriptive statistics is used. But it can be analyzed quantitatively by ranking the ideas.

SUMMARIZE

- Commonly employed consensus group methods such as Delphi and NGT are a systematic means to measure and develop consensus on a topic.
- These methods are suitable when empirical evidence is insufficient, inconsistent or not present.
- Consensus methods are especially useful in medical education research where there are still many areas of studies where there is not much authentic literature to make evidence-based decisions.
- The Delphi method involves six stages, participants never meet or interact directly. It is possible to include a large number of experts who are spread around the world. Takes time to arrive at consensus, depending on the number of rounds conducted.
- NGT is a face-to-face interactive method, number of participants are limited to 5-12. It involves minimal discussion among the participants. Advantage of NGT lies in possibility of clarification and debate if consensus is not arrived at initially. Disadvantage being the consensus is obtained from only a small number of participants.

EVALUATE

We hope you have understood the similarities and differences in both the methods. Take a minute on the key learning from this chapter. Now try to apply it for the following scenario.

Scenario 2: You wish to develop competencies for a course in Medical Education Research and Publication along with entrustable professional activities (EPAs) so as to ensure that the stated competencies are achieved by the participants of the course. Select appropriate method/s for deciding the competencies and the EPAs so that the various stakeholders can agree upon them. It is expected that the formulated competencies are rationally based, feasible, measurable and observable. Sequence the EPAs in terms of increasing difficulty or sophistication. Justify your selection of method/s and outline the process which you wish to follow.

ROAD AHEAD

Apart from Delphi and NGT, a third method, RAND appropriateness method has been developed by the RAND Corporation and the David Geffen School of Medicine at UCLA, which is a hybrid of the Delphi and NGT methods (Fitch et al., 2001). In this method the experts meet between the rounds face-to-face. Interested readers can read an article by Davies et al (2011)., This negates the principle of anonymity, but the personal interaction has shown to exert positive influence in some studies (Boulkedid et al., 2011). It is preferable that such face-to-face meeting is held at the end of last round to clear misinterpretations if any or when consensus has not been achieved (Belton et al., 2019).

Another variation is dissent-oriented Delphi studies. They are conducted for exploring systematically viewpoints of heterogenous groups regarding various aspects of a specific policy. It is termed as Policy Delphi (De Loë et al., 2016; Steinert, 2009). Such Delphi can be incorporated in scenario planning involving multiple stakeholders to surface "structured conflict" and to judge the future scope using this multi-modality approach (Nowack et al., 2011; Schmalz et al., 2021).

Recently, online survey systems (e.g. SurveyMonkey, Qualtrics) or online web-based tools, which are either custom-made or those available commercially like RAHS, e-Delfi, GFIS, Surveylet are used. Automatic updates are possible as soon as an entry is made by the expert and immediate feedback is provided with respect to the median and justification, which allows more flexibility and multiple chances to the experts to modify the response. This real-time update limits the Delphi to only single round ("roundless" Delphi) (Aengenheyster et al., 2017; Belton et al., 2019; Geist, 2010; Gordon & Pease, 2006).

Thus, one may come across lot of variations in implementation of the Delphi or NGT or in reporting them (Belton et al., 2019; Humphrey-Murto & de Wit, 2019; Rowe & Wright, 2011). It is essential for any researcher to carefully examine these varied designs and confirm that the basic principles of Delphi or NGT are not over-ruled while modifying them. Whenever such modifications are done, the details of the modification should be detailed in the publication.

REFERENCES

Abdullah, M. M. B., & Islam, R. (2011). Nominal group technique and its applications in managing quality in higher education. Pakistan Journal of Commerce and Social Sciences (PJCSS), 5(1), 81–99.

Aengenheyster, S., Cuhls, K., Gerhold, L., Heiskanen-Schüttler, M., Huck, J., & Muszynska, M. (2017). Real-Time Delphi in practice—A comparative analysis of existing software-based tools. Technological Forecasting and Social Change, 118, 15–27.

Belton, I., MacDonald, A., Wright, G., & Hamlin, I. (2019). Improving the practical application of the Delphi method in group-based judgment: A six-step prescription for a well-founded and defensible process. Technological Forecasting and Social Change, 147, 72–82.

Boddy, C. (2012). The nominal group technique: An aid to brainstorming ideas in research. Qualitative Market Research: An International Journal.

Boulkedid, R., Abdoul, H., Loustau, M., Sibony, O., & Alberti, C. (2011). Using and reporting the Delphi method for selecting healthcare quality indicators: A systematic review. PloS One, 6(6), e20476. https://doi.org/10.1371/journal.pone.0020476

Chalmers, J., & Armour, M. (2019). The delphi technique.

Dajani, J. S., Sincoff, M. Z., & Talley, W. K. (1979). Stability and agreement criteria for the termination of Delphi studies. Technological Forecasting and Social Change, 13(1), 83–90.

Davies, S., Romano, P. S., Schmidt, E. M., Schultz, E., Geppert, J. J., & McDonald, K. M. (2011). Assessment of a novel hybrid Delphi and nominal groups technique to evaluate quality indicators. Health Services Research, 46(6pt1), 2005–2018.

De Loë, R. C., Melnychuk, N., Murray, D., & Plummer, R. (2016). Advancing the state of policy Delphi practice: A systematic review evaluating methodological evolution, innovation, and opportunities. Technological Forecasting and Social Change, 104, 78–88.

Delbecq, A. L., & Van de Ven, A. H. (1971). A group process model for problem identification and program planning. The Journal of Applied Behavioral Science, 7(4), 466–492.

Delbecq, A. L., Van de Ven, A. H., & Gustafson, D. H. (1975). Group techniques for program planning: A guide to nominal group and Delphi processes. Scott, Foresman,.

Devaney, L., & Henchion, M. (2018). Who is a Delphi 'expert'? Reflections on a bioeconomy expert selection procedure from Ireland. Futures, 99, 45–55.

Dunham, R. B. (1998). Nominal group technique: A users' guide. Madison: Wisconsin School of Business, 2.

Fitch, K., Bernstein, S. J., Aguilar, M. D., Burnand, B., & LaCalle, J. R. (2001). The RAND/UCLA appropriateness method user's manual. Rand Corp Santa Monica CA.

Foth, T., Efstathiou, N., Vanderspank-Wright, B., Ufholz, L.-A., Dütthorn, N., Zimansky, M., & Humphrey-Murto, S. (2016). The use of Delphi and Nominal Group Technique in nursing education: A review. International Journal of Nursing Studies, 60, 112–120.

Gaba, D. M. (2007). The future vision of simulation in healthcare. Simulation in Healthcare: Journal of the Society for Simulation in Healthcare, 2(2), 126–135. https://doi.org/10.1097/01.SIH.0000258411.38212.32

Gallagher, M., Hares, T. I. M., Spencer, J., Bradshaw, C., & Webb, I. A. N. (1993). The nominal group technique: A research tool for general practice? Family Practice, 10(1), 76–81.

Gary, J. E., & Heiko, A. (2015). The future of foresight professionals: Results from a global Delphi study. Futures, 71, 132–145.

Geist, M. R. (2010). Using the Delphi method to engage stakeholders: A comparison of two studies. Evaluation and Program Planning, 33(2), 147–154.

Gordon, T., & Pease, A. (2006). RT Delphi: An efficient, "round-less" almost real time Delphi method. Technological Forecasting and Social Change, 73(4), 321–333.

Green, R. A. (2014). The Delphi technique in educational research. Sage Open, 4(2), 2158244014529773.

Hasson, F., Keeney, S., & McKenna, H. (2000). Research guidelines for the Delphi survey technique. Journal of Advanced Nursing, 32(4), 1008–1015.

Hegedus, D. M., & Rasmussen, R. V. (1986). Task effectiveness and interaction process of a modified nominal group technique in solving an evaluation problem. Journal of Management, 12(4), 545–560.

Heiko, A. (2012). Consensus measurement in Delphi studies: Review and implications for future quality assurance. Technological Forecasting and Social Change, 79(8), 1525–1536.

Horton, J. N. (1980). Nominal group technique: A method of decision-making by committee. Anaesthesia, 35(8), 811–814.

Hsu, C.-C., & Sandford, B. A. (2007). The Delphi technique: Making sense of consensus. Practical Assessment, Research, and Evaluation, 12(1), 10.

Humphrey-Murto, S., & de Wit, M. (2019). The Delphi method—More research please. Journal of Clinical Epidemiology, 106, 136–139.

Humphrey-Murto, S., Varpio, L., Gonsalves, C., & Wood, T. J. (2017). Using consensus group methods such as Delphi and Nominal Group in medical education research. Medical Teacher, 39(1), 14–19.

Humphrey-Murto, S., Varpio, L., Wood, T. J., Gonsalves, C., Ufholz, L.-A., Mascioli, K., Wang, C., & Foth, T. (2017). The Use of the Delphi and Other Consensus Group Methods in Medical Education Research: A Review. Academic Medicine: Journal of the Association of American Medical Colleges, 92(10), 1491–1498. https://doi.org/10.1097/ACM.0000000000001812

Landeta, J., & Barrutia, J. (2011). People consultation to construct the future: A Delphi application. International Journal of Forecasting, 27(1), 134–151.

List, D. (2001). The consensus group technique in social research. Field Methods, 13(3), 277–290.

McMillan, S. S., King, M., & Tully, M. P. (2016). How to use the nominal group and Delphi techniques. International Journal of Clinical Pharmacy, 38(3), 655–662. https://doi.org/10.1007/s11096-016-0257-x

Mullen, P. M. (2003). Delphi: Myths and reality. Journal of Health Organization and Management.

Murphy, M. K., Black, N. A., Lamping, D. L., McKee, C. M., Sanderson, C. F., Askham, J., & Marteau, T. (1998). Consensus development methods, and their use in clinical guideline development. Health Technology Assessment (Winchester, England), 2(3), i–88.

Niederberger, M., & Spranger, J. (2020). Delphi Technique in Health Sciences: A Map. Frontiers in Public Health, 8, 457.

Nowack, M., Endrikat, J., & Guenther, E. (2011). Review of Delphi-based scenario studies: Quality and design considerations. Technological Forecasting and Social Change, 78(9), 1603–1615.

Rowe, G., & Wright, G. (2001). Expert opinions in forecasting: The role of the Delphi technique. In Principles of forecasting (pp. 125–144). Springer.

Rowe, G., & Wright, G. (2011). The Delphi technique: Past, present, and future prospects—Introduction to the special issue. Technological Forecasting and Social Change, 78(9), 1487–1490.

Schmalz, U., Spinler, S., & Ringbeck, J. (2021). Lessons Learned from a Two-Round Delphi-based Scenario Study. MethodsX, 8, 101179.

Sinha, I. P., Smyth, R. L., & Williamson, P. R. (2011). Using the Delphi technique to determine which outcomes to measure in clinical trials: Recommendations for the future based on a systematic review of existing studies. PLoS Medicine, 8(1), e1000393.

Spickermann, A., Zimmermann, M., & Heiko, A. (2014). Surface-and deep-level diversity in panel selection—Exploring diversity effects on response behaviour in foresight. Technological Forecasting and Social Change, 85, 105–120.

Steinert, M. (2009). A dissensus based online Delphi approach: An explorative research tool. Technological Forecasting and Social Change, 76(3), 291–300.

Toma, C., & Picioreanu, I. (2016). The Delphi technique: Methodological considerations and the need for reporting guidelines in medical journals. Int J Public Health Res.[Internet], 4(6), 47–59.

Trevelyan, E. G., & Robinson, N. (2015). Delphi methodology in health research: How to do it? European Journal of Integrative Medicine, 7(4), 423–428.

Uhl, N. P. (1983). Using the Delphi technique in institutional planning. New Directions for Institutional Research, 1983(37), 81–94.

Vella, K., Goldfrad, C., Rowan, K., Bion, J., & Black, N. (2000). Use of consensus development to establish national research priorities in critical care. Bmj, 320(7240), 976–980.

Williamson, P. R., Altman, D. G., Bagley, H., Barnes, K. L., Blazeby, J. M., Brookes, S. T., Clarke, M., Gargon, E., Gorst, S., & Harman, N. (2017). The COMET handbook: Version 1.0. Trials, 18(3), 1–50.

Chapter 12

Observation Schedules, Checklists and Rating Scales

Shital Bhandary

ABSTRACT

Observation schedule is a particularly useful tool to observe and assess performance of students as well as teachers in medical education. This tool can be created or compiled for a specific trait/construct like history taking, physical examination, communication, procedures, preparation, participation, teaching, skills etc. using structured items and pre-define scoring rule. Observation schedule is used as a checklist or rating scale widely in medical education. You must gather evidence of validity and reliability before using observation schedule in the high-stake setting. The content validity of the observation schedule must be established using iterative discussions and/or through consensus indices from the content experts. Pre-test is used to gather evidence of face validity using debriefing with the volunteers and observers whereas pilot-test is used to gather the evidence of internal consistency reliability using alpha coefficient and, inter-rater and test re-test reliabilities using linear/non-linear correlation coefficients. The "what if" analysis of alpha coefficient should be used to establish tentative construct validity of the tool, but factor analysis must be done to confirm it. G theory-based decision studies can also be done with well-planned pilot studies to find number of items, observers, stations/sessions/encounters required to achieve minimum level of generalizability. Quality assurance of the observation schedule tool in terms of difficulty level, discrimination level, fairness etc. is done using classical item analysis and item response theory methods. The mean/standard deviation or median/inter-quartile range is used to summarize the bell shaped and skewed item/total scores respectively. Similarly, parametric tests (T-Test/ANOVA, etc.) are used to compare scores following normal distribution whereas non-parametric tests (Mann-Whitney/Kruskal-Wallis/Median test etc.) are used to compare skewed scores.

Key Words: observation schedule, checklist, rating scale, validity, reliability, construction, analysis

ASSESS NEED

Observation schedule is made up of observation and schedule. Observation is the process in which individuals observe the events in a pre-defined situation and record them according to a prior plan. So, you need to plan, execute, record and interpret the scores with justification for various levels of observations (Patton 1990). Schedule, on the other hand, is a tool consisting of a set of questions (items) asked and/or filled by one or more individuals. So, observation schedule is a bit different from a questionnaire as it contains a focused list of structured items to collect information of an underlying trait using a specified scoring rule in a short form (1-page).

A checklist is a simple tool consisting of parallel lists of items which are constructed or compiled by an individual or group of individuals relevant to the construct or trait under consideration. Here each item is measured on a binary scale (e.g. yes/no, done/not-done, etc.) which draws attention of the observer to the items and enables him/her to record the data quickly and systematically. Thus, checklist responses are a record of the observed "facts" rather than the "judgements". Checklist can be of four forms but observation schedule checklist uses the form where all the items are given in a list and the observer is asked to check in all the items found in a situation with done/not done, yes/no, etc. (Kempfer 1960).

Rating, on the other hand, is used to express judgement regarding the situations, objects and persons and the judgements are usually expressed on a scale. It can be observed and recorded using numerical, graphic, standard, forced choice and cumulative points scales (Guilford 1954). Numerical rating scale e.g. "1-Unacceptable, 2-Needs improvement, 3-Good, 4-Very good, 5-Excellent" is commonly used to score the attributes related to a trait/construct during observation in medical education. This means rating scale provides the opportunity to the observers to use his/her own judgment on the items included in the observation schedule like Objective Structured Clinical/Practical Examination (OSCE/OSPE). However, you need to train the observers if you need objective, valid and reliable scores from an observation schedule based on numerical rating scales e.g. Mini Clinical Evaluation Exercise (Mini-CEX) and Direct Observation of Procedural Skills (DOPS) (Norcini et. al. 2003, Norcini and Burch 2007). Thus, it is necessary to decide *a priori* about the scoring methods for the observation schedule to use it as a checklist or rating scale in medical education.

Once you compile the items and decided on the scoring method for the observation schedule then it requires evidence of validity e.g. face validity from pre-tests, content validity with expert consensus and construct validity with factor analysis (Ruel et. al. 2015). It also requires evidence of internal consistency, inter-observer and test re-test reliabilities. G theory can be used to determine the number of items, observers, encounters to achieve minimum level of generalizability (Webb and Shavelson 2005). You can use appropriate descriptive statistics to summarize and suitable inferential statistical methods to compare item/scale score with sex, age, observers etc. in medical education (Yudkowsky, Park and Downing 2019).

BRIEF

- Observation schedules are useful to observe the performance of students as well as teachers using checklists or rating scales in medical education
- Observation schedule contains focused and structured items that are used to observe certain trait/construct under consideration using certain scoring rules

- You must gather evidence of reliability and validity for a new observation schedule developed in the local setting and the observation schedules developed in the other settings before using the local setting
- Classical test/item analysis is used to assess the quality of the observation schedule scores and descriptive statistics helps to summarize them
- Item response theory is used to evaluate the fairness of the observed item/scale score with age, sex and other important background variables
- Inferential statistics helps to compare item/scale scores with important predictors

CONTEXTUALIZE

Scenario 1

You are the coordinator of the Medical Education Unit/Committee. You decided to evaluate the didactic sessions (lectures) of the faculty using an observation schedule to provide feedback and improve the didactic teaching learning sessions. You decided to compile a new observation tool and validate it *a priori*, evaluated by at least two faculty in each session. The committee members compiled various observation schedules currently in use for this purpose. You now need to gather evidence of validity and reliability of this tool so that it can be used effectively in your college.

Scenario 2

You are the problem based learning (PBL) coordinator of your college and plan to introduce a process assessment tool to assess the soft skills (e.g. preparation, presentation, participation, self-directed learning, leadership, communication and sensitivity) of the students in the PBL tutorial sessions. You have decided to compile a new tool from a literature review, validate it and use for formative as well as summative assessment of affective domain in your college. You also planned to develop, validate and use student assessment of tutors to assess facilitation skills of the PBL tutors and use it for formative purpose.

Scenario 3

You are the clinical year coordinator of a medical college implementing a new competency based medical curriculum. You need to use OSPE/OSCE with observation schedules to assess non-certifiable competencies and Mini-CEX/DOPS to certify competencies. You have decided to conduct a half-day/full day workshop to write OSPE/OSCE stations with at least two faculty members from each department to establish face and content validity of these stations. You also decided to convene a separate workshop to write rubrics (benchmarks) for the pre-validated Mini-CEX/DOPS rating scales to use them effectively in your college as you found problems using these tools without the benchmarking.

DESCRIBE

Purpose

You can use an observation schedule as checklists or rating scales to assess online and offline classroom teaching skills of faculty for formative as well as summative purpose. Similarly, you can use them to assess the performance (psychomotor domain) of the students for formative as well as summative purpose. You can also use observation schedules to assess the performance (affective domain) of the students in the small group tutorials, clinical clerkships, community postings etc. and use them for formative as well as summative purpose in medical education.

Advantages and disadvantages

Observation schedule is a very useful tool based on focused and structured list of items related to a particular construct. This tool with binary scale scoring (checklist) is used widely to conduct formative and summative assessment in undergraduate levels due to its scoring simplicity whereas observation schedule with rating scale is common in the formative and summative assessment of post-graduate levels due to its scoring complexity.

Observation schedule requires at least one trained observer for each encounter, and this presents a logistic problem in many situations. Further, it cannot be used for the constructs that do not require observation such as interpretation skills. Observation schedule with binary scale scoring (checklist) is prone to measurement errors as the candidates can fake it/guess the items included in the tool whereas observation schedule with numerical rating scale scoring without rubrics can produce a biased score if the observers are not experienced and/or trained personnel.

When to use?

You must use observation schedules as checklist or rating scale when you need to get objective, defendable and generalizable score of a particular construct/trait though a structured item and scoring system. This can be a high-stake situation like selection of students using Admission OSCEs or low stake situation like providing feedback to students after a PBL tutorial session and to the faculty after a large group session. You can also use this tool for getting objective, valid and reliable scores of applicants/students on the history taking, physical examination, communication, counselling, procedural skills etc. that require direct observation. This can be a single or multiple *in-vitro* OSCE stations and Mini-CEX or DOPS tools with single or multiple *in-vivo* encounters.

Construction

You can construct the observation schedule from scratch using focus group discussions with experts or compile it using various published and unpublished sources. You can ask a single or multiple person to compile/construct it but validity requires process documentation of discussions and content validity indices. So, you will face difficulty to establish face and content validity of the tool constructed by a single person. Iterative discussions among the content experts must be done to ensure content validity.

Once the observation schedule is tentatively agreed by the content experts then you must do a pre-test with 5-10 volunteers involving other experts as the observers (Bisits 2014). This must be followed by debriefing with the volunteers and experts involved in the pre-test to establish the face validity(difficulty, confusion and sensitivity of the items) of the tool. This process must be properly documented and analyzed using qualitative data analysis methods like content/thematic analysis. Pre-test results must be discussed among the same group of content experts and modified for the pilot test in consensus. And, once the revised tool is available for the pilot study then it must be pilot tested with a large number of candidates to compute the internal consistency reliability, inter-observer reliability, test re-test reliability to gather evidence of the tool reliability and generalizability coefficient to gather evidence for its generalizability (Tavakol and Dennick 2012).

Administration

Administration of observation schedule is different for pre-test, pilot-test and final administration. Observation schedule can be delegated to individual level for the diagnostic assessment, as validation of the tool is optional whereas observation schedule should be delegated to a group/concerned department for formative assessment, as tool validation is desirable here. The observation schedule must be done at the central/experts level for summative assessment as pre-validated tools must be used for this type of assessment in medical education. Thus, you must promote the micro-teaching session in the faculty development workshops and follow it up systematically if you are plan to evaluate teaching skills of the faculty using observation schedule (Ramesh 2013). You must use a valid process assessment tool like Tutor Assessment of Student (TAS-tool) to longitudinally monitor and evaluate the affective domain of students in small group tutorials (Upadhyay et al 2017). You can also utilize Self-Assessment of Student (SAS-tool) and Peer Assessment of Student (PAS-tool) to validate (triangulate) the TAS-tool scores obtained from the same sessions as shown in Figure 1.

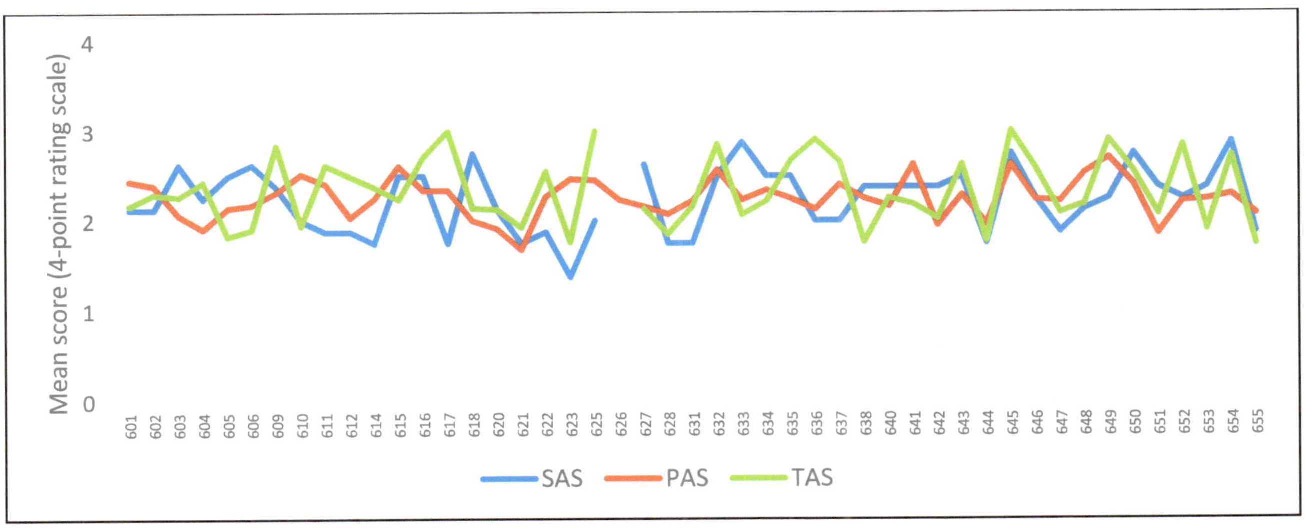

Figure 1: Mean SAS, PAS and TAS Scores, Integrated GI Block, Basic Sciences, MBBS Program, Nepal

Analysis

An observation schedule as a checklist/rating scale is analyzed using individual item or the scale scores as unit of analysis. Firstly, the internal consistency reliability (alpha coefficient) of the observation schedule must be obtained as shown in Figure 2. It shows the alpha reliability coefficient of 0.7642 for a 12-item observation schedule with 5-point rating scale from a pilot test with 35 students using the R statistical software. As the reported alpha coefficient is greater than 0.70 (Nunally 1978), you can say that the 12 items are internally consistent (hanging together) to measure of the satisfaction construct.

Output

```
Alpha reliability =  0.7642
Standardized alpha =  0.7792

Reliability deleting each item in turn:
      Alpha Std.Alpha r(item, total)
q1  0.7355     0.7488          0.5428
q2  0.7489     0.7631          0.4017
q3  0.7284     0.7452          0.5982
q4  0.7356     0.7509          0.5194
q5  0.7377     0.7529          0.4842
q6  0.7394     0.7539          0.5017
q7  0.7597     0.7695          0.3630
q8  0.7688     0.7858          0.2142
q9  0.7646     0.7820          0.2429
q10 0.7480     0.7663          0.4041
q11 0.7571     0.7718          0.3302
q12 0.7517     0.7699          0.3683
```

Figure 2: Alpha reliability coefficients and what-if analysis of 12-item observation schedule, Nepal

You must extend this result with "what if" alpha reliability analysis where alpha coefficient is assessed by removing one item at a time from the scale as shown in the "Reliability deleting each item in turn" result in the Figure 2 (Gliem and Gliem 2003). If the alpha coefficient decreased after removing certain items from the original alpha value (e.g., q1, q2, q3, q4, q5, q6, q7, q10, q11 and q12in Figure 2), then those items must be retained in the scale. In addition, if alpha coefficient increased after removing a certain item then those items can be removed from the scale (e.g., q6, q7, q8 and q9, q10, q11 and q12 in Figure 2).

This also means that q1, q2, q3, q4, q5, q6, q7, q10, q11 and q12 are related to the construct under consideration whereas q8 and q9 seems to be not related to the construct. However, it requires further "what if" analysis by dropping 'items giving higher alpha reliability after its removal' or the 'items with a low item-total (item-construct) correlation i.e. below 0.3' one-by-one from the scale. This helps establish tentative construct validity of the tool but it must be confirmed using the factor analysis techniques (Pett, Lackey and Sullivan 2003).

```
Alpha reliability =  0.7836
Standardized alpha =  0.7921

Reliability deleting each item in turn:
      Alpha Std.Alpha r(item, total)
q1  0.7529     0.7605          0.5535
q2  0.7725     0.7814          0.3951
q3  0.7488     0.7584          0.5752
q4  0.7492     0.7589          0.5651
q5  0.7648     0.7686          0.4660
q6  0.7546     0.7625          0.5402
q10 0.7630     0.7779          0.4686
q11 0.7813     0.7880          0.3660
q12 0.7784     0.7885          0.3680
```

Figure 3: Final what-if alpha reliability coefficient of the 12-item observation schedule, Nepal

Figure 3 shows that alpha reliability does not improve further after removing q8, q7 and q9 from the scale. Further, item-total correlation is now greater than 0.3 for all the remaining 9-items so you can accept the training satisfaction scale with the highly internally consistent 9 items now. This was a 12-item observation schedule used to measure satisfaction of the 7-day research methodology and data analysis workshop where q7, q8 and q9 were related to logistics. The trainees gave less importance to these three items than others and "what if" alpha analysis traced it well and removed them from the scale.

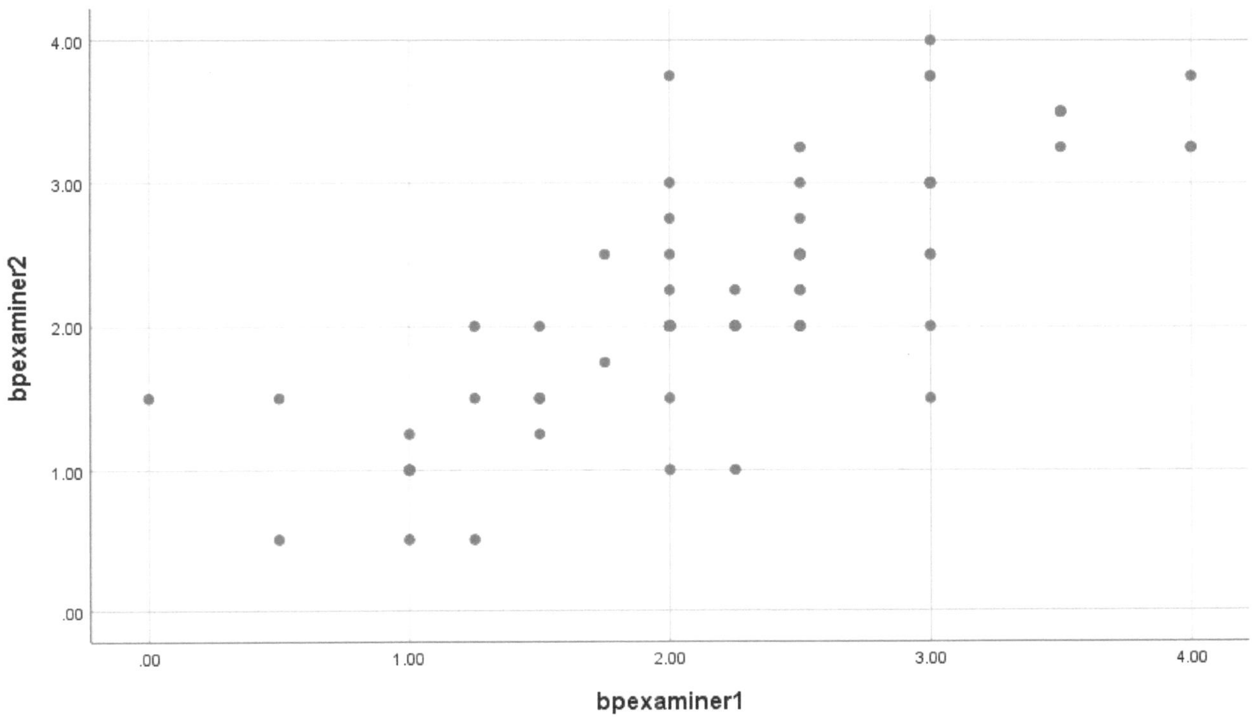

Figure 4: Scatterplot of total score of observer 1 and observer 2 in an OSPE station, Pilot-Test, India (N=81)

Secondly, you must assess the inter-observer reliability of the observation schedules using scale/total score of two raters with correlation coefficient as they provide measurement of relationship for two continuous variables i.e. scale/total score of rater 1 and rater 2. Nonetheless, you must assess the linearity of these scale/total scores using a scatterplot and if they show linear relationship as in Figure 4 then you can use Pearson's correlation coefficient otherwise you must use Spearman's rank correlation coefficient as shown in Table 1 (Mindrila and Belentyne 2013).

Thirdly, you must also gather evidence of test re-test reliability for the observation schedules. So, you must do the test and re-test of the observation schedules within short period of time e.g. after a tea/snack break so that you can control the contamination and fatigue among the students and observers (Table 1).

Table1: Internal consistency, Inter-observer and Test Re-Test reliabilities of OSPE stations, Pilot Test, India

Station	Internal consistency	Inter-observer	Test Re-test	Remarks
Pulse measurement	0.575	0.79[a], p-value<0.001	0.976[a], p-value<0.001	N=81
Blood Pressure measurement	0.717	0.83[a], p-value<0.001	0.856[a], p-value<0.001	N=81
Vital Capacity measurement	0.149	0.29[b], p-value=0.110	0.932[a], p-value<0.001	N=31
Note: a = Pearson's linear correlation coefficient, b = Spearman's non-linear rank correlation coefficient				

Table 1 shows the pilot-test result of a 3 physiology OSPE stations done in India. Blood pressure measurement station shows a good internal consistency, very good inter-observer as well as test re-test reliabilities whereas pulse measurement station shows an acceptable internal consistency due to few items included in the observation checklist, good inter-observer and excellent test re-test reliability. However, vital registration measurement station shows unacceptable internal consistency and inter-rater reliability but it shows an excellent test re-test reliability. So, you can accept pulse and blood pressure measurement stations for the summative assessment in such situation. The findings of Table 1 and Figure 5 must be discussed in a team of experts so that you can also apply the contemporary approaches to validity argument using the Kane's framework (Cook, Brydges, Ginsburg and Hatala 2015).

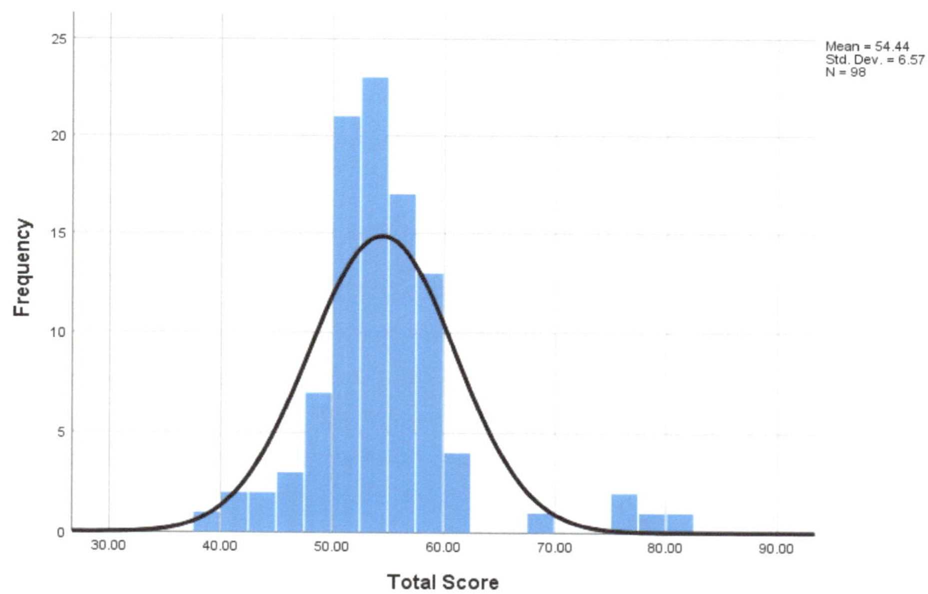

Figure 5: Histogram of total OSCE score, S-PEST module, Nepal (N=98)

Figure 5 shows the distribution of a total score of students from 13 OSCE stations used to assess Structured Physical Examination Skills Training (S-PEST) module piloted for the early clinical exposure course in a private medical college of Nepal (Piryani et al 2013). Distribution of this 13-station OSCE score is tentatively bell-shaped so you can use mean and standard deviation to summarize it and use parametric tests (e.g., T-test, One-way ANOVA etc.) to compare it with gender, age groups etc. for its fairness and/ or discrimination indices.

Once the psychometric evaluation of the observation schedule is complete and the observation schedule is deemed valid and reliable (Tavakol and Dennick 2012) then you can move to the statistical analysis of scale using descriptive and inferential statistics. You can use the mean of the checklist items and weighted mean of the rating scale items to assess the item-wise difficult level and/or consensus indices (Ghimire and Bhandary 2015).

When you find an outlier/extreme item score then it must be assessed by gender, age and other predictor variables as they will provide you evidence of the fairness or discrimination power of the tool. You can use a special item response theory technique called differential item functioning to conduct this type of analysis (Martinková et al 2017) or use common statistical test such as T-Test/Mann-Whitney/Median test to compare item score for variables with two categories (e.g. male/female). You can use One-way ANOVA/Kruskal-Wallis/Median test to compare items score for variables with more than two categories (e.g. <20/20-22/>22 years) depending on the distribution of the item score (Rosner 2015).

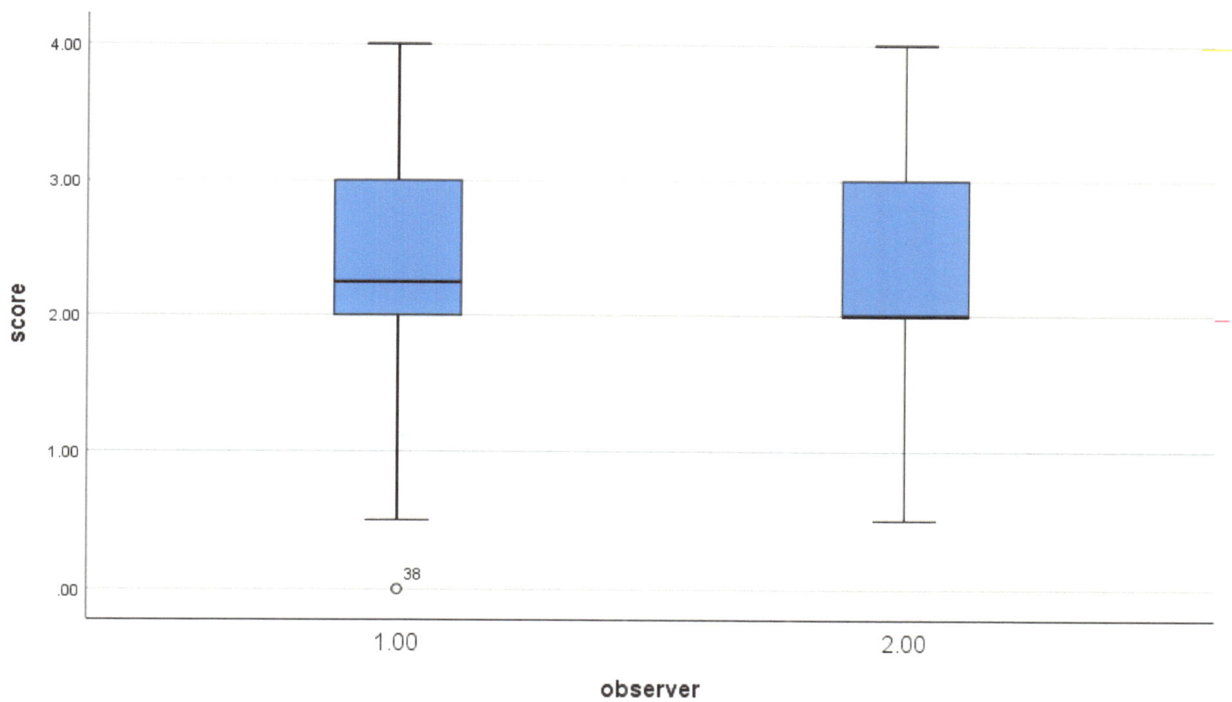

Figure 6: Boxplot of total blood pressure measurement score by two observers, Pilot Test, India (N=81)

The main use of the valid and reliable observation schedule tool is the scale score as it represents the value of the trait/construct. You can summarize the scale score with mean and standard deviation if it is bell shaped like Figure 5 and with median and inter-quartile range if it is skewed to the right or left. The scale can be assessed using a reference range of mean ± 2 times standard deviation for the bell-shaped distribution or median ± 1.5 times inter-quartile range for skewed distribution. You can label the scores beyond this range as outliers/extreme values like student 38 shown with "o" in Figure 6. This comes handy to assess students with poor and good performance (discrimination power of the tool) and/or the observers with leniency or stringency traits (measurement error) (Bartman et al 2013).

The other main use of the scale score is to compare it with the socio-demographic and educational variables to confirm or refute the research questions using estimation theory (non-overlapping 95% confidence interval statistical significance) or hypothesis testing (p-value< 0.05 a statistical significance) approach (Rosner 2015). For instance, you can test whether the median score between observer 1 and observer 2 in Figure 6 is statistically different or not using estimation theory if it is a cross-sectional study and, hypothesis testing if it is a comparative study like non-experimental, quasi-experimental and experimental designs.

SUMMARIZE

The observation schedule is a very useful tool to observe and assess the performance of students as well as teachers for formative as well as summative purposes in medical education. This tool can be created or compiled for a specific construct using structured items and pre-define scoring rule (binary scale or rating scales). It is required to gather evidence of validity and reliability before using it in the high-stake setting.

Quality assurance of the observation schedule tool can be done using classical item analysis and item response theory methods. The mean/standard deviation or median/inter-quartile range is used to summarize the bell shaped and skewed item/total scores. Similarly, parametric tests are used to compare bell shaped scores whereas non-parametric tests are used to compare skewed scores.

EVALUATE

Imagine that you have decided to use standardized patients in the OSCE stations in your college to assess the performance of the students using observation schedules. You now need to create multiple parallel OSCE stations and you need to ask how am I going to establish the content validity of these parallel OSCE stations? Who will be involved in the compilation of the items and deciding on the scoring rule? You also need to think how to gather evidence of face validity as well as internal consistency; inter-observer and test re-test reliabilities of the parallel OSCEs.

Who will be the standardized patients? You also need to think whether you are going to use staff/faculty of the college/hospital or professional actors as standardized patients. Depending on the local context, you need to decide on using staff/faculty in the summative assessment or not. In both the cases, you need to think about the training of the standardized patient and the observers. You need to pay the standardized patients and may end up paying a huge amount of money as professional actors charge per encounter or per day basis. Thus, some medical colleges enroll standardized patients from the community, train them and put them in the payroll. Can you do this in your college?

During the training, as well as formative and summative assessments, you need to have multiple standardized patients for the assessment of the same construct so how are you going to organize the trainings of the standardized patients for the particular stations and switch them after certain rounds. Who will be involved in the training and what logistics are needed for it? Also, decide if standardized patients can score the performance of the students on the station or not and, how to control the communication/contamination between standardized patients and students prior to the assessments.

ROAD AHEAD

- Cut-off score (pass marks) of performance assessment with observation schedule checklist or rating scales must be based on the sound standard setting methods
- Criterion-referenced method must be used to determine the pass marks of the performance tests instead of a fixed criterion of 50% or 60% pass marks widely used
- Borderline, Borderline regression or contrasting group methods must be used to standard set the performance tests like OSCE/OSPE and Mini-CEX/DOPS

The criterion-referenced cut-off score of performance test with observation schedules tool like OSCE/OSPE, Mini-CEX and DOPS must be based on the performance on the objective checklist/rating scale along with the holistic global rating (Bhandary 2011). Comparison of checklists, checklists with global ratings and rating scales only in the same OSCE stationsis described here:

https://qa1.simmedical.com/sites/wiser/ns10/presentations/Berg-Howard-AssessmentTools-Checklists1.pdf

This will provide different pass marks than the 50% or 60% pass marks used in the undergraduate and post-graduate medical education in South Asia and considered defendable.

Three criterion-referenced methods have been used widely for the performance-based assessments around the globe. They are contrasting group method, borderline method and borderline regression method where a 2-point (Fail/Pass), 3-point (Below average/Average/Above Average) and 5-point holistic global rating (Very Poor/Poor/Average/Good/Very Good) is used to find the pass mark of the objective checklist/rating scale score. This paper describes the various criterion-referenced methods for OSCE:

https://www.ceesvandervleuten.com/application/files/9214/2875/7755/A_Comparison_of_Standard-setting_Procedures_for_an_OSCE_in_Undergraduate_Medical_Education_2000_.pdf

What do you think about these methods? Is this applicable, feasible and acceptable in our setting? How to include them in our settings?

REFERENCES

Bartman, I., Smee, S., & Roy, M. (2013). A method for identifying extreme OSCE examiners. *The Clinical Teacher*, 10(1), 27-31.

Bhandary, S. (2011). Standard setting in health professions education. *Kathmandu University Medical Journal*, 9(1), 3-4.

Bisits, P. (2014). How to pretest and pilot a survey questionnaire. Available from: *https://www.tools4dev.org/wp-content/uploads/how-to-pretest-and-pilot-a-survey-questionnaire.pdf*

Cook, D. A., Brydges, R., Ginsburg, S., & Hatala, R. (2015). A contemporary approach to validity arguments: a practical guide to K ane's framework. Medical education, 49(6), 560-575.

Ghimire, S., & Bhandary, S. (2015). Students' Perception and Preference of Problem Based Learning During Introductory Course of a Nepalese Medical School. *Journal of Patan Academy of Health Sciences*, *1*(1), 64-68

Gliem, J. A., & Gliem, R. R. (2003). Calculating, interpreting, and reporting Cronbach's alpha reliability coefficient for Likert-type scales. Midwest Research-to-Practice Conference in Adult, Continuing, and Community Education.

Guilford, J. P. (1954). Psychometric methods (2nd ed.). McGraw-Hill.

Kempfer, H. (1960). Tools for evaluation. Indian Journal of Adult Education, XXI (7), 15-39.

Martinková, P., Drabinová, A., Liaw, Y. L., Sanders, E. A., McFarland, J. L., & Price, R. M. (2017). Checking equity: Why differential item functioning analysis should be a routine part of developing conceptual assessments. CBE—Life Sciences Education, 16(2), rm2.

Mindrila, D. & Balentyne, P. (2013). Scatterplots and Correlation. Available from: *https://www.westga.edu/academics/research/vrc/assets/docs/scatterplots_and_correlation_notes.pdf*

Norcini, J. J., Blank, L. L., Arnold, G. K., & Kimball, H. R. (1995). The mini-CEX (clinical evaluation exercise): a preliminary investigation. Annals of internal medicine, 123(10), 795-799.

Norcini, J., & Burch, V. (2007). Workplace-based assessment as an educational tool: AMEE Guide No. 31. Medical teacher, 29(9-10), 855-871.

Nunnally, J. C. (1978). Psychometric theory (2nd ed.). New York: McGraw-Hill.

Patton, M. Q. (1990). Qualitative evaluation and research methods (2nd ed.). Sage Publications, Inc.

Pett, M. A., Lackey, N. R., & Sullivan, J. J. (2003). Making sense of factor analysis: The use of factor analysis for instrument development in health care research. Sage.

Piryani, R. M., Shankar, R. P., Piryani, S., Thapa, T. P., Karki, B., Khakurel, M. P., & Bhandary, S. (2013). Conducting Integrated Objective Structured Clinical Examination: Experiences at KIST Medical College, Nepal. Archives of Medicine and Health Sciences, 1(2), 166.

Remesh, A. (2013). Microteaching, an efficient technique for learning effective teaching. Journal of research in medical sciences: the official journal of Isfahan University of Medical Sciences, 18(2), 158.

Rosner, B. (2015). Fundamentals of biostatistics (8th ed). Cengage learning.

Ruel, E., Wagner III, W. E., & Gillespie, B. J. (2015). Pretesting and Pilot Testing (Chapter 6). The practice of survey research: Theory and applications. Sage Publications. Available from:*https://us.sagepub.com/sites/default/files/upm-assets/68507_book_item_68507.pdf*

Tavakol, M., & Dennick, R. (2012). Post-examination interpretation of objective test data: monitoring and improving the quality of high-stakes examinations: AMEE Guide No. 66. Medical teacher, 34(3), e161-e175.

Upadhyay, S. K., Bhandary, S., Ghimire, S. R., Maharjan, B. R., Shrestha, I., Joshi, M., & Vaidya, S. (2017). Validating a problem-based learning process assessment tool in a Nepalese medical school. Journal of Patan Academy of Health Sciences, 4(2), 65-72.

Webb, N. M., & Shavelson, R. J. (2005). Generalizability theory: overview. Encyclopedia of statistics in behavioral science.

Yudkowsky, R., Park, Y. S., & Downing, S. M. (Eds.). (2019). Assessment in health professions education. Routledge.

Chapter 13

Focus Group Discussions

Pathiyil Ravi Shankar, Medha A. Joshi, Savita Ravindra

ABSTRACT

During a focus group discussion (FGD) a group of individuals selected and assembled by the researchers, discuss and express their opinion on the research topic. FGD can generate rich data during a short time, and its strength lies in the interaction among the group members. Discussion takes place among a group who feel they are equals and share common interests. Online FGDs are becoming more common during the ongoing pandemic.

FGD can be used for preliminary exploration of a topic helping to develop a questionnaire or can be used to explore in detail issues identified using other methods. Ethical challenges may need redressal, especially if faculty members conduct FGDs among students. Participants may communicate sensitive matters discussed, outside the group. FGDs should be arranged in a neutral venue and the atmosphere should be relaxed..

The concept of data saturation is used to decide on the number of FGDs to be conducted. A FGD guide is necessary. The moderator plays a vital role in the FGD and should ensure that the discussions are balanced. The other important member is the note taker. There is a definite sequence of activities to be followed while conducting an FGD. FGDs are usually audio or video recorded.

Transcribing the FGD, coding, reporting of findings are subsequent steps, which are similar to other qualitative data analysis and reporting. Software is available to help the process. FGD like other research methods have both advantages and limitations.

Key Words: education, focus groups, qualitative, research, research design

ASSESS NEED

Focus group discussions can be used as a preliminary exploration of topics in educational research which can be further used to create a questionnaire or to explore in detail, issues that need further clarification that were raised in a survey questionnaire. For example, a preliminary focus group can be used to explore the attitudes of medical students towards economic migrants and develop a questionnaire. Or if a study of the educational environment using a validated questionnaire found very low scores among a particular subgroup of students, then a focus group can be used to explore this further.

What is a focus group discussion?

A focus group discussion (FGD) has been defined by Powell and co-workers as 'a group of individuals selected and assembled by researchers to discuss and comment on, from personal experience, the topic that is the subject of the research'(Powell & Single, 1996). FGD uses guided, interactional discussion to generate rich details of complex experiences and the reasons behind actions, beliefs, perceptions, and attitudes. The focus could be a collective activity engaging the group ranging from watching a movie, examining a health education message, or debating and discussing a particular set of questions (Kitzinger, 1994).

What are their advantages and disadvantages?

FGDs have advantages over other qualitative data collection methods. The method can generate rich data in a relatively short time. FGDs can collect information and insights about a variety of phenomena. In a FGD about six to ten participants discuss a set of predetermined questions and the discussion is facilitated by a trained moderator.

The strength of FGD lies in the interaction between the group members generating rich data and insights. The interactions should be mainly among the participants and to enable this the facilitator/moderator should create a comfortable, non-threatening atmosphere where participants feel encouraged to freely express their opinions (Acocella, 2012). The discussion should take place among a group who feel equal and share common interests. FGD does not require many resources for data collection and can be recorded using a voice recorder or a video camera or smartphone. The moderator can dive more deeply to obtain in-depth insights into the researched topic (Barrows, 2000). Online FGDs can be conducted using a variety of platforms like Zoom and Microsoft Teams which also allow for recording the discussions. The analysis can be facilitated using software packages which we will discuss later. The software is expensive but recently cheaper alternatives may be available. A major point to consider is that since only a limited number of individuals are chosen, the group/s chosen may not be representative of the population and the outcomes cannot be generalized (Barrows, 2000; Davies, 1999)

BRIEF

This chapter will discuss FGDs under the following points

- What is a FGD?
- Where can we use FGDs in educational research?
- Ethical issues to be considered in FGDs
- Arranging an FGD
- Creating a FGD guide
- Role of the FGD moderator

- Conducting a FGD
- Role of note taker
- Recording a FGD
- Analysing and Reporting findings of a FGD
- Use of software
- Strengths and Limitations of FGD

CONTEXTUALIZE

The first author (PRS) started using FGDs in education research nearly two decades ago. One of the challenges he faced was the absence of skilled colleagues who could provide insights and guidance. His major source of knowledge was through books. In the early 2000s, videos explaining technics were scarce. E-books were still not common, and the major method of communication was through e-mail and snail mail. Smartphones were still in the future and researchers had to invest on special devices to record the discussions. He prepared a FGD guide, read as much about the process as possible and along with a colleague decided to conduct an FGD.

His colleague acted as the note taker and observer and he was the main facilitator. They obtained written informed consent from the participating students. One of the challenges is that the student-teacher relationship is an unequal one and students may find it difficult to say 'no' to their teachers. The other challenge was to find a 'neutral' venue. This was difficult as most places in the institution are used for teaching-learning activities where the teacher is the dominant person. The cafeteria and the mess are noisy and unsuited for conducting and recording FGDs. We arranged some light refreshments and tea/coffee to encourage interactions and get people relaxed. One of the first author's major worries was whether the recording was going on smoothly and whether it could be played back loud and clear.

Have you conducted FGDs?

What was your experience facilitating your first FGD?

What challenges did you face?

What is a focus group discussion (FGD)?

Early in the chapter we had looked at the definition of FGD. As mentioned before in an FGD the emphasis is on the interaction between the group members and the technique of information gathering is based on apparently informal discussion among a group of people (Acocella, 2012). The moderator leads the discussion while the observer takes notes and observes participants' on-verbal behaviour integrating it with the discussion. Focussed group discussion has also been described as '*a group of interacting individuals having some common interest or characteristics, brought together by a moderator, who uses the group and its interaction as a way to gain information about a specific or focused issue.*'*(Mary & Sewell, 2007).*

Where can we use FGDs in educational research?

FGDs can be used to explore a variety of areas in educational research. They have been used for a wide range of purposes in education ranging from development of learning tools which appeal better to students, evaluation of students' knowledge and attitudes about curricular issues, enhancing results obtained through surveys and developing new marketing strategies for educational programs (Williams & Katz, 2001). They have been used to explore topics as diverse as nutrition, AIDS, sex education and technology. The possible impact of increasing female medical student admissions was studied in Nepal using FGDs (Shankar et al., 2012). A variety of issues including student perception about artificial intelligence (AI) in health professions education and in practice, student perception about disadvantaged populations, their opinions about different issues like various facilities in the institution including support facilities for students and staff among others can be studied using FGDs. One of the challenges is students may be reluctant to share negative feedback especially if faculty members are facilitating FGDs or if students think that the FGD recording may be shared with the faculty and the administration and their confidentiality and anonymity is not guaranteed. They can be used to study faculty perspectives for example on problem-based learning, curricular changes like the Attitude, Ethics and Communication skills module in India, their perception about online learning among others.

Ethical issues to be considered in FGDs

Several ethical challenges may arise while conducting an FGD. Predicting what will happen during a FGD may be problematic as the discussion and the group interactions may be unpredictable (Sim & Waterfield, 2019). Once the FGD starts it may be difficult for the participant to revoke the consent. Participants may communicate what was discussed during the FGD with persons outside the group creating confidentiality and anonymity issues. The potential of over disclosure by some participants of sensitive topics may be a challenge.

In educational research the issue of the power imbalance between the teacher/faculty and student may be an issue if the faculty is facilitating the FGD. Students may feel compelled to participate and they may not be comfortable sharing sensitive information or negative opinion. Students in hierarchical organizations (most educational institutions) have been classified as a vulnerable population and could be unjustifiably influenced by the positive expectations associated with participating (Shivayogi, 2013). In some countries, faculty members cannot be involved as FGD facilitators, and a person not directly associated with teaching-learning facilitates the FGDs. Finding a neutral venue for the FGD may not always be easy as mentioned before.

Arranging an FGD

The group should not be too diverse that demographic differences and differences in professional status and class impact the deliberations. At the same time, the group should not be so homogeneous that the diversity of opinion is not revealed. Ensuring a proper group composition can often be difficult. Wherever possible, the FGD should be arranged in a neutral venue and a relaxed atmosphere created. The facilitator/moderator and observer should be present at the venue before the participants so that they can welcome them to the session. Informal interaction before the actual FGD can help create a coherent group and ensure the members are comfortable with each other. Snacks and light refreshments can help. If the FGD is being held online, then the moderator and observer should be present at the virtual venue before the participants. Table 1 summarizes important steps and challenges while conducting an FGD.

The participants should be seated in a circle in a face-to-face FGD to ensure appropriate eye contact and interactions. The venue should be comfortable, and the recording equipment should be unobtrusive so that the participants are not inhibited. The ground rules should be discussed and agreed on before the start of the session. Consent should be obtained from the participants and this should include consent for recording the session. If the FGD is being done face-to-face, two copies of the consent form should be available, one copy be kept with the investigator and the other with the participant. Participants should be fully informed about the confidentiality of the recordings, with whom they will be shared and what data will be published. The moderator should be friendly and unbiased. Recruiting participants may be time consuming and can often be difficult.

Size of the group: Ideally, the number of participants per FGD should not be too large or too small. Adequate participation of all the group members may not be possible if the group is too large and too small a group may not generate adequate discussion and diverse opinions. Generally, the group size is limited to six to 12 members (Escalada & Heong, 2014).

The number of FGDs to be held depends on the type and complexity of the research topic. FGDs should generate sufficient data to allow for comparisons and to generate and test theoretical ideas (Barbour, 2005). Like in many other types of qualitative research, the concept of 'saturation' is very useful. Reaching saturation means reaching a point where subsequent group discussions no longer provide new insights or outcomes. Saturation can determine the number of FGDs to be held. Generally, the duration of the FGD should be less than two hours for a face-to-face session (Escalada & Heong, 2014)

Creating a FGD guide

To ensure that the discussions remain focussed on the topic of interest while at the same time allowing the participants to talk freely, the moderator uses a discussion guide. This moderator's guide is prepared to cover the main topics or research questions in the session. The purpose of the discussion guide is to provide a framework for the moderator to ask questions to cover all research questions, without missing out on any critical points. Use of the guide helps in collecting the data efficiently and covering the entire topic. The guide is not a survey instrument, and the questions need not be followed in the order written but should be covered sometime during the discussion (Wong, 2008). The number of questions in the guide is generally kept to a minimum to leave enough time for in-depth discussion. The sequence of questions in the guide usually moves from general to specific. In a particular discussion topic, the initial questions should be general, and as the discussion continues, the questions should be more specific and focused. Questions should be open-ended, simple, unbiased, and not leading. The guide should be flexible enough for the moderator to follow any relevant but unexpected points that come up during the discussion (Wong, 2008). All the members of the research group should be involved in preparing the questions.

The suggested steps for developing the FGD guide are:

- Specify the objectives and research topic for which responses are sought from the FGD. These should not be the direct research question/s, but the inference drawn from responses of the participants should help the researcher to answer the principal research question (van Eeuwijk & Angehrn, 2017).
- The main items/questions should be between 6-12 (to be able to discuss in 45-90 minutes) (Wong, 2008)

- The main question should be broken down into smaller discussion points or themes.
- Be ready with probe questions if needed to get in-depth information.
- Pre-test the guide with a "mock" FGD
- Review, revise and delete questions based on the feedback received from pilot testing the questions in the "mock" FGD.

Table 1 summarizes important steps and challenges while conducting an FGD.

Role of the FGD moderator

The success of the FGD depends on the skills and experience of the moderator in conducting an FGD. As per Lewis the moderator should be "thinking, listening and managing time at the same time" (Lewis, 2003). S/he should be familiar with the discussion topic, should be polite, empathetic and allow the participants to interact freely, keeping in mind the facets of group dynamics. S/he should ensure participation from all the group members, handle the dominant participants tactfully and encourage the non-responders. The moderator should be friendly and sensitive to cultural and gender issues (Escalada & Heong, 2014). The moderator should ensure that the topic is introduced correctly, and the discussions are balanced and at the same time should not dominate the discussion or be judgmental or biased (van Eeuwijk & Angehrn, 2017).

Conducting an FGD

Generally, a team consisting of two to three members, a moderator, also called facilitator or the discussion leader, a note-taker, and an observer (optional) are involved in conducting the FGD. The FGD typically follows these steps (Dawson et al., 1993)

1. The moderator starts the discussion with a welcome, followed by self-introduction and introduction of the note-taker. This is followed by a round of self- introduction by the participants.
2. Next, the moderator explains the overall research question and the objectives of the FGD. This can be done orally, by projecting them or putting it up as a poster on the waal.
3. The ground rules are explained including the duration of the discussion (generally 45 to 90 minutes) and permission is taken for note taking and audio/video recording.
4. The moderator reiterates that each participant should contribute, and all the contributions are valued. Also reassures that the discussions will remain confidential and anonymous,
5. The moderator then starts the discussion by asking the questions listed in the guide, asking probing questions if required. The discussion can flow freely between the participants, moderator ensuring that all the participants have a chance to express their views.
6. It is a good practice to summarize the major points discussed in one question before moving on to the next question. This will help clarify any doubts and to make sure that all viewpoints are recorded.
7. At the end of the discussion, the moderator should summarize the salient points to ensure correct interpretation as well as to allow the participants to elaborate their points further, if any have been left out.
8. The moderator thanks the participants and concludes the interview.

Role of the note taker

Next to the moderator, the other crucial member of the FGD team is the note taker. The quality of the notes determines the quality of the collected data. A note taker does not participate in the discussion. The note taker must take detailed notes on what is being discussed. This is not limited to just verbal conversation but even the nonverbal communication (tone, body language) and where the participant pauses or hesitates before responding. The notes add to the audio or video recording of the session. The notes are critical for focus group transcription to clarify and add contextual details to what the participants said during the focus group session (Barbour, 2005). If the discussion is recorded on audiotape, a sketch of the sitting arrangement with assigned numbers will help later while transcribing the tapes to ensure the information is matched accurately (Wong, 2008).

A few strategies to help improve the note taking include-

- **Use a Form** – Develop a standard form that can record each entry with name, date, and time. Maintain their inputs and leave space to add additional points when necessary.
- **Prepare Notes** – It will help to use key words or phrases to record instead of noting each word. This will help when doing the transcription.
- **Document Both Questions and Responses** – You should record both questions and responses in your notes.
- **Differentiate Participant Comments and Your Own Observations** – You should distinguish clearly between participant comments and your own observations. Use a column in your form to write down the quotes or the main ideas of what a speaker said and, in another column, write down your observations. Either use your own initials or 'MO' indicating 'My Observation'.
- **Cover a Variety of Observations** – Apart from documenting what people say during a session, record their body language, moods or attitudes, the general environment and other information that could be relevant for the session.

Once the initial notetaking and expanding the notes is completed, a debriefing session with the focus group moderator and note taker should be held to add any additional information, discuss any issues or comments that require clarification, any questions that did not work well, and new topics that came up during discussion. Also, one should try to identify missing information. After completion of this task the notes can be used for effective transcription along with the recorded discussion. It is, however, important to summarize main ideas and points of view that are presented during the conversation. It is also helpful to include any impression or observations made during the discussion. For instance, note takers can note who was most talkative, which questions made people uncomfortable, or which questions were the hardest to answer.

Recording an FGD

FGDs are usually either audio or video recorded. In case of an audio recording it would be helpful to get each speaker identify themselves either using a pseudonym or by serial number assigned to them which helps during transcription. If using a video recording, the videographer should stand at a place that will not obstruct the flow of discussion. The process of transcribing a **focus group discussion** begins with the audio or video recording.

Points to keep in mind while recording the FGD:

1. **Speaker Identification**
   In case of audio recording, it would be critical, while using video recording the identification may not be difficult, however it is useful.
2. **Location for FGD**
   The choice of location is critical in case of recording. One must look for a quiet place where recording has clarity.

Analysing and reporting findings

Analysing the FGD data is like analysing any other qualitative data. So, the initial step is to prepare a verbatim transcription of the discussion. The transcript is then compared with the notes taken by the note taker to ensure completeness of the transcript.

The next step after transcription, is the process of analysing and reporting the findings.

Step 1- Coding of the information

After the FGD transcripts, one can begin coding and organizing the information in categories. These crucial tasks can be difficult and sometimes tedious. They are very important, though, because coding helps in identifying patterns, relationships, and meaning in the information. In addition, coding reduces the quantity of information that must be analyzed (by focusing only on the categories that are relevant to the research question and it helps to quickly retrieve segments of the information as needed). Coding can be done manually using letters, words, numbers, and different colored pens. Usually, a team decides on the coding method (De Negri & Thomas, 2003). Now a days software packages like (NUDIST, NVivo, Atlas/ti, QRS Int, Melbourne, Australia), and Ethnography (Qualis Research Associates, Colorado, USA) are available that make qualitative data analysis, starting from coding the transcript easier.

Table 1 summarizes important steps and challenges while conducting an FGD. Once the information is coded, one will be able to see themes evolving. For example, if a FGD is being conducted on barriers to family planning, after coding the responses, some of the responses can get categorized under stigma, or beliefs, or practices etc.

Finally, these themes will give a narrative that can be represented as diagrams, tables, or response rates depending on the research group decision. The data then can be further analyzed at the basic level where a descriptive account of the data is presented, giving just the explanation of what was said with no assumption being made. The second interpretative level of analysis is one which involves the understanding of the themes, creating links between the themes, revealing how those themes emerged and generating a theory grounded in the data (Basit, 2003; Hancock et al., 2001).

Generally, several FGDs are conducted till there is data saturation. Hence the data reporting is done in the context of all the FGDs and not individual group discussions (Wong, 2008). The reporting is usually done using undetailed terms and is full of statements such as "many students expressed.....", "few of the faculty members disagreed...." Direct quotes should be included to support these statements.

As for using quantitative data analysis, simple statistical frequencies may be used to describe the themes or categories. As the FGDs are conducted with a small sample size, it is not possible to generalize the results hence detailed statistical analysis is not appropriate for reporting FGD data (Wong, 2008)

Use of Software

There are several software available to transcribe and analyze the data. Example of the some of the commonly used software:

- MAXQDA- The art of Data Analysis, tool for both transcription as well as data analysis.
- COLLABITO - An online focus group chat. It has an app-based option as well.
- Asynchronous focus groups using a Facebook or Learning Management System (LMS) platform is another option.
- Focus group-it is a software that is easy to use and is used when the participants are at different geographic locations and can connect online for an FGD.
- Software use in Qualitative Data Analysis has been elaborated in a separate chapter in this book.

Strengths and Limitations of FGD

A few of the strengths **quoted in literature** include:

- It is comparatively easy to conduct·
- It can be conducted as a standalone methodology or may be used along with another quantitative research method
- It allows to explore topics and to generate hypotheses·
- The participants can build upon each other's opinions, thus providing a broader view
- It has high "face validity" (data).
- It allows us to collect an appropriate amount of data in a short period of time
- It gives speed in the supply of the results (in terms of evidence of the meeting of the group)·
- It allows the researcher to increase the size of the sample of the qualitative studies by increasing the number of FGDs (Krueger, 2014).

Limitations include

1. The researcher has less control over the data that are generated·
2. The data analysis is more tedious to perform.
3. The interaction of the group forms a social atmosphere, and the comments should be interpreted within this context
4. It requires a carefully trained moderator
5. It takes effort to assemble the groups
6. The discussion should be conducted in an atmosphere that facilitates dialogue
7. The discussion may be influenced by a dominant participant and others may just echo his/her opinion.
8. Moderator by expressing his/her own opinions or the dominant individual opinions may result in biased outcomes.

SUMMARIZE

FGD is a qualitative data collection technique that uses guided, interactional discussion to generate "the rich details of complex experiences and the reasoning behind their actions, behaviour perceptions and attitudes". A focus group can be employed either as a single data gathering method to explore complex phenomena not suitable for quantitative research or it can be conducted prior to, simultaneously with, or after a quantitative study such as survey questionnaire to get in-depth views from diverse groups.

Recruitment of the participants is a crucial step to ensure that the group discussion will generate meaningful data.

The number of participants per FGD is restricted to 6-12, duration of each session between 45-90 minutes and not exceeding beyond 120 minutes. The number of FGDs to be conducted is generally decided once the data saturation occurs and no further new ideas/opinions are generated. The success of the FGD also depends on the skills of the moderator to facilitate the group, using a moderator's guide and keeping in mind the principles of group dynamics. The recorded discussion along with the notes taken by the notetaker are then transcribed, analysed and reported.

Analysis and reporting are time consuming and arduous part of the focus group study and very similar to other qualitative research methods. The major advantage of FGD is the that the researchers are able to get full range of perspectives held by the participants in a relatively short time. The interactions between the participants allows for clarification and expansion of the ideas. At the same time, it is likely that a participants' contributions may be influenced by the "group effect". The purpose of FGDs is to elicit varied ideas and experiences and not to look for a consensus.

EVALUATE

India has a high Prevalence of Diabetes Mellitus (DM) with the numbers increasing at an alarming rate. An initiative was undertaken to make the integrated diabetes care available at urban health centers in the city of Bangalore to enable a comprehensive care pathway for individuals. This would reduce the burden on tertiary care hospitals and enable them to provide more complex care.

A multi-disciplinary team was sent at two urban health care centers in the city as a pilot study to plan, initiate and deliver this service. Individuals of the locality and ward were screened for diabetes and after taking consent for treatment. The services were offered three days a week at the centers. To develop a clinical care pathway, it was decided to obtain all stakeholders' opinions at the planning stage (Chambers et al., 2013).

Questions.... Please identify the stakeholder groups. How many stakeholder groups could you identify?

1. What is the ideal method that could be used to gather stakeholder opinions?
2. What are the ethical issues involved?
3. If you think FGD could be a method, who are the participants to be considered?
4. Identify the number of participants to be included for each group.
5. If you are the moderator planning the activity, list the questions that you would like to get opinions at the start of the program (**Hint** – Frame questions based on people involved in service, process and expectation of the service)

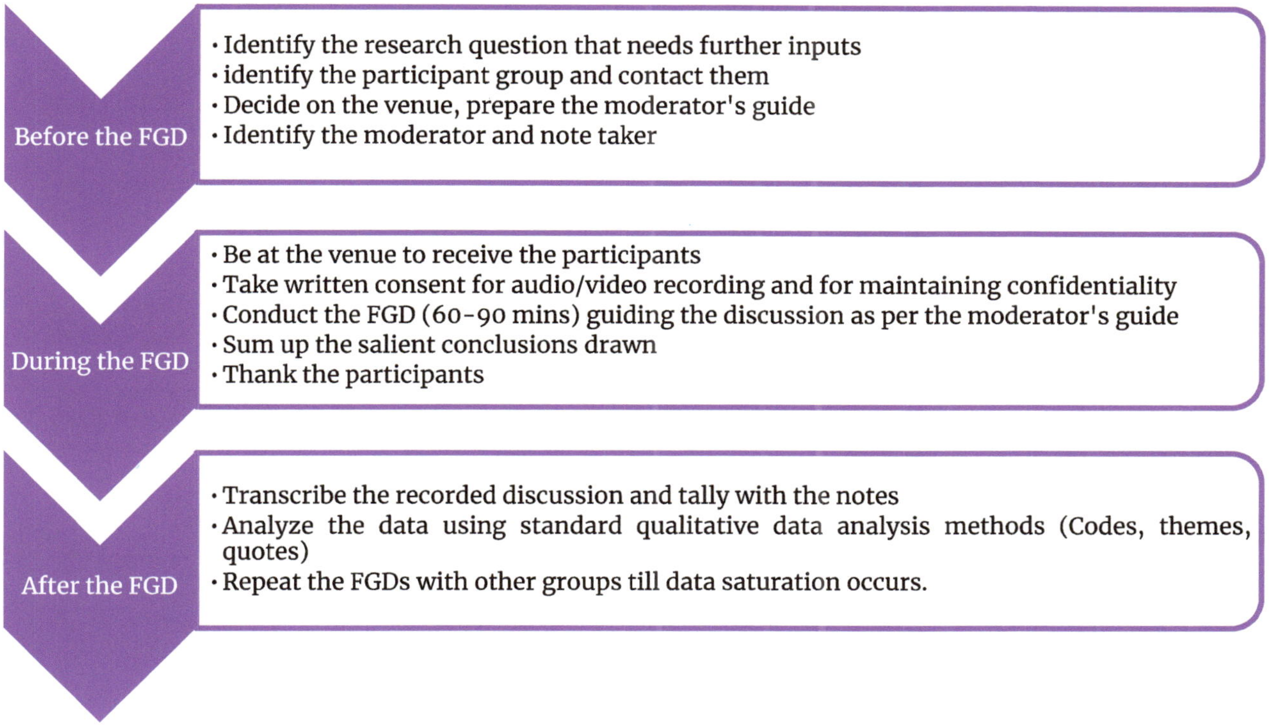

Figure 1: Would you like to conduct your first FGD? Then this might help you.

Table 1: Steps in carrying out an FGD and associated challenges

Step	Challenge	Possible solution
Arranging the FGD	Ensuring a proper group composition.	Consider differences of rank, social classes, economic group, and caste while choosing participants. Have enough diversity to ensure diversity of opinions.
	Create a welcoming and relaxed atmosphere.	Be present at the venue (physical or virtual) before the participants. Select a neutral venue and ensure supply of light refreshments and snacks in physical FGDs. Icebreaker in virtual FGDs.
	Select a proper group size.	The recommended size is six to 12 for physical FGDs and around five for virtual FGDs.
	Be mindful of time.	The duration is less than two hours (physical) and 90 mins (virtual FGD).
	Develop and test the FGD guide.	The FGD should answer the principal research question Pretest the FGD guide with mock participants.

Step	Challenge	Possible solution
Moderating the FGD	Ensure all individuals participate.	Be polite, empathetic, encourage non-responders, handle dominant participants and be aware of sociocultural issues.
	Summarize the discussions.	The discussion of one question is summarized before moving on to the next. At the end, the main discussion is summarized. This keeps participants on track, and they can elaborate where required.
	Take detailed notes during the FGDs.	Adds to the recording. Important during transcription to clarify and add contextual details. Separate note taker required.
Analyzing and reporting the findings	Prepare the transcript.	Professional help to transcribe the recordings can be used. Free and paid online transcription software is also available.
	Qualitative data analysis should be done.	Can be done manually. A variety of platforms are available both paid and free.

ROAD AHEAD

FGDs are a powerful tool to explore a variety of topics in health professions education and require expertise to conduct and analyze. Analyzing and interpreting FGDs is time consuming. We will attempt to explore recent changes in how FGDs are conducted, transcribed, and analyzed.

What changes have taken place in how FGDs are conducted?

FGDs are increasingly being conducted online both due to the ongoing COVID-19 pandemic and due to the ease of involving participants from different regions. A blended approach to FGDs, face-to-face sessions for participants located in the same place as the facilitators and online for remote participants is expected to continue even post-pandemic. Specialized software for conducting online FGDs are available and web-conferencing tools can also be used.

Certain modifications to how a FGD is conducted are recommended for online FGDs (UXalliance, 2020). The number of participants to be involved is only four to five, Confidentiality agreement can be signed online. Incentives can be provided through online transfer or through gift vouchers. The session time should be between 60 to 90 minutes. Some participants may want to use an avatar and features like video blurring and audio masking may be useful to protect participant identity if required. The discussion topics are usually reduced to four to five. If the FGD participants speak multiple languages then simultaneous translation services may be required. Both the moderator and the participants should be familiar with the online platform. It is recommended to log in about 10 to 15 mins before the start of the session. Some of the professional platforms also allow for transcribing.

Free transcribing tools for FGDs

Transcribing an FGD is a labor-intensive process. Different transcribing services are available online and most charge a fee. A recent article examines three free transcription software ('3 Free Transcription Tools You Can Try', 2020). Among those recommended are OTranscribe, Express Scribe and the FTW Transcriber.

Free qualitative data analysis software

This software can carry out transcription analysis, coding, text interpretation, content analysis, discursive analysis, among others. The software enables content search, data visualization and reporting, storing and coding, data linking and data mapping (Top 19 Free Qualitative Data Analysis Software in 2021 - Reviews, Features, Pricing, Comparison, 2020). Among the software mentioned are coding analysis toolkit, General architecture for text engineering (GATE), FreeQDA, QDA Miner Lite, TAMS, among others.

FGDs and chatbots

Chatbots are software applications using artificial intelligence and natural language processing to understand what a human wants and guide them to their desired outcome (Chatbots - The Beginners Guide to Chatbot Technology, 2019). Chatbots can be used to filter, select and group individuals in a conversation by using condition and options in the chatbot scripts (Chatbots for Market Research: Automate Surveys, Focus Groups and Interviews by Chat or Phone, n.d.). These individuals can then be directed toward FGDs. A chatbot has been developed to facilitate group discussions by managing the discussion, time, encouraging even participation of the members, and organizing members' opinions (Kim et al., 2020).

What are the different types of FGDs?

FGDs have been divided into:

- single FGD, mini FGD,
- two-way FGD (with two groups, with one group observing the other group during their discussion),
- dual moderator FGD (with two moderators taking charge of one group),
- dueling moderator FGD (with the two moderators examined opposite sides of an issue),
- respondent moderator FGD (with one of the respondents temporarily assuming the role of a moderator) and
- a remote FGD (which we have discussed already) (Research, n.d.)

REFERENCES

3 Free Transcription Tools You Can Try. (2020, May 4). Ai-Media. https://www.ai-media.tv/the-best-free-transcription-software/

Acocella, I. (2012). The focus groups in social research: Advantages and disadvantages. Quality & Quantity, 46(4), 1125–1136.

Barbour, R. S. (2005). Making sense of focus groups. Medical Education, 39(7), 742–750.

Barrows, C. W. (2000). An exploratory study of food and beverage training in private clubs. International Journal of Contemporary Hospitality Management.

Basit, T. (2003). Manual or electronic? The role of coding in qualitative data analysis. Educational Research, 45(2), 143–154.

Chambers, N., Harvey, G., Mannion, R., Bond, J., & Marshall, J. (2013). Health services and delivery research. National Institute for Health Research, 1(6).

Chatbots for market research: Automate surveys, focus groups and interviews by chat or phone. (n.d.). Retrieved 31 May 2021, from https://www.chatcompose.com/marketresearch.html

Chatbots—The Beginners Guide to Chatbot Technology. (2019, August 2). Drift. https://www.drift.com/learn/chatbot/

Davies, R. (1999). Focus groups in Asia. Orient Pacific Century.

Dawson, S., Manderson, L., & Tallo, V. L. (1993). A manual for the use of focus groups. Boston: international Nutrition foundation for developing countries.

De Negri, B., & Thomas, E. (2003). Making sense of focus group findings: A systematic participatory analysis approach. AED.

Escalada, M., & Heong, K. L. (2014). Focus group discussion. Retrieved from ricehoppers.net: http://ricehoppers.net/wp-content/uploads ....

Hancock, B., Ockleford, E., & Windridge, K. (2001). An introduction to qualitative research. Trent focus group.

Kim, S., Eun, J., Oh, C., Suh, B., & Lee, J. (2020). Bot in the Bunch: Facilitating Group Chat Discussion by Improving Efficiency and Participation with a Chatbot. Proceedings of the 2020 CHI Conference on Human Factors in Computing Systems, 1–13.

Kitzinger, J. (1994). The methodology of focus groups: The importance of interaction between research participants. Sociology of Health & Illness, 16(1), 103–121.

Krueger, R. A. (2014). Focus groups: A practical guide for applied research. Sage publications.

Mary, M., & Sewell, M. (2007). Using Focus Groups for Evaluation. Online:< https://Cals. Arizona. Edu/Sfcs/Cyfernet/Cyfar/Focus. Htm>(11/2018).

Powell, R. A., & Single, H. M. (1996). Focus groups. International Journal for Quality in Health Care, 8(5), 499–504.

Research, C. for. (n.d.). What are the Different Types of Focus Groups? Retrieved 6 June 2021, from https://www.cfrinc.net/cfrblog/what-are-the-different-types-of-focus-groups

Shankar, P. R., Singh, K. K., & Singh, S. (2012). Possible impact of increase in female medical student admissions in Nepal: Findings from a qualitative study among medical undergraduates. The Australasian Medical Journal, 5(3), 184.

Shivayogi, P. (2013). Vulnerable population and methods for their safeguard. Perspectives in Clinical Research, 4(1), 53.

Sim, J., & Waterfield, J. (2019). Focus group methodology: Some ethical challenges. Quality & Quantity, 53(6), 3003–3022.

Top 19 Free Qualitative Data Analysis Software in 2021—Reviews, Features, Pricing, Comparison. (2020, December 17). PAT RESEARCH: B2B Reviews, Buying Guides & Best Practices. https://www.predictiveanalyticstoday.com/top-free-qualitative-data-analysis-software/

UXalliance. (2020, June 11). Conducting remote online focus groups in times of COVID-19. Medium. https://uxalliance.medium.com/conducting-remote-online-focus-groups-in-times-of-covid-19-ee1c66644fdb

van Eeuwijk, P., & Angehrn, Z. (2017). How to... Conduct a Focus Group Discussion (FGD). Methodological Manual.

Williams, A., & Katz, L. (2001). The use of focus group methodology in education: Some theoretical and practical considerations, 5 (3). IEJLL: International Electronic Journal for Leadership in Learning, 5.

Wong, L. P. (2008). Focus group discussion: A tool for health and medical research. Singapore Med J, 49(3), 256–260.

Chapter 14

Introducing In-Depth Interviews

Savita Ravindra, Medha A. Joshi

ABSTRACT

The Interview is one of the commonest qualitative data collection methods used in healthcare research. Interviews are considered when the interviewer wishes to explore the interviewee's feelings and perspectives on a research topic.

In-depth interviews (IDI) are useful when one wishes to ask open-ended questions to obtain a depth of information from relatively small number of respondents (as compared to surveys, which tend to be more quantitative and are conducted with large number of people). Interviews generate rich information that can be used to understand a problem or issue in detail. They are used for a variety of purposes, including needs assessment, and to identify gaps in a program, or situation. It involves one-on-one engagement with the participant, usually done face-to-face or occasionally over the telephone. An in-depth interview duration usually ranges between 60-120 minutes depending on the subject matter and the context.

An interview could be structured, semi structured or of unstructured format. There are four steps involved in conducting in-depth interviews (1) developing a sampling strategy; (2) writing an in-depth interview guide; (3) conducting the interviews; (4) analyzing the data.

Interviews require a highly skilled interviewer to conduct an interview, one with considerable knowledge and experience. In depth Interviews are usually audio recorded or written down as notes verbatim. The transcribed data is coded, analyzed and findings are reported. The process of data analysis and reporting is similar to other qualitative data analysis and reporting process. Software are available to help in the Process of analysis.

In-depth interviews have both advantages and limitations. Data obtained cannot be generalized to the population. It can be combined with other research methods.

Key Words: qualitative research, in-depth interview, semi-structured interviews, unstructured interviews, education, health science

ASSESS NEED

Interviewing is a paradox. From a distance, it appears deceptively simple. In depth interview (IDI) method is used to delve deep into the human experiences, views, and perceptions on one or two issues to understand human behavior. The rationale for using interviews in health care practice is to produce empirical data or evidence that can help healthcare professionals develop better healthcare practices (Parahoo, 2014). Use of IDI helps the researcher and clinician to understand the views, opinions and practices of the patients and care givers on health care issues. This qualitative input can help develop a comprehensive clinical care pathway that is holistic in approach (Britten, 1995).

In medical education research, IDI can be used to understand student views, perceptions, and experiences of a newly introduced curriculum, to identify the strengths, and gaps as perceived by the students enabling the faculty to bring in change in delivery if needed.

In this chapter, we have used the terms interviews and in-depth interviews interchangeably.

BRIEF

- In this method, one or two issues are discussed in detail.
- The purpose of IDIs is to collect a rich individual experience that helps in understanding the perception of the interviewee on the research topic.
- Interviews are usually conducted with small number of respondents.
- Experienced interviewer with active listening skills will be able to capture the underlying beliefs, attitudes, and feelings of respondents on a particular subject.

CONTEXTUALIZE

It was observed that the stress levels in the nursing staff posted in COVID wards in a private hospital, where the first author (SR) works, were very high. The head of the Psychiatry department decided to conduct IDIs with few of the nurses who were posted in COVID wards during both COVID waves. Twelve nurses were interviewed, to understand their thoughts, perceptions and beliefs with the intention to address the issue of coping with the stress. All the interviews were conducted by a single researcher. The outcome of these interviews was, development of coping strategies by the department of Psychiatry. All the nurses who were posted for COVID ward duty during the pandemic were then trained to handle the stress, using short experiential modules.

Have you conducted an IDI any time? For what purpose did you use this qualitative data gathering technique? Did you face any difficulties while conducting the interviews?

DESCRIBE

What is an In-Depth Interview method?

IDI is a data gathering technique intended to present interviewee's standpoint or perspective on the research topic. We need to differentiate a research interview from that of a journalistic interview. In the later, the respondent often controls the presentation of information, while the interviewer has his own agenda to get what they can get out of it (Lune & Berg, 2017).

Interviews are generally conducted with small number of participants, on one-to-one basis. It is not a question and answer session. Rather, the interviewee is considered as being knowledgeable on the topic and the interviewer a novice trying to learn from the interviewee. Thus, the interviewee contributes to making a meaning instead of responding to the views and perceptions of the researcher as happens in structured surveys or questionnaires. IDIs are conducted using mostly open-ended questions in conversational style, many a times followed by ***why* and *how*** to get deeper understanding of the interviewee's perception.

When are In-Depth Interviews Appropriate in Educational Research?

IDIs are very commonly used for program evaluation input process. It offers an opportunity to gain insight into how individuals interpret a particular issue. IDIs are commonly conducted to understand the perceptions of patients, care givers or healthcare providers on diverse research questions such as how is pain perceived by patients in palliative care? Why do general practitioners prescribe antibiotics for common cold or flu? Why do students miss out on assignment dates? (Dicicco-Bloom & Crabtree, 2006).

This method of data gathering could be used alone when you:

- want to get individual member's thoughts with open ended questioning
- are not sure of getting honest answers from participants during a focus group discussion.
- are seeking information on sensitive personal issues
- seek inputs from various key stakeholders on one-to-one basis while conducting program evaluation

Or IDIs could be useful in mixed method research either to add depth or to supplement other research approaches. For example, IDIs could be conducted

- prior to developing a survey or finalizing on FGD questions
- post survey when some close ended questions generate unexpected results
- if, after drafting a survey questionnaire, you realize that important questions cannot be effectively addressed without more open ended questions and extended probing (Boyce & Neale, 2006).

What are the Types of In-Depth Interviews?

Interviews have been loosely classified as unstructured, semi structured or structured interviews (Crabtree & Miller, 1999; Fontana & Frey, 2005). Structured interviews generate quantitative data whereas semi-structured and unstructured interviews are suitable in generating qualitative data and will be the focus of discussion in this chapter. Though called unstructured, no interview could be totally devoid of any structure. The major difference among these different interview types is their degree of rigidity with regard to presentational structure (Lune & Berg, 2017).

Table 1: Shows salient differences between these three types of interviews.

Type of Interview	Structured Interviews	Semi-structured Interviews	Unstructured Interviews
Format	Completely structured, strict adherence to question order, similar to a survey questionnaire.	Somewhat structured, interviewer can change the order of questions.	Completely free of any structure, interviewer has full freedom to ask any questions in any order.
Questions format	Questions to be asked exactly as written in the guide, no change of words allowed.	Words of the questions flexible and may be altered to make the interviewee understand the question.	No set wording to any question.
Process of interview	No additional clarification questions allowed.	Interviewer may respond to questions from interviewee and clarify the doubts.	Interviewer may answer questions and give clarifications during the interview.
Process of Interview	No additional questions may be added during the interview.	Interviewer may add or delete probes during subsequent interviews.	Interviewer may add or delete questions during interviews.
Type of data	Generates mostly quantitative data.	Generates narrative, qualitative data.	Generates descriptive, qualitative data.
Analysis of Data	Easy to analyze and possible to generalize.	Tedious data analysis process, results not generalizable.	Tedious data analysis process, results not generalizable.

Structured Interviews: In this type of interviews, the interviewer has a set of structured questions for which she/he is looking for answers in terms of thoughts, opinions, and attitudes from the interviewees about study-related issues. The interviewer cannot chance the order or the wording of the questions, nor can she/he is ask any probing questions, she/he has to strictly follow the "scripted questions" in the guide. The rationale here is to offer each interviewee almost the same stimulus so that responses to questions, ideally, will be comparable (Babbie, 2007). The researchers have a fairly good idea about the information that is expected to emerge from these interviews (Flick, 2018; Merriam, 1998).

Semi-structured Interview: This type of interview is commonly the singular data source for the qualitative research question. The semi-structured interview is a preplanned event, with time and venue decided in advance in contrast to unstructured interviews, which happen anywhere and anytime as the interviewer is observing the interviewee in the field. These semi- structured, IDIs are based on a few open-ended questions, which may be expanded, modified or further probed based on the interviewee's responses. The duration of the interview varies anywhere between 30 minutes to several hours and are most often conducted once with one interviewee. IDIs with an individual allows the interviewer to delve deep into personal and social matters. It enables interviewees to "speak in their own voice and express their own thoughts and feelings" (Lune & Berg, 2017).

The questions for IDIs needs to be adequately focused such that a relatively identical group would have shared the experiences about the topic (Crabtree & Miller, 1999). Based on the main research question, which may be a good question to start the interview, anywhere between five and ten more specific questions are usually developed to explore more deeply into different aspects of the research topic. These questions may be modified or even deleted and new questions added depending on the responses obtained and also on the results seen as the data is simultaneously analyzed as it is collected, the iterative process, which is a typical feature of qualitative research (Dicicco-Bloom & Crabtree, 2006). The interview guide helps in keeping the discussion in right direction.

Unstructured interviews: Can also be called as guided conversations. This technique is more commonly used by anthropologists for ethnography research (Williams et al., 1994) During the process of participant observation and taking field notes, the researcher identifies a few "key informants" based on their knowledge and role in the research settings, and their ability and willingness to contribute as a mentor or a commentator for the researcher (Poggie Jr, 1972). Unstructured interviews are generally conducted along with observations and field notes as a method to add meaning to the observed behavior. Interviewers begin with the assumption that they do not know in advance what all the necessary questions are. Hence it is not possible to preplan a complete list of questions to ask. Here the interviewee determines the flow of the topic rather than the interviewer (Lune & Berg, 2017).

What are the steps Involved in Conducting a IDI?

Step 1: Develop an interview guide

The purpose of drafting the questions and an interview guide is to ensure that all the topics for which inputs from the interviewee are sought, are covered during the interview. This guide is essential when a number of interviews are conducted, especially when conducted by different research team members. The questions should be flexible and serve as a trigger for the interviewee to delve deep in the research topic. Sufficient time should be spent in writing, refining and pretesting the questions and the guide. It is advisable to prioritize the questions and mark them as critical, others can be categorized as optional or secondary, and can be asked if time permits. Always consider the interview guide as work in progress and depending on the feedback received in the field, adjustments in the questions will have to be considered (Galletta, 2013).

Box 1: Tips for drafting Interview Questions

- Questions should be open-ended. Example, instead of asking "Do you know about the curricular changes?" ask "Please describe what you know about the curricular changes."
- Start with simple direct question before moving on to perception/opinion questions. For example, ask, "What events were conducted as a part of this change?" before asking, "What did you think of the events?"
- Use probes as and when required. Some questions that could be used as probes include
    - Would you explain this further?
    - Can you give an example?
    - Would you explain that a bit, I'm not sure I understand what you're saying.
    - Is there anything else that you would like to add?

Step2: Identify and select interviewees

Once the target group or groups have been identified based on the research question, interviewees can be selected by random or stratified random sampling if the group is large, if the target group is small and if time and resources are not limiting factors then all members could be interviewed.

As mentioned earlier, in-depth interviews are conducted to know the shared perception or feelings of a fairly homogenous group. So, the interviewees should be selected from a similar cohort with respect to the research topic. Generally, a purposeful sampling method is followed to optimize the richness and depth of the data obtained. Based on the iterative data analysis, if gaps ae found in the responses obtained, additional interviewees may be included at a later stage.

Once the interviewees are selected, they need to be informed about the purpose of the interview, a brief introduction about the research project and approximate time that will be needed. This information can be shared either through a telephonic call or by mail. At this stage it would be a good idea to mention about the voluntary nature of participation, confidentiality and anonymity issues.

Step 3: Develop a rapport with the interviewee

Developing a rapport with the interviewee is a fundamental requirement. Unlike unstructured interviews of ethnography research where the interviews are conducted over a few days thus giving ample time for the interviewer to gain the trust and develop rapport with the interviewee, in IDI, the rapport has to be developed quickly. Having a relaxed and safe environment helps in the process. Four stages of rapport building have been described by Spradley and others. These include: apprehension, exploration, co-operation and participation (Briggs, 2002; Crabtree & Miller, 1999; Spradley, 1979). These steps have to be kept in mind while building a rapport with the interviewee.

Step 4: The Interview Process

After the initial welcome and formal introduction, interview is started with few general, even a closed ended question which can be then further probed with “why do you feel so?” or “can you explain why?” Once the interviewee moves from apprehension to exploration stage of developing rapport, you could start asking direct critical questions. As the agenda for the interview is always flexible, if the dialogue moves from question one to question three, let it go in that direction. You can always come back to the questions that were missed out. The potentially uncomfortable, controversial, or awkward questions should come toward the end (Newcomer et al., 2015).

By this time the interviewee would have reached the final stage of rapport, the participation where sharing of such information comes without hesitation. General demographic information can be filled in a standard form provided to the interviewee before or after the interview.

With the consent of the interviewee the interview can be recorded using a digital audio recorder. This will allow the interviewer to actively listen to the interviewee instead of trying to take complete notes. Interviewer may note down certain expressions or hesitancy shown while answering sensitive questions.

On completion of the session, review the interview guide to check that no key questions were missed out. The interview can then be concluded with a cordial greeting for having spent their valuable time and shared their personal views and perceptions with you.

It is a good practice to complete the interview notes by the end of the day so that the same can be shared with other members of the research team. Raw notes should be edited, reviewed and entered in a computer file while it is fresh in the mind.

What are the Ethical Issues to be Considered in Conducting IDIs?

Following four ethical issues may be considered while conducting IDIs:

1. Risk of unanticipated harm to the interviewee: When the interviewer listens actively and repeats the information back to the interviewee, sometimes this may trigger unexpected reaction from the interviewee leading to unintended harm. For example, while talking about their life experiences, some respondents may feel unexpected intense feelings ending in grief. Hence remember as an interviewer you may have to provide psychological support if the interviews create undue stress or cause psychological complications (Dicicco-Bloom & Crabtree, 2006).
2. Maintaining the interviewee's information confidential: It is very important to maintain anonymity of the interviewee's information shared with you during the interview. Many a times, interviews may lead to venting out frustrations towards higher ups in the organization. If this information leaks out, it may put the position of the interviewee in jeopardy. Hence maintaining anonymity of the interviewee while reporting is most critical.
3. Informing the interviewee about the nature of the research accurately: This is sometimes an issue when the investigator may not initially know what the preliminary interviews may reveal. The interviewee should be informed beforehand about this and given a choice to withdraw from the study anytime.
4. Chances of exploitation: Personal gain should not be a motive for conducting interviews. The contribution made by interviewees to the success of the research should be acknowledged and their efforts should be compensated in various ways (Anderson, 1991).

How are In-Depth Interviews Analyzed?

Ideally, qualitative data analysis occurs parallel with data collection. This will help the investigators to advance their understanding of the research question, which in turn will influence the sampling size and further modification of the interview questions and the guide. This reiterative process of data collection and data analysis, which is a characteristic of qualitative research analysis, eventually reaches a stage when no new categories or themes emerge. This is called the saturation of the data and is a sign that data collection is complete (Kuzel, 1992).

The first step in analysis of in-depth interview is to transcribe the data collected either from the audio recording or the hand written notes. It is important to take into account nonverbal communication as well like body language, gestures, tone of speech while transcribing the audiotapes.

Computer-assisted qualitative data analysis software such as Atlas ti, Folio Views, and NVivo is now available for data coding and theme generations.

Box 2: Steps for analysing data of In-Depth Interview
• Read a few times the transcribed notes. Observe if there are any common threads or themes emerging in the notes. • Note down the themes as you read through. • Group the responses of each participant under a theme, if similar. • While analysing, observe for any emerging new information based on demographic data. Like does gender make a difference in beliefs, experiences, could that be grouped? • Observe and note body language, eagerness to share information against mono syllabi response.

How are In-Depth Interviews Presented in a Paper?

When presenting the results of interview analysis, the format is a descriptive writing. The findings can be presented under the themes or narratives that emerged in analysis. These are then written down as a descriptive expression of the experiences narrated by the interviewee. An in-depth description of participant perspectives is shared. In interview research, the participant's words are your data (DeJonckheere & Vaughn, 2019).

What are the Potential Advantages and Disadvantages of IDIs?

Table 2: Advantages and disadvantages of interviews

Advantages	Disadvantages
Sharing the perceptions/opinions may serve as a release for the interviewee.	Time-consuming with regard to both data collection and data analysis.
Possible to get answers to all questions.	Usually done on a small scale.
Possible to get clarifications for both interviewee and interviewer.	Not possible to maintain 100% anonymity.
Comparatively less expensive, less man power required.	Potential for possible bias.
Interviews grant a sense of empowerment, and self-awareness to the interviewee.	interviewees will only give what they are willing to reveal about their perceptions and opinions.
Gives voice to the unrepresented and marginalized people.	These perceptions, being subjective might change over time and situations.

SUMMARY

The Interview is one of the commonest qualitative data collection methods used in healthcare research. It is a data gathering technique intended to present interviewee's standpoint on the research topic. IDIs are useful when one wishes to ask open-ended questions to obtain a wealth of information from relatively small number of respondents. Interviews are classified broadly into three types structured, semi structured and unstructured. Structured interviews generate quantitative data, while semi structured and unstructured are formats used in in-depth interviews to obtain qualitative data. The steps involved in conducting in-depth interview consists of four steps:

- Develop an interview guide
- Identify and select interviewees
- Establish a rapport with the interviewee
- Finally, the interview process.

A skilled interviewer will actively listen to what is being said without interruption to hear what the participant is saying. They may occasionally prompt, or request the participant to expand on an experience or belief, noting at the same time, expressions, body language, tone of voice and gestures. All these together enables the interviewer a deeper understanding of rich qualitative data (Davies et al., 2020).

The process could be preferably audio recorded to enable the interviewer to concentrate on the active listening, with occasional noting down any specific expressions or body language that may contribute to the richness of the information. The data is then transcribed. These notes can be categorized into themes that will have rich data under each area. Computer assisted software can also be used for data analysis. The presentation of this is usually in a descriptive format. The narration is usually done under themes. The observations of tone, body language noted during the interview are also described to enable a clear capture of qualitative information.

EVALUATE

India has 8.6% of the population in geriatric category as per Census 2011, with the numbers increasing at 3% per year. Of this 71% reside in rural India and 29% in urban settings (Malik et al., 2021) An initiative was undertaken to understand the health issues faced by the elderly in rural areas where access to health care is limited.

A team of five research assistants was set up to meet the elderly citizens in the Chintamani taluka in Karnataka. With 30 villages under it as a pilot study to understand their needs and issues faced by them.

Five senior citizens from each village were selected to participate. The outcome of the interactions would enable the researcher to give feedback to the health care service provider of the strengths and gaps in delivery of health care.

Question:. Please identify the stakeholder groups that could be included. How many stakeholder groups could you identify?

1. What is the ideal method that could be used to gather stakeholder opinions?
2. What are the ethical issues involved?
3. If you would like to use in-depth interview method, what are steps in preparation?
4. If you are the interviewer, List the questions that you would like use to obtain perceptions, views and beliefs of the interviewee.

ROAD AHEAD

Though face-to-face interviews are traditionally considered ideal, many a times geographical distances and selecting a suitable time may force the interviewer to look for other possible alternatives. These could be telephonic interviews, computer assisted interviewing which could be either done synchronously using various e platforms such as Zoom, MS teams, Google meet or asynchronous such as though emails or social media such as WhatsApp. COVID -19 pandemic has introduced us to many electronic virtual media that could be conveniently used to conduct interviews from the comfort of one's home.

Table 3: Briefly describes advantages and disadvantages of some of these unconventional modes of conducting interviews

Criteria	Telephonic Interviews	Virtual Media	Email/WhatsApp/Messenger
Time	Synchronous communication.	Synchronous communication.	Synchronous or asynchronous communication.
Place	Asynchronous communication.	Asynchronous communication.	Asynchronous communication.
Accessibility of the interviewee	Wide geographical access. People from all over the globe can be interviewed	Wide geographical access. People from all over the globe can be interviewed.	Wide geographical access. People from all over the globe can be interviewed.
Type of population	Possible to get hard to reach population such as duty doctors, nursing mothers, people with special needs.	Should have access to the virtual platforms.	Should be able to express fluently (language proficiency), access to smartphones or computers.
Social Clues	Body language, appearance clues lost, but voice and intonation are still available.	With video on, social clues can be easily captured.	No social clues can be picked up.
Response time	Interviewee can directly react to the question leading to more spontaneous responses.	Interviewee can directly react to the question leading to more spontaneous responses	Interviewee can reflect on the questions asked and respond after deliberation.
Data collection	Interview can be recorded and then transcribed.	Both recording and transcription of the interview is possible.	Direct transcription is available saving on time.

Further details can be obtained from the following sources.

Brinkmann, S. and Kvale, S. (2014). Interviews': Learning the Craft of Qualitative Research Interviewing. London: SAGE.

Edwards, R. and Holland, J. (2013). What Is Qualitative Interviewing? London: Bloomsbury

Howard Lune, Bruce L. Berg (2017) Qualitative Research Methods For Social Sciences, Chapter 4 A Dramaturgical Look Of Interviewing. www.downloadslide.com

Raymond Opdenakker (2006). Advantages and Disadvantages of Four Interview Techniques in Qualitative Research **DOI:** *https://doi.org/10.17169/fqs-7.4.175*

REFERENCES

Anderson, J. M. (1991). Reflexivity in fieldwork: Toward a ferninist epistemology. Image: The Journal of Nursing Scholarship, 23(2), 115–118.

Babbie, E. (2007). Tile Practice of Social Research. Belmont: Thompson Wadsworth.

Boyce, C., & Neale, P. (2006). Conducting in-depth interviews: A guide for designing and conducting in-depth interviews for evaluation input.

Briggs, C. L. (2002). Interviewing, power/knowledge, and social inequality. Handbook of Interview Research: Context and Method, 911–922.

Britten, N. (1995). Qualitative research: Qualitative interviews in medical research. Bmj, 311(6999), 251–253.

Crabtree, B. F., & Miller, W. L. (1999). Doing qualitative research. 2nd edn. Thousand Oaks, California: Sage 1999;18–20. 8

Davies, L., LeClair, K. L., Bagley, P., Blunt, H., Hinton, L., Ryan, S., & Ziebland, S. (2020). Face-to-face compared with online collected accounts of health and illness experiences: A scoping review. Qualitative Health Research, 30(13), 2092–2102.

DeJonckheere, M., & Vaughn, L. M. (2019). Semistructured interviewing in primary care research: A balance of relationship and rigour. Family Medicine and Community Health, 7(2).

Dicicco-Bloom, B., & Crabtree, B. F. (2006). The qualitative research interview. Medical Education, 40(4), 314–321. https://doi.org/10.1111/j.1365-2929.2006.02418.x

Flick, U. (2018). An introduction to qualitative research. 6th Edition, sage. Publications Inc. Thousand Oaks, California

Fontana, A., & Frey, J. H. (2005). The interview. The Sage Handbook of Qualitative Research, 3, 695–727.

Galletta, A. (2013). Mastering the semi-structured interview and beyond: From research design to analysis and publication (Vol. 18). NYU press.

Kuzel, A. J. (1992). Sampling in qualitative inquiry. In B. F. Crabtree & W. L. Miller (Eds.), *Doing qualitative research* (pp. 31–44). Sage Publications, Inc.

Lune, H., & Berg, B. L. (2017). Qualitative research methods for the social sciences. Ninth edition, Global edition, Pearson.

Malik, C., Khanna, S., Jain, Y., & Jain, R. (2021). Geriatric population in India: Demography, vulnerabilities, and healthcare challenges. Journal of Family Medicine and Primary Care, 10(1), 72.

Merriam, S. B. (1998). Qualitative Research and Case Study Applications in Education. Revised and Expanded from" Case Study Research in Education.". ERIC.

Newcomer, K. E., Hatry, H. P., & Wholey, J. S. (2015). Handbook of practical program evaluation. John Wiley & Sons. Incorporated, 2015. ProQuest Ebook Central, http://ebookcentral.proquest.com/lib/umanitoba/detail.action?docID=2144898.

Poggie Jr, J. J. (1972). Toward quality control in key informant data. Human Organization, 23–30.

Spradley, J. (1979). Asking descriptive questions. The Ethnographic Interview, 1, 44–61.

Williams, R. L., Snider, R., & Ryan, M. J. (1994). A key informant 'tree' as a tool for community oriented primary care. The Cleveland COPC Group. Family Practice Research Journal, 14(3), 273–280.

Chapter 15

Qualitative Data Analysis of Interviews

Amol R Dongre

ABSTRACT

Medical educators are often required to handle text data in the form of interview transcripts, feedbacks, free list of responses, posts on social media platforms or description of observations. Often, there is a lack of clarity on how to carry out qualitative data analysis in a systematic and scientific manner. The purpose of the present chapter is to introduce the basic terms used in qualitative data analysis and to offer robust and practical tips to thematic analysis of the text data generated during interviews. This chapter will elaborate steps in conducting qualitative data analysis such as - deciding the approach to data analysis based on theoretical underpinning, transcription, selecting the meaningful unit relevant to research questions for coding, categories, and theme generation, writing memos and reflexivity, presentation of results and steps to ensure rigor in qualitative data analysis. In the end, some resources have been suggested for further exploration.

Key Words: qualitative data analysis, transcription, codes, categories, themes

ASSESS NEED

Educational institutions are complex social environments due to mutual interaction among students, teachers, parents, society, and regulating\ accrediting agencies (Ringsted et al., 2011). Decision making in such dynamic environments require understanding and accommodation of diverse views of its stakeholders. The educational processes such as curriculum development, implementation, evaluation of educational intervention, and change management after accreditation require qualitative processes such as exploration of perspectives, understanding the problem from stakeholders' point of view, and systematic consensus building for change management. All this is best achieved through qualitative research methods.

Medical educators are required to handle text data in the form of interview transcripts (focus groups, one-to-one interviews), feedback in the form of words or short phrases, group discussions, posts on formal Learning Management System, and social platforms, and description of free observations etc. Though the basic qualitative data analysis revolves around codes and categorization, the overall approach to qualitative data analysis depends on the theoretical underpinning of research and the purpose of research (Bernard et al., 2017; Adu P., 2019). Often the qualitative findings are felt as less defensible owing to lack of transparency and robustness in qualitative analysis processes. There are ways to ensure rigor in qualitative research to generate the evidence to facilitate decision making. Hence, the purpose of the present chapter is to offer robust and practical tips to content and thematic analysis to text data generated during interviews.

BRIEF

The chapter will elaborate Qualitative Data Analysis under the following heads
1-Deciding the approach to data analysis based on theoretical underpinning
2- Steps in Qualitative Data Analysis

- Transcription,
- Selecting the meaningful unit (empirical indicator) relevant to research questions for coding,
- Categories and theme generation,
- Writing memos and reflexivity.
- Presentation of results
- Steps to ensure rigor in Qualitative Data Analysis

CONTEXTUALIZE

Imagine a situation where you as an educational researcher have interview data from your students and faculty which answers to a 'why' types of questions (Why students\faculty do the thing in the way they do so?) to explain some phenomenon. Being a novice, you get overwhelmed and feel that there is too much chaos in the text data. Now you want to find out the order in that chaos and make sense of what is going on. To make the process systematic and scientific, you must decide the approach to data analysis, transcription, coding, categorization and finally the presentation of results. The present chapter aim to offer practical tips on technical know-how of these steps. Let us begin the journey.

DESCRIBE

Deciding the approach to data analysis based on theoretical underpinning

The first step in data analysis is to decide the data analysis approach which is in alignment with the theoretical underpinning and purpose of the research. Theoretical underpinnings are philosophical assumptions about the nature of truth and reality which guides the research. Qualitative research assumes truth as multiple and subjective realities (Creswell and Clark., 2011). There are two major approaches to qualitative data analysis:

1) ***Descriptive approach*** – where the purpose is to describe and summarize information under codes and categories. It is less abstract and less iterative design. This approach is useful for less complex data. For example, it involves summarization of text data on opinion\reasons\feedbacks.

2) ***Interpretative approach*** (phenomenology, grounded theory, and ethnography) where the purpose is to make the meaning by reflecting on what does it mean? (Elliot and Timulak., 2005). Phenomenological approach helps to understand the "lived-in" experiences of the participants. In this approach, participants are asked to share their experiences with the phenomenon (van der Mescht., 2004). For example – What is lived-in experience of students undergoing a course. Vimal et al interviewed learners with problems, parents, and teachers to explore their current experiences to develop the model of student support system (Vimal et al., 2021). According to Oktay (2012), in grounded theory, the purpose is to develop a middle-range theory to explain the phenomenon of interest. It offers plausible explanation to observed behavior. Ommering et al (2020) used the grounded theory approach to know how first year medical students perceive research and which factors motivates and demotivate them. Ethnography aims to understand the culture in its natural environment from participants' point of view (Reeves et al., 2008). Becker and Hughes (1961) carried out an ethnographic study to know "how medical students progress through their first year of medical school to build their own student culture" (cited in Wilson., 1977). Being interpretative in nature, both grounded theory and ethnography are more flexible and more abstract in nature.

In both the approaches, there is a risk of influence of researchers' background and biases on the way coding, categorization and interpretations are done. Hence, researcher needs to be aware and acknowledge these influences during analysis and interpretations (Adu P., 2019). Though the basic steps in data analysis for both the approaches involves creation of codes, bring similar codes together to form categories and themes, the approach to codes and categorization for each of them varies a little. The basic steps in data analysis are – 1) Transcription, 2) Selecting the meaningful unit (empirical indicator) relevant to research questions for coding, 3) Categories and theme generation, 4) Reporting and reflexivity.

Transcription

After interviews are conducted, the next step is to transcribe the data. It can be seen as data entry phase in quantitative research. Transcription is the process of transforming spoken conversation (audio or video) to written language. It may also involve translation from regional language to English if the team involves people from diverse regions or when there is a plan to use software in data analysis. As there is conversion of spoken language into written and translation from regional languages, there is risk of loss of information. Hence, a great care is required to ensure the representation of what has been said in the interview (Gibbs., 2007).

Adu (2019) noted the benefit of traditional listen-and-type method by the researcher himself\herself. It offers the opportunity to researcher to understand the data well. This step is seen as beginning of analysis as it involves extracting the meaning of what is being said in the interview. Software programmes such as Express Scribe, Audacity and ATLAS-ti helps in transcription. Verbatim transcript is prepared to exactly capture the spoken words or lines in the interview. As transcription is a time-consuming process, it is advised to start it as soon as possible preferably same day or within a week. It might take more than three to four hours or even more to transcribe the content of a one-hour conversation. It is the responsibility of the researcher to accurately represent the thoughts of the participants in transcript. Early transcription offers an opportunity to reflect on the interview process and questioning and improve it with the subsequent interviews (Gibbs., 2007). Box 1 demonstrate a sample verbatim transcript for response to one question. Please note that it is a simulated response to a question for understanding and exercise purpose.

Box 1: Verbatim transcript (response to one question)
Interviewer: In what way, has the Covid Pandemic changed the teaching and learning for you all as a group? **Respondent (student)**: "*As a part of our routine teaching, we used to have group discussions where we used to discuss on the assigned topic. It used to help us to know what others think about it, thus help us learn from each other. After pandemic it is no longer happening. One of our most favorite was field visits to centres and nearby villages. Anything which would take us out of the campus was our favorite. It used to help us see people, their houses and interact with them. In addition to that we all would get an opportunity to closely interact with each other. Due to lock down measures, it is also not happening now. In current time, we have online lecture sessions on various online learning platforms. Sometimes teachers host quiz and MCQ tests for us.*"

Storage of data

Qualitative research involves in-depth study on a small sample size. It is researcher's responsibility to take measures to ensure confidentiality of their participants. To begin with, decide who all in the research team will have access to data. As sample size is small, it is easy to identify who said what, particularly when researchers know the participants. Hence, it is advised to anonymize the transcript by using pseudo names. The audio file, transcript and consent form for each group interview or one-to-one interview should be kept in one folder for easy retrieval. Name the files and folders to avoid the confusion. The soft copy of data should be kept in a password protected system and hard copies of transcripts should be kept in a locked cabinet.

Coding

If the research involves single data source such as interviews, small amount of data (less than 10 interviews or total less than 30 pages of transcripts) and the researcher is trained to handle the codes manually, then manual approach to coding is best (Adu P., 2019). However, if the data is large (more than 10 interviews or total more than 30 pages of transcript), and researcher is skilled and familiar with software assisted data analysis, then software (Licensed version, trial version or free software) may be used for analysis. One can use pencil or colored pens for coding on transcripts. Alternatively, one can use "new comment" function in Microsoft word (right click on selected line) to tag the relevant portion in the transcripts with the codes (Adu P., 2019). The choice of method depends on researcher's comfort and familiarity with the approach and tools used.

In content and thematic analysis, the basic meaning making tactics includes counting, clustering, linking, comparing, and summarization (Vaismoradi., 2013). A quantitative approach to qualitative data is called as content analysis. It includes counting (example - free listing, content analysis of newspaper articles) and clustering (example – use of item-by-respondent proximity matrix to get cluster analysis or network analysis). A qualitative approach to text data is called as thematic analysis where the major purpose is coding, categorization, and description of its summary (Vaismoradi., 2013; Saldana., 2009).

There are more than 32 types of coding and more than 15 types of qualitative data presentation. Descriptive and interpretative type of coding are most basic and commonly used for codes and categorization of interview data. In descriptive coding, the portion of text data which is explicitly relevant to research questions is coded or indexed. The word or the phrase for code is taken from the text itself. Descriptive coding is easy as it is less abstract. It is usually written in two to three words. In interpretative coding, the researcher has to infer the underlying meaning which is hidden in the text data. It is more abstract as it requires interpretation. Hence, there is a risk that researchers' background and prior knowledge about the subject have influence the way things are seen and interpreted (Adu P., 2109).

A sample codebook for interpretative coding exercise is given in Table-1. It is common to use both descriptive and interpretative type of coding in a single analysis process. Most of descriptive and even inferential type of qualitative data analysis revolves around this basic step of codes, categorization, and theme generation.

Table 1: Codebook development

Unit of transcript	Meaning of the unit	Code	Memo

Category and theme generation

Once the coding is done, next step is categorization. It includes the examination of characteristics of codes, its similarities and differences and then clustering the related or similar codes to form the categories. Thus, a cluster of similar codes is called as categories These categories need a label to be given. Subsequently, cluster of similar or related categories can form the theme or concept. Thus, a shift from codes to categorization and themes leads to data reduction from more specific to general. Meanings of units and memos in codebook can help in categorization and theme generation (Bernard et al., 2017; Adu P., 2019)

To bring interpretative credibility, qualitative data analysis is done by a team of two or more researchers. The exercise can be done by two investigators together, where they build the codes and categories in consensus. Secondly, one researcher does the coding and categorization, and other informed researcher reviews it. In another option two researcher do the codes and categorization independently and then review it together. Any discrepancies between the two can be resolved by mutual discussion or by consulting another researcher (Petticrew and Roberts., 2003). The researcher undertaking the coding should be aware about the literature so that s\he do not miss the new information.

Demonstration on descriptive codes and categorization

Let us code the above paragraph (not from real interview). Steps involved in thematic analysis are – 1) Transcription, 2) Code the relevant text data, 3) Bring the similar units (codes) together to form categories, 4) Summarize, describe, and report. Assume that the purpose of coding is to understand the changes in teaching and learning due to covid pandemic. Let us do the descriptive coding where the main purpose is to index what we explicitly find in the data which is relevant to our research question. Please refer to Table-2 for demonstration of codes and categorization.

Table 2: Demonstrations of codes and categorization

Transcript (Unit of analysis)	Descriptive code	Categories
Interviewer: In what way, Covid Pandemic has changed the teaching and learning for you all as a group?		
Respondent (student): "*As a part of our routine teaching, we used to have group discussions where we used to discuss on the assigned topic. It used to help us to know what others think about it, thus help us learn from each other. After pandemic it is no longer happening.*	*Group discussion*	**Teaching activities ceased.**
One of our most favorite was field visits to centres and nearby villages. Anything which would take us out of the campus was our favorite. It used to help us see people, their houses and interact with them. In addition to that we all would get an opportunity to closely interact with each other. Due to lock down measures, it is also not happening now.	*Field visits*	**Teaching activities ceased.**
In current time, we have online lecture sessions on various online learning platforms.	*Online lectures*	**Teaching activities ongoing.**
Sometimes teachers host quiz and MCQ tests for us."	*MCQ test\Quiz*	**Teaching activities ongoing.**

Thus, we got four descriptive codes – group discussion, field visits, online lectures and MCQ test\quiz. On comparison of codes with each other, you will note that codes 'group discussion' and 'field visit' are similar in the way that these activities are no longer happening. Other two codes 'online lectures' and 'mcq test/quiz' are those activities which are still ongoing. We can categorize these four codes into two categories – 1) teaching activities ceased and 2) teaching activities ongoing. You may note that the codes are closer to data as compared to categories. It is important to note that it is the content that is captured by the code is important than the words selected for the code. The length of unit coded (text in transcript) should be long enough for researcher to make out meaning when it is de-contextualized. As we move from codes to categories and themes, we tend to shift from more specific to general become more abstract in nature. In large data, one may get a greater number of categories which may be hard to summarize and describe. In such situations, a pile sort of categories may be done to form clusters of related categories, which is called as theme. When themes are linked with each other to explain the phenomenon, then it is called as theory. Following figure-1 summarize the journey from codes to a theory.

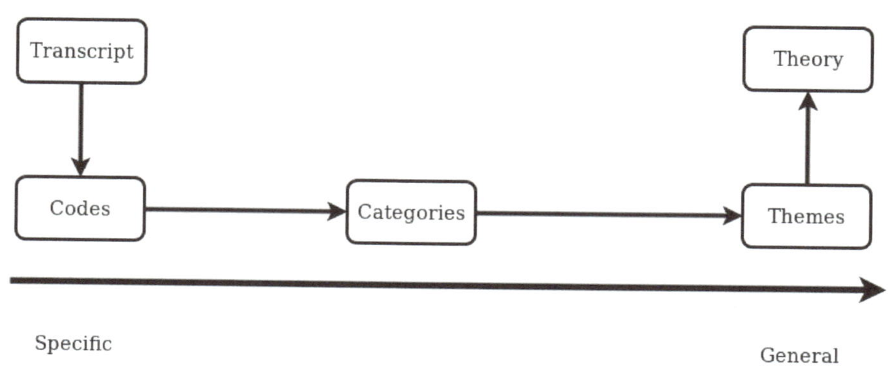

Figure 1: Journey from codes to a theory

Writing memo and reflexivity

In complex data with statement having latent meanings, it is important to document the researchers' thought or reflections about codes and yet-to-be examined ideas – known as memos (Gibbs., 2007). The documentation of memos helps to hold the transient thoughts emerged during coding and subsequently bring more direction and clarity to categorization process. In addition, the act of comparison of codes, themes and theories help discover new ideas. These analytic memos help to link themes (concepts) to form a theory to explain the phenomenon of interest. Hence, its explicit documentation during the coding process is an essential step.

When the meaning of statements to be coded is explicit, then descriptive coding is close to intended meaning of the participants. However, in interpretative coding, as researcher has to think of implicit meaning hidden in the lines, there is a risk of influence of researchers' background, subject knowledge, and perspectives. In such cases, bracketing i.e., setting aside the researcher's biases and perspectives while coding is crucial to accurately make out the meaning of what has been said in the interviews (Newman, 2010 cited in Adu P., 2019). It is advised that researchers think, and document their preconceptions about study topic, its sources, and their response to the research questions before embarking on the coding exercise.

The memo i.e., reflective thoughts about code can be documented on margin of the transcripts, in a separate diary or as audio memo which ever methods is convenient for researcher to retrieve and refer. This exercise of documenting brings their perceptions to the level of consciousness. It is to be kept in mind that the purpose is not to ignore researcher's perceptions if supported by data, but to allow coding of data other than these perspectives to capture diversity.

Presentation of results

At descriptive level, the results can be presented as description of themes and categories. You may provide representative quotes under each description. You can examine the number and frequency of codes to get its 'groundedness' in the data. The frequency of codes may help in comparison and discovery of themes. One may present complex data in visual form such as a conceptual framework, pathway, or a network diagram for better explanation. The results can also be presented as non-hierarchical typology. It is to be kept in mind that the output should be presented in such a manner that it answers the research questions.

At inferential level, a code-by-respondent proximity matrix may be obtained for carrying out analysis by using visualization techniques such as correspondence analysis or network analysis (Bernard et al., 2017). These data reduction techniques help to identify the salient or central codes. Such proximity matrix can be easily obtained in software assisted qualitative data analysis. The steps in data analysis and reporting have been presented in the following figure. The findings of qualitative study can be reported using established checklist such as Consolidated Criteria for Reporting Qualitative Research (Tong et al., 2007). One has to make the best efforts to illuminate the context, methods chosen, rational for choices and decision taken, so as to help the readers to make decision on applicability of findings to their settings. Figure-2 summarizes the basic steps in data analysis and measures required to ensure rigor in study findings.

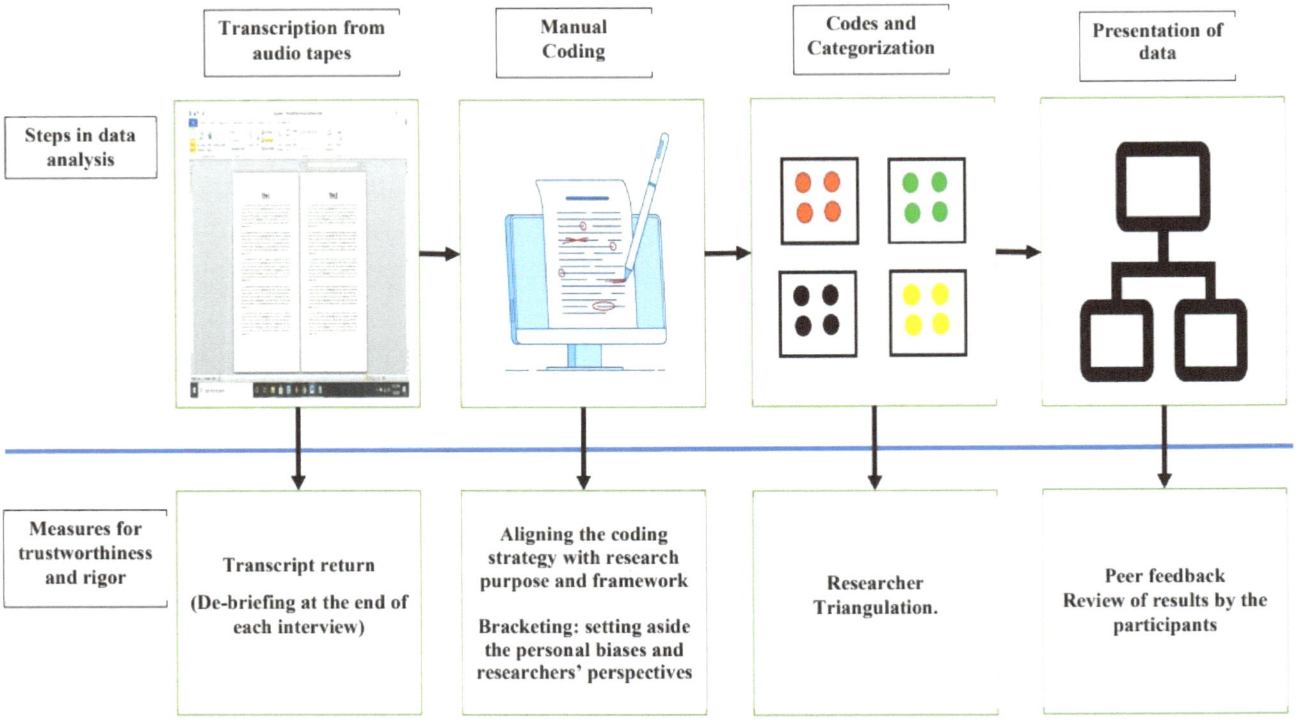

Figure 2: Steps in data analysis and corresponding steps to ensure rigor in results

Measures to improve the rigor in QDA

In quantitative research, the quality of evidence is decided by internal and external validity. The generalizability in quantitative research is of decided by statistical generalizability model. In qualitative research, it decided by the transferability model of generalizability and credibility. The credibility of qualitative research can be enhanced by ensuring congruency between study findings and reality (Merriam., 2009, cited in Gerber et al., 2017). It is achieved by measures such as – participant validation, where the interviewer checks his\her understanding with the participants so that s\he can accurately represent what participant has said. Participants may be given the transcript to review and edit before subjecting it for analysis (Saldana., 2009). The researcher may share findings with the peers, or externals for their review and comments. Denzin (1978) has proposed four strategies for triangulation – 1) using more than one source of data collection (method triangulation), 2) using more than one source for data collection (source triangulation), 3) use more than one researcher in data analysis and interpretation (researcher triangulation) and 4) use of multiple theories to confirm the findings (Cited in Gerber et al., 2017). Among the various ways to ensure credibility, researcher may choose two to three approaches which are feasible and relevant to the research purpose.

Transferability refers to extent to which the findings of the present study can be applied to other similar settings (Munn et al., 2014, Gerber et al., 2017). The researcher should illuminate the context in which the present study was undertaken. It should include details on back background of the setting, number of participants, their demographics, sampling, tools used for data collection, methods, duration of interviews and duration of the study. Researcher should explain the logic of inquiry and should describe the methods in detail. This detail of the context is expected to help the readers to decide on suitability of findings to their own circumstances (Ringsted et al., 2011). Theories or models developed to explain the phenomenon of interest may have analytic generalizability. Hence, findings of qualitative research may be considered for generalizability using transferability and analytic generalizability model (Polit and Beck., 2010).

SUMMARIZE

1. Review the study objectives\purpose\research questions
2. Review the theoretical underpinning used for study design and data collection
3. Decide the approach to data analysis which is congruent to research questions and theoretical underpinning used for guiding the study
4. Decide the type of coding required
5. Document your thoughts about the research questions, and its sources for bracketing
6. Undertake coding and categorization
7. Report the findings
8. Ensure credibility – member checking, peer review of results, triangulation
9. Illuminate the context and procedures used for data collection for transferability
10. Report the findings in such a way that it answers the research questions
11. Findings of qualitative research can be generalized using transferability and analytic generalizability model.

EVALUATE

Try your hand at coding and then categorizing the codes from these interviews. You may select a paragraph or transcript for hands-on practice line-by-line coding. Apply the lessons learned. You may do this activity in a pair. Decide the objective and start the coding and categorization.

ROAD AHEAD

There are several ways to approach to qualitative data analysis. It depends on the purpose and type of data one has. It is always better to be focused and offer clarifications for the choices made in data analysis approach. As each data is unique, one needs to be flexible and creative to meet the purpose of analysis. The emerging output is thus, influenced by theoretical sensitivity of the researchers and their approach to the research questions. You may go through following YouTube video - "What to do with your qualitative data?" (Dr. Philip Adu) - *https://www.youtube.com/watch?v=QnbX55u1J7k.*

Suggested reading

Adu P. A step-by-step guide to qualitative data coding. New York: Routledge; 2019.p.1-444.

Green, J., and Thorogood, N. Qualitative Methods for Health Research. In Silverman, D (Ed). London: The SAGE Publications; 2014.

REFERENCES

Adu, P. (2019). *A step-by-step guide to qualitative data coding.* New York, Routledge, p.1-444.

Bernard, H. R., Wutich, A., Ryan, G. W. (2017). *Analysing qualitative data: systematic approaches.* 2nd ed. New Delhi: SAGE Publications, p.1-576.

Creswell, J.W., Clark, V.L.P. (2011). *Designing and conducting mixed methods research.* 2nd ed. New Delhi: Sage Publications, p.1-275.

Elliot, R., Timulak, L. (2005). *Descriptive and interpretative approaches to qualitative research.* Accessed from:*http://nideffer.net/classes/GCT_RPI_S14/readings/interpretive.pdf.*

Gerber, H.R., Abrams, S.S., Curwood, J.S., Magnifico, A.M. (2017). *Conducting qualitative research in learning in online spaces.* London: SAGE Publications, p.1-232.

Gibbs, G. (2007). Data preparation. In Flick U. (Ed.), *Analyzing qualitative data.* London: The SAGE Qualitative Research Kit.

Gibbs, G. (2007). Analytic quality and ethics. In Flick U. (Ed.), *Analyzing qualitative data.* London: The SAGE Qualitative Research Kit.

Miles, M.B., Huberman, A. M., Saldana, J. (2014). *Qualitative dataanalysis: a methods source book.* 3rd ed. University of Michigan: Sage Publications, p.1-263.

Munn, Z., Porritt, K., Lockwood, C., Aromataris, E., Pearson, A. (2014). *Establishing confidence in the ouput of qualitative research synthesis: the ConQual approach.* BMC Medical Research Methodology, 14:108.

Oktay, J.S. (2012). *Grounded theory: Pocket guide to social work research methods.* New York: *Oxford University Press*, p.1-192.

Ommering, BWC., Wijnen-Meijer, M., Dolmans, D.H.J.M. et al (2020). Promoting positive perceptions of and motivation for research among undergraduate medical students to stimulate future research involvement: a grounded theory study. *BMC Med Educ*, 20(1), 204.

Petticrew, M., Roberts H. (2003) Evidence, hierarchies, and typologies: horses for courses. *J Epidemiol Community Health*, 57(7), 527-529.

Polit, D.F., Beck, C.T. (2010). Generalization in quantitative and qualitative research: Myths and strategies. *International J of Nursing*, 47, 1451-1458.

Reeves, S., Kuper, A., Hodges, B.D. (2008). Qualitative research methodologies: ethnography. *BMJ*, 337, Accessed from doi: *https://doi.org/10.1136/bmj.a1020*

Ringsted, C., Hodges, B., Scherpbier, A. (2011).'The research compass': an introduction to research in medical education: AMEE Guide No. 56. *Med Teach*, 33(9), 695-709.

Saldana J. (2009). The coding manual for the qualitative researchers. London: *The SAGE Publication*, p.1-260.

Tong, A., Sainsbury, P., Craig, J. (2007). Consolidated criteria for reporting qualitative research (COREQ): a 32-item checklist for interviews and focus groups. *Int J Qual Health Care*, 19(6), 349–357.

Vaismoradi, M., Turunen, H., Bondas, T. (2013). Content analysis and thematic analysis: Implications for conducting a qualitative descriptive study. *Nurs Health Sci*, 15(3), 398–405.

Van der Mescht, H. (2004). Phenomenology in education: a case study in educational leadership. *Indo-Pacific Journal of Phenomenology*, 4(1), 1-16.

Vimal, M., Dongre, A.R., Nishanti, A., Kagne, N. (2021). Student support system for medical undergraduates: A qualitative exploration of stakeholder perspectives. *J Edu Health Promot*, 10(1), 150.

Wilson, S. (1977). The Use of Ethnographic Techniques in Educational Research. *Rev Educ Res*, 47(1), 245-265.

Chapter 16

Principles of Software use in Qualitative Data Analysis (QDA)

Amita Ray, Harshal Sabane

ABSTRACT

Quantitative and qualitative analysis is akin to swimming in the pool as against the ocean. One may find swimming in a pool easier as the pool provides a structured environment where there is a labeled entry, exit and a track to follow. This is what most medical education researchers are accustomed to with quantitative research. With its iterative and looping approach, qualitative analysis may feel like a dip in the ocean with multiple ports of entry, exit and depths of analysis. Since the advent of computer assisted qualitative data analysis (CAQDA) managing voluminous datasets with a variety of data inputs has been rendered a relatively less arduous task. In this chapter we will introduce the reader to the principles of software use for qualitative analysis with examples and screenshots of the step-by-step process.

Key Words: qualitative analysis (QDA); computer assisted qualitative data analysis (CAQDA)

ASSESS NEED

Qualitative research is a methodological approach which aims to understand the participant's point of view, and their social context on a given theme as interpreted by the investigator. (Trena M. et al., 2016; Camargo et al., 2013) Until the mid-80s quantitative research was considered the only reliable way of collecting data. Since 1977, Bardin popularized a method of qualitative data analysis (QDA) by content analysis. This had many advantages, however certain challenges remained like the lack of methodological rigor and difficulty in handling extensive databases. (Schlosser et al., 2011; Franzosi R et al., 2013) This need led to the development of software packages for assisting in QDA which have since become widespread. (Souza et al., 2018; Niedbalski et al., 2017)

Qualitative data refers to non-numeric information such as interview transcripts, notes, video and audio recordings, images, and text documents. Qualitative research in medical education usually answers the question "how" an educational intervention works in contrast to quantitative research in medical science which "compares" a medical intervention with another to ascertain which would give better health care results. Unlike quantitative analysis it does not deal with numbers rather it deals with themes and codes. Allotting codes and themes to qualitative data manually is a tedious and time-consuming endeavour. Since the advent of computer assisted qualitative data analysis (CAQDA) managing voluminous datasets with a variety of data inputs has been rendered a relatively less arduous task. Another case for use of software in QDA is that it has demonstrated increased reflectivity in the researcher by increasing reflective consciousness (Woods et al., 2015; Schlosser et al., 2019).

Reflective consciousness is the awareness that enables a person to reflect on his own activities. Reflecting on our own activities while doing qualitative analysis is essential to increase the robustness and rigor of the analysis. As qualitative investigators, we need to be aware of our contribution to the construction of meanings and of life experiences.

Presently there are dozens of CAQDAs available and each of them have their own strengths and weaknesses. Having said that, most of them work on the function of descending hierarchical classification (Camargo et al., 2013). In this chapter we will introduce the software used for qualitative data analysis focusing on the common workflow and procedures.

BRIEF

After reading this chapter the reader should be able to understand and emulate the following steps in the use of software for qualitative data analysis.

- Creating a Project
- Importing data
- Understanding the workstation
- Creating quotations in the document
- Coding
- Categorization of codes and theme generation
- Querying the data
- Generating a report

It is important to remember that these steps do not necessarily follow a linear progression.

CONTEXTUALIZE

Madame Quantity in High Grade Medical College is a medical teacher, a practitioner and a researcher all rolled in one. She had done a lot of research in her own specialty and had 50 publications in indexed journals. Since she read about qualitative research, she felt that her resume would be enhanced if she could do qualitative research. So, she chose a research topic and did 20 interviews of students.

Having completed the interviews Madame Quantity is deluged with information and does not know how to code, analyze, interpret, and document the results of her study.

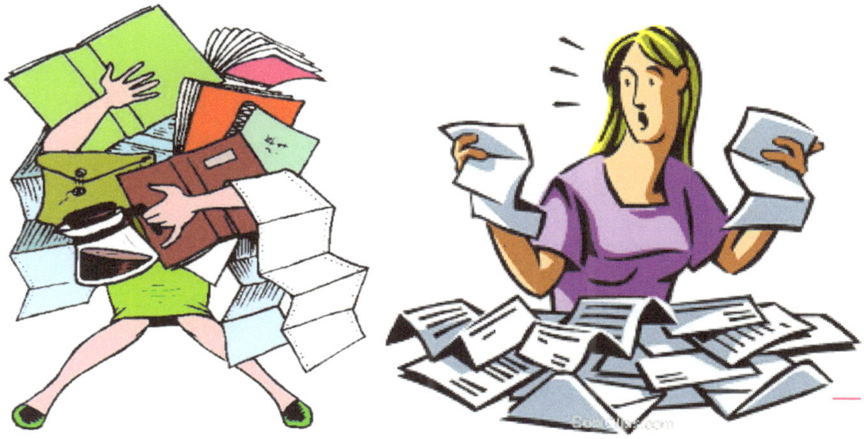

DESCRIBE

The generic workflow in the CAQDAs is discussed below. It is assumed that the reader is familiar with preliminary glossary and steps in QDA. For the neophyte as well as the veteran alike, it would benefit to read the chapter on QDA preceding this chapter before starting with the software. Bear in mind that unlike quantitative, qualitative analysis does not flow from point A to B and then to C. Barring few obvious exceptions such as grouping codes before coding, many steps in the analysis can be done simultaneously or one before the other. We will be using references to ATLAS.ti and NVivo in the chapter but most other software doing QDA would have comparable features and the generic flow of the analysis presented in the chapter can be used in them as well.

Downloading the software

The trial versions of the software are available on their respective websites. At the time of writing of this chapter, ATLAS.ti can be downloaded from atlastti.com and NVivo from qsrinternational.com. The installation is straightforward and mimics software installations like most other software. There are scores of other software for QDA and some of them are free. Expectedly, the free software has limitations in comparison with the paid software.

Creating a “project”

Next is the creation of a project with a specific name which will store your data. This ensures that you have all the data in one place and the software is ready to help guide you to the next step. You might already have a project created in the software and want to work on it further. In that case, click on “open an existing project”. Be sure to give a name to your project for an appropriate and easy identification. A helpful tip would be to periodically create a back-up of the project in a secure location on your desktop to avoid loss of work.

Importing your data

Now that you have created a project the next step is importing all your research materials including word documents of interviews, focus group discussion, PDFs, datasets, audio, video, pictures, memos etc. into the created folder. All data that you would like to analyze should be imported into this project. The supported formats are:

- *Text*:.doc;.docx,.rtf,.odt,.htm,.html,.txt and.ooxml. A plethora of transcripts prepared by transcribing software like Easytranscript, f4 & f5 transcript, Transcribe, Inqsribe, Transana, ExpressSribe are supported. Apart from these auto-generated transcripts in SRT and VTT format from practically all sites are also import compatible with Atlas.ti.
- *Image:* bmp, gif, jpeg, jpg, png, tif and tiff.
- *Audio file formats*: aac, m4a, mp3, mp4, wav.
- *Video file formats*: 3g2, 3gp, 3gp2, 3gpp, asf, avi, m4v, mov, mp4, wmv
- *Reference manager data*: Endnote XML (Atlas.ti quick tour - Windows., n.d)

When you click on the project icon you will get the screen below and you can click on the import files to bring all your files which you require for the analysis.

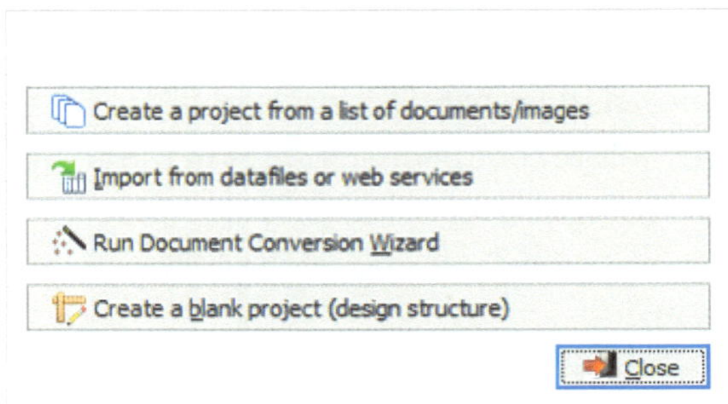

Figure 1: The dialog box for common starting options

Once you click on the import files it will show you the files you have in your PC as below. You could select the one you need or if you require several you can press the control button as you would do for other computer processes.

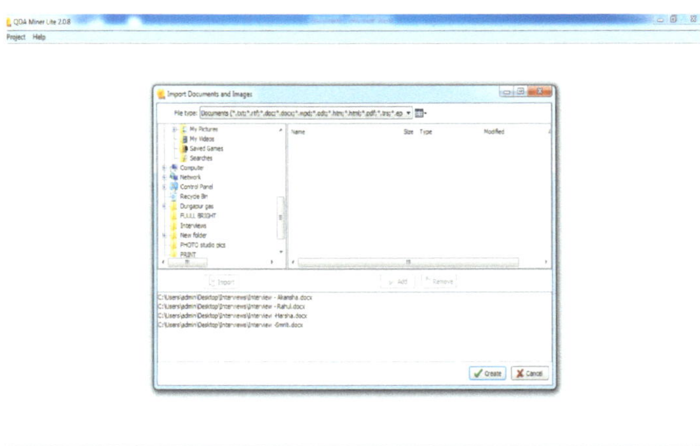

Figure 2: Document import screen

Overview of the Workstation in QDA software

Each software available for QDA has a different set of features and utilities. We will be using a sample of the landing page to get familiar with the sections after creating a new project. Every software has a different set of features and utilities. We have shown below a screen shot to illustrate this. Remember this screen will appear only after you have imported your transcripts into a project folder.

The features of this workstation are:

1. Menu bar at the top.
2. Case window, which contains the list of available cases in the project. These cases are displayed either as a list or grouped as a tree. This window is used mainly to browse through cases and select the active case on which to work.
3. Variables window, which displays and allows editing of values for any variable associated with the currently active case. Example of variable could be the age, gender, or years of experience.
4. Codes window, located in the lower left corner of the screen, contains all codes currently defined in the codebook.
5. Document window is the large window on the right side of the screen and is the main working space. This window is used to view and edit documents and images and assign codes to text segments or image areas. The document that is to be coded is opened in this window by clicking the desired document icon in the project folder. When a case contains more than one document or image, you can switch between them by selecting the document/image tab located in the top left corner of this window.
6. To the right of the document window is an area used to display the codes assigned to text segments and image areas. A second area is displayed below the images. Colored brackets are used to indicate the physical limits of the coded segment. This area is used to review coding, remove, or change assigned codes, and attach notes to any coded segment.

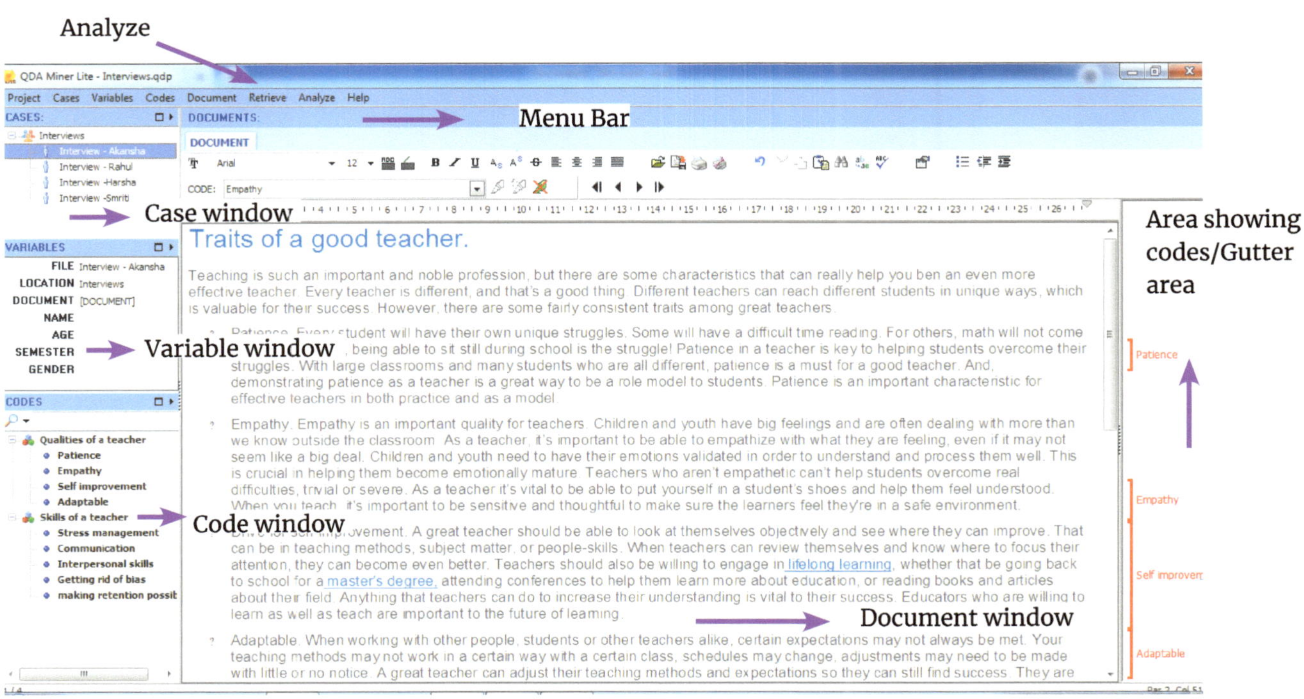

Figure 3: The Workstation

Creating Quotations in text documents

This is the process of selecting interesting segments of data relating to the phenomenon under study. Once a quotation is made it can be retrieved or reviewed later. This is typically done when the researcher is perusing the data and getting a "feel" of it. One can name the quotation and add description in memo on the quotation. This is like working on a whiteboard canvas in pen-and-paper setup where the researcher would typically place post-it notes defining or describing the code that will go with the quotation. The researcher may choose to code the quotations right away but should steer away from this pressure if the codes are not ready. It is advisable to come back to coding quotations once a bird's eye view of the transcripts is captured.

Coding

Coding is the strategy that moves data from diffuse and messy text to organized ideas about what is going on. It is the assignment of conceptual tags to segments of information that are of interest to the research objective. Ultimately these quotations and codes will shape the framework which will scaffold the theory emerging from the project. (Archer et al., 2017). Its importance cannot be overstated.

Coding can be done by various attributes but the thing that remains the same is that all quotations labeled with a particular code share a commonality. The common denominator is dependent on the research question and there are no set guidelines for it. For example, selecting a paragraph about water quality and coding it at the node 'water quality'. Node is the word used by the software to denote a container for the codes.

Steps to follow:

1. Select a phrase or word that you would like to code.
2. Go to the Top Menubar and press "code"/Right click
3. Drop-down menu shows create code or add code. When you click on that the following dialogue box appears.

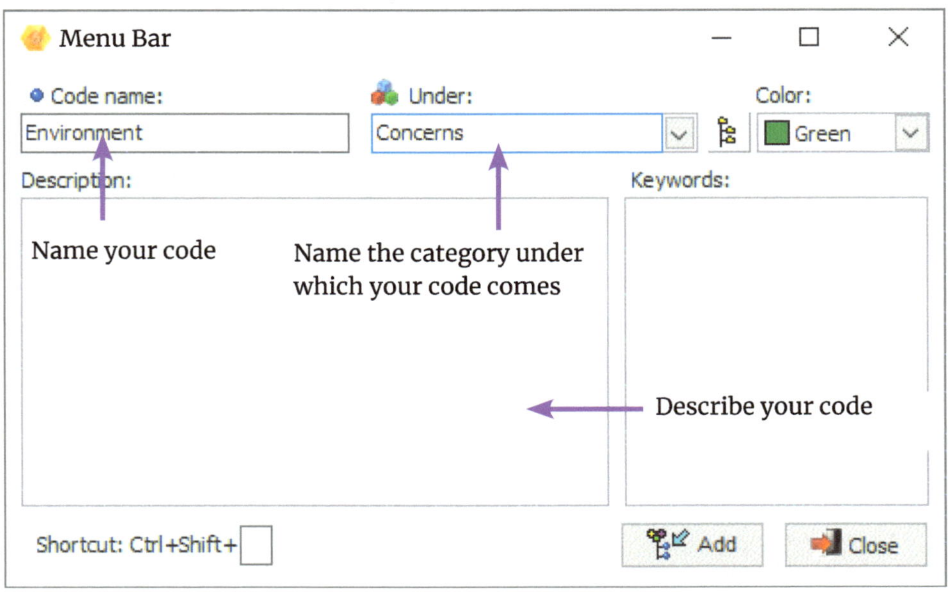

Figure 4: Coding window and its description

Once this is done the new code will show up in the code box under a specific category. In the gutter area there will appear flower brackets at the spot where this code (phrase or word) is quoted (Image 3). The next time when you want to assign the same code, select the area of the graphic/text you want to code and double-click the code in the code list.

Here is an example:

> We have interviewed 5 students. We asked them to express their views on what they think are the qualities of a good teacher and the skills required for effective teaching. One of these interviews is coded as shown below.

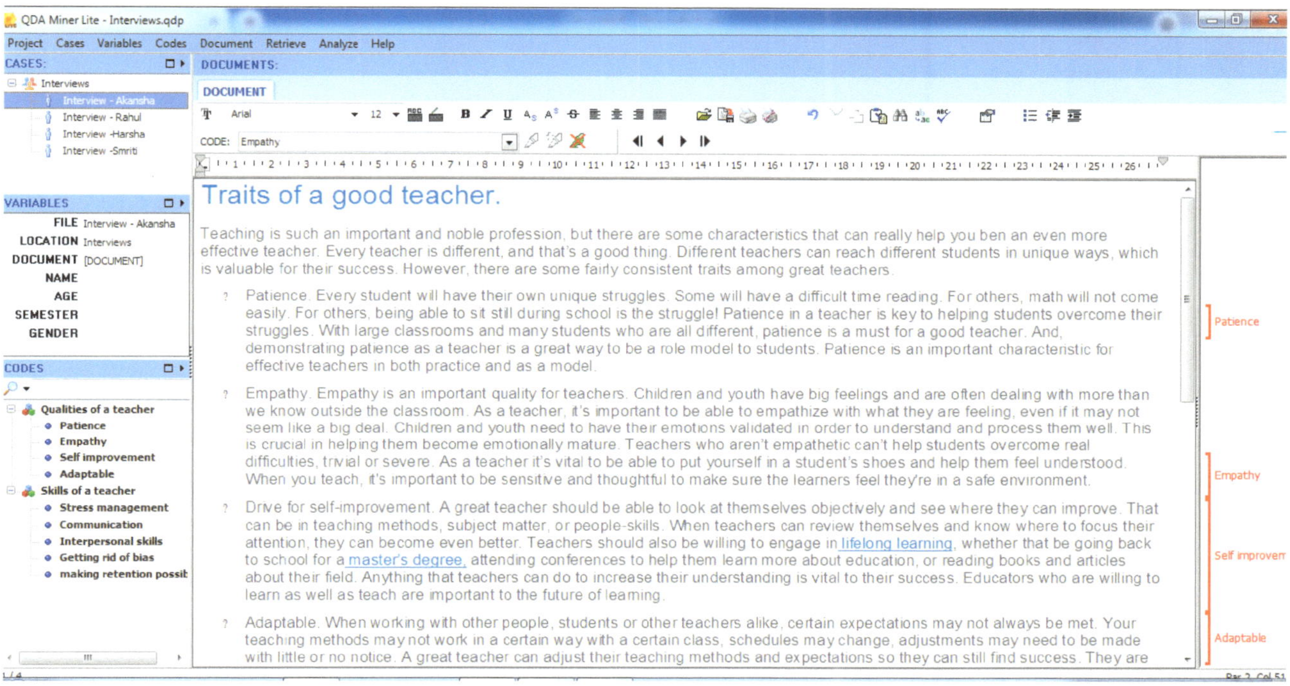

Figure 5: Document view showing codes.

After all your coding is done it is advisable to go through all your transcripts and have a rethink on whether you would like to merge, delete, change category or edit your codes.

If so, you need to click on the Code button and select the appropriate action from the drop-down menu shown below:

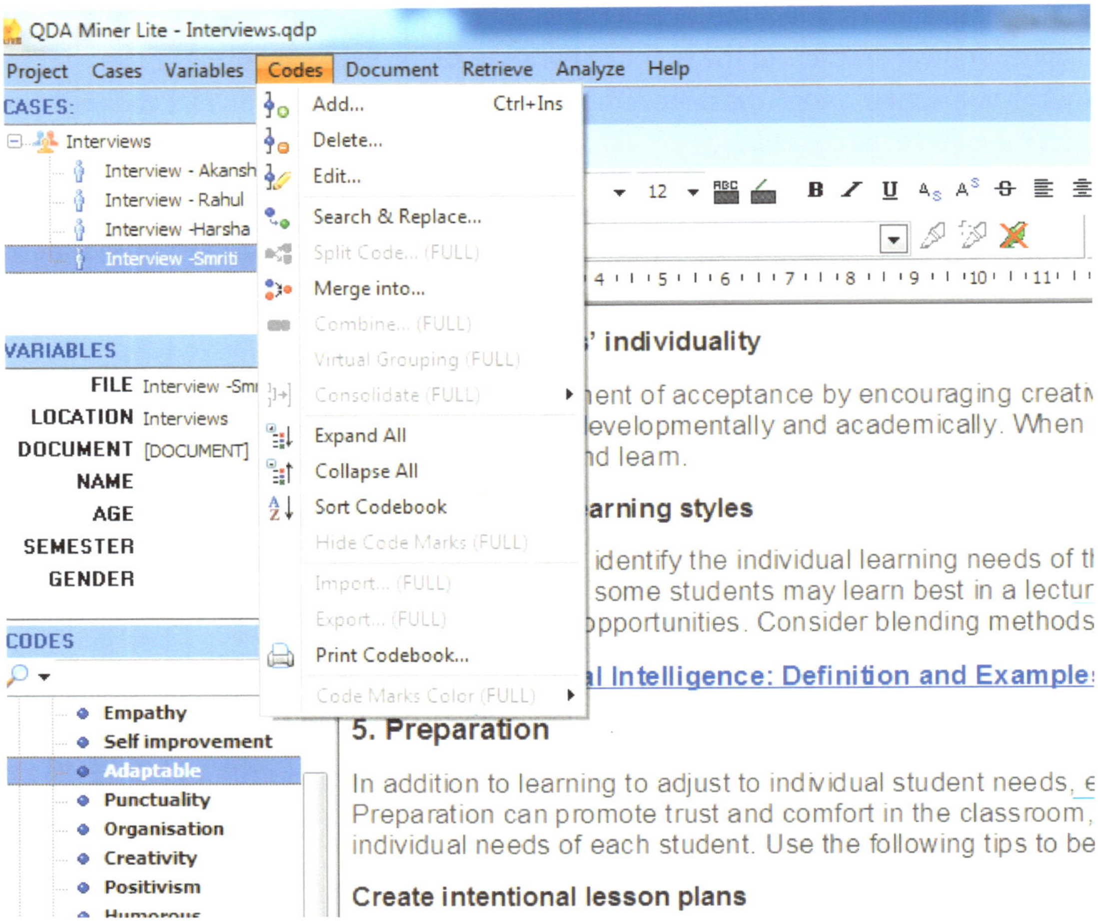

Figure 6: Common operations available for codes.

A priori and Emergent coding

The researcher can prepare a skeleton of codes even before starting the qualitative data collection. Superficial codes pertaining to chief socio-demographic factors are examples of codes that can be present a-priori (before-the-fact). Sometimes the researcher anticipates some conceptual connections in the resource documents and creates codes beforehand to label when these connections are spotted.

Emergent coding is the more classical approach where codes are generated after the researcher has completed "feeling" the data. It might be worth reiterating that coding can be skipped until a significant number of transcripts are read, else one runs the risk of generating too many codes without any thought-out function.

Grouping Codes

The process of grouping codes is remarkably like that of grouping documents. In addition, to being used as local filters (used to visualize all grouped codes) and global filters (used to run a query on one or more selected codes), code groups are also used in the code document table discussed later in the chapter.

Merging codes

If one ends up having too many codes or would like to combine granular codes together to a higher abstract level, one may merge codes. Sometimes two codes will share a similar meaning and can be merged.

Categorizing codes

Categorization is simply the process of reviewing everything that is coded and then **creating code categories** that can be used to guide future analysis. In other words, it is about creating categories for the set of codes. A practical example could be as follows: If different types of animals in a particular habitat is the topic of the interview, initial codes may be "monkeys", "snakes" and "lions". During categorization, the categories could be reptiles, amphibians, or mammals. This helps the data to be more organized and enriched in that new connections are generated between different groups of codes. The codes also go from specific to general.

The next step is to identify the themes in the data.

Theme identification\Theme generation

From categorization emerges the themes. The coding and categorization processes will reveal the theme of the narrative and therefore the next step would be to identify the themes in the data set. When determining themes, the coding and categorization must be kept in focus and one should logically flow into the other i.e., from codes to categories and onto themes. If we take the above example, we could say that an emerging theme from the above would be the "fauna" in a particular habitat. And another theme that could go with it could be "flora" although not described above.

This is how meaningful inferences and conclusions can be drawn from data. The inferences that are drawn would be crucial in generating a report or a narrative from the data and the nature of which would depend on the research aims and objectives. This narrative should be able to answer the research question that was posed at the beginning of the qualitative study as explained in the previous chapter.

Querying the data

After the coding is done the next step would be to query the data or analyze it.

In the software top bar there will be a button which says query or analyze which will give a drop-down menu for a lot of query or analysis options.

Some of the data querying tools available in QDA software:

Coding frequency

This is a simple table showing the frequency distribution of the applied codes in the document.

	Count	% Codes	Cases	% Cases
Qualities of a teacher				
Creativity	15	20.5%	4	100.0%
Empathy	3	4.1%	2	50.0%
Humorous	2	2.7%	1	25.0%
Organisation	5	6.8%	3	75.0%
Patience	1	1.4%	1	25.0%
Punctuality	2	2.7%	2	50.0%
Role modelling	6	8.2%	2	50.0%
Self improvement	9	12.3%	4	100.0%
Skills of a teacher				
Communication	17	23.3%	4	100.0%
Ethical Practice	4	5.5%	2	50.0%
Getting rid of bias	4	5.5%	2	50.0%
Interpersonal skills	2	2.7%	1	25.0%
making retention possible	2	2.7%	1	25.0%
Stress management	1	1.4%	1	25.0%

Figure 8: Frequency distribution table of codes applied.

Code document table

It is a cross tabulation of codes or code groups within documents or document groups. It depicts the frequency of appearance of a code in a document or document group.

	Effects of p... 4 8	Gender::fe... 13 26	has children... 9 18	has children... 15 30	Totals
Positiv... 6 41	4	2	2	3	11
RQ 2 14 117	4	5	5	9	23
Totals	8	7	7	12	34

Figure 9: The code document table

The Sankey Diagram

This is a visual representation of the code document table. The rows and columns of the table are presented as the nodes and edges in a Sankey diagram. Each node on the diagram represents a number in a cell of the table. The thickness of the node is proportional to the co-occurrence frequency.

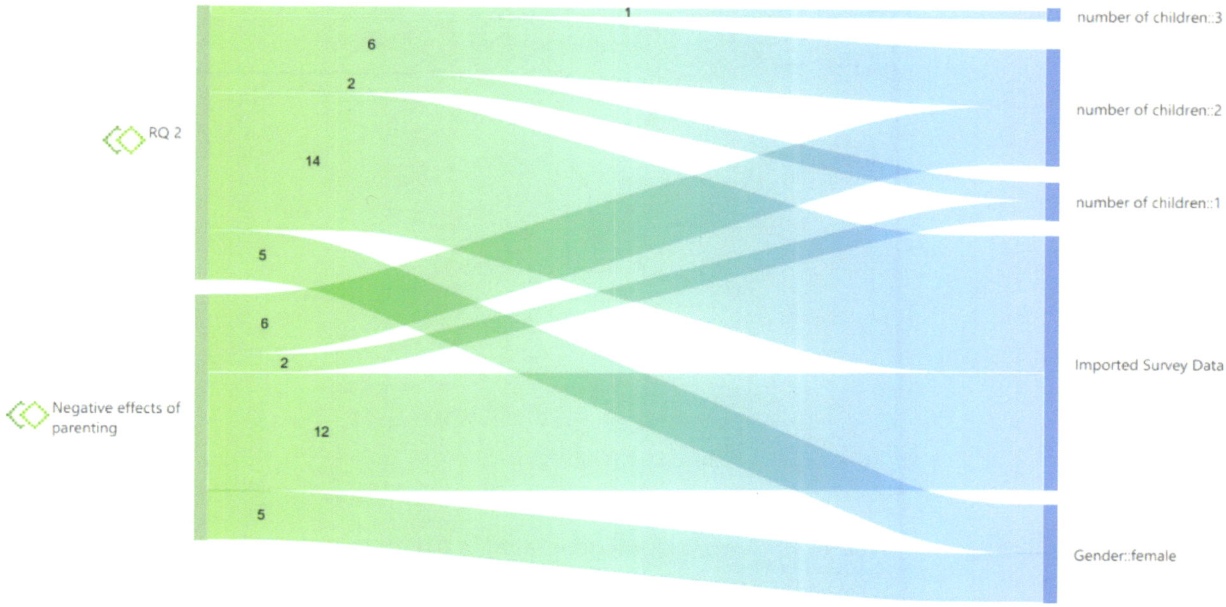

Figure 10: The Sankey diagram

Let us study the Sankey diagram shown above. It shows us the co-occurrence of 2 codes (on left) with 5 document groups (on right). The darker line adjacent to the names of the codes and documents is the "node". The thickness of codes shown on the left is almost equal. This is because the document groups mention these 2 codes with approximately equal frequency. From the diagram it can be inferred that the documents generated from couples having 3 children were least and most documents came from imported survey data. Finally, the number on the band between two nodes shows the numerical frequency of the co-occurrence of the two entities.

Code Co-occurrence analysis

If you have a reason to believe that 2 or more codes will occur simultaneously then this can be further explored by the code co-occurrence analysis. It also sets the stage for interesting chance occurrence findings. It presents result for codes that have been applied to same quotations. This is useful when there are passages that have content that is thematically in close proximity to others.

Like the code-document table, a Sankey diagram for code co-occurrence is also generated.

Word cloud

Word cloud is an interesting method to depict the frequently used words in the transcripts. Words with the maximum frequency revolve around the central theme of the research. (Wiltshier et al., 2011) A flip side of generating word cloud is the frequent usage of articles such as "a", "the", "is", "was" etc. which invariably are the most frequently used words. To suppress counting of these words, a stop list can be given to the software. All words entered in the stop list will be excluded from being measured. The cloud can be exported as an image file to be used in other documents.

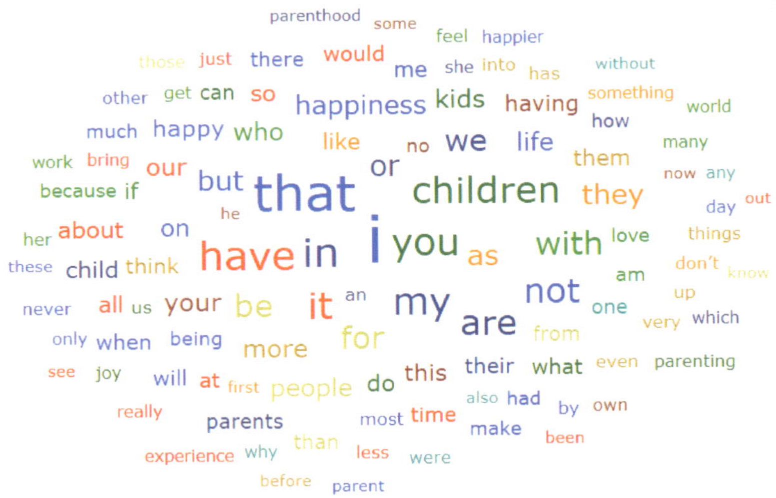

Figure 11: A word cloud generated in ATLAS.ti

The Network

The network is the most analogous to the whiteboard work of a qualitative researcher. It gives the flexibility of plotting codes, documents, quotations and memos in a visual landscape. It may be intuitive for representing complex relations by graphical means.

Once a blank network is created elements to be visualized in the network can be added by simply dragging and dropping them on the workspace. Each entry on the workspace is now a standalone, called as a "node". The nodes are connected to form a network. To do this select the node to be connected. A white dot appears on the left side of it. Drag and drop this dot on the node to be connected and select a relation between the 2 nodes from a drop-down list.

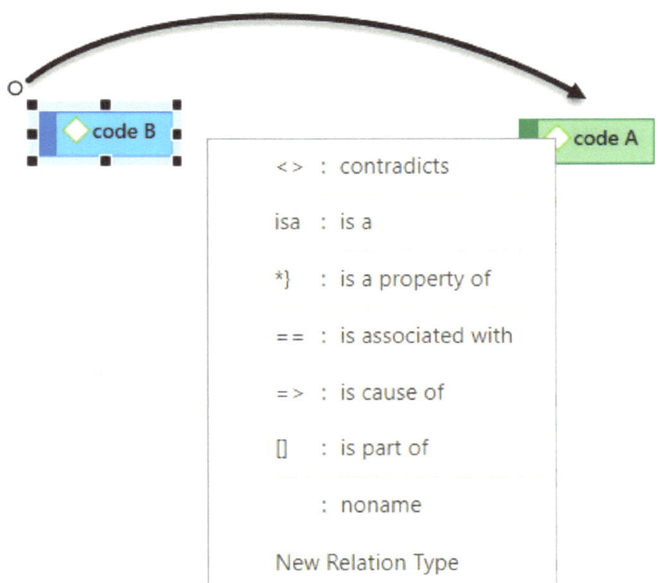

Figure 12: Connecting the nodes in a network

Creating a report

After the analysis and querying, comes the final step of creating a report which answers the research question. Keeping this in mind the researcher can chose to represent the data in the various forms described above namely a code frequency table, a code document table, a Sankey diagram, a word cloud showing predominance, a network showing relationships etc. Besides these analytical features that have been described above there are several others depending upon the software used. Whatever may be the analytical or querying tool it should adequately answer the research question.

SUMMARIZE

The three stages below summarize the principles of software use in qualitative data analysis.

Stage I

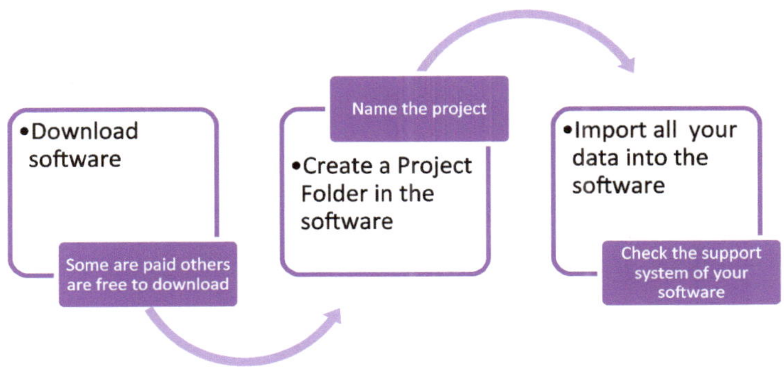

Stage II

Understand your work-space

- 1 What each section represents
- 2 What are the icons in the top bar
- 3 What are the functions that you can perform using both the above

Stage III

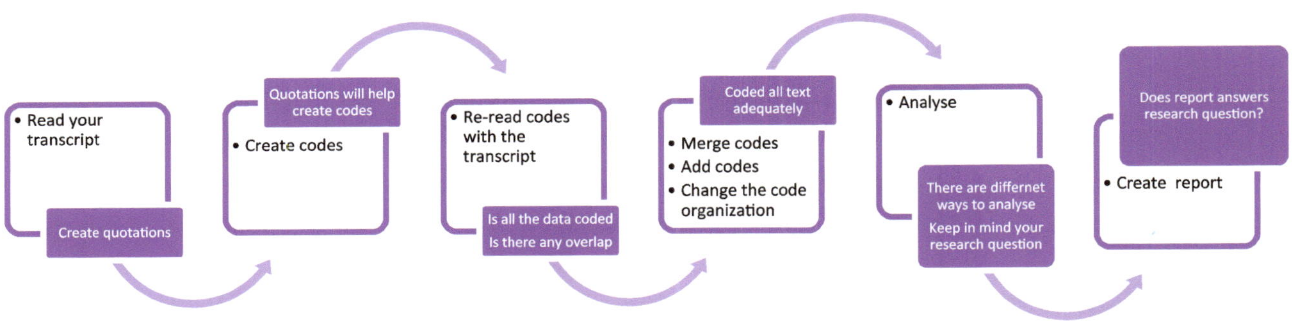

EVALUATE

Ponder on the following questions. These will help strengthen the use of CAQDAs in your own qualitative research.

- In your own work as a researcher have you ever felt drowned by qualitative data and wished there were more assistance?
- Have you avoided conducting qualitative research because of challenges with data analysis?
- Reading the chapters on qualitative data analysis and CAQDAs do you now feel more confident about your ability to deal with this arm of research?
- Please give us your feedback as well as your suggestions on how we could help you.

ROAD AHEAD

Each software available for CAQDA deserves a book of its own. The authors are aware that this chapter is an introduction to the vast possibilities to be availed by the qualitative researcher to free up his/her time for more abstract and higher-level analysis. If not already using one or more software as discussed above, the interested reader can use a vast online resource bank for further reading according to the software selected for use. Some of the recommended sources are:

- ATLAS.ti quick tour available at *https://doc.atlasti.com/ManualWin.v9/ATLAS.ti_ManualWin.v9.pdf*
- A ton of free training on qualitative analysis in general and ATLAS.ti is available at *https://atlasti.com/learning/free-training/*. This page includes demo webinars, demonstrations, methodology discussions etc.
- An excellent accompaniment after reading this chapter for the time constrained would be *https://atlasti.com/video-tutorials/atlas-ti-9-videos/*. It has video resources on the procedures discussed in the chapter and will kickstart the hands-on with the software.
- Free sample projects for practicing working with ATLAS.ti are available at*https://atlasti.com/learning/sample-projects/*.
- For NVivo their official YouTube channel provides excellent introductory videos for the software at *https://www.youtube.com/c/NVivobyQSR/playlists*.

REFERENCES

Archer, E., Janse van Vuuren, H. H., & Van der Walt, H. D. (2017). *Introduction to Atlas.ti: Basic operations, tips, and tricks for coding* (6th Edition). Pretoria: Research Rescue.

ATLAS.ti 9 Quick Tour - Windows. (n.d.). Retrieved from *https://doc.atlasti.com/QuicktourWin.v9/Intro/IntroductionPrefaceQuickTour.html*.

Camargo, B. V., & Justo, A. M. (2013). IRAMUTEQ: Um software gratuito para análise de dados textuais. *Temas Em Psicologia, 21*(2), 513-518. doi:10.9788/tp2013.2-16

Franzosi, R., Doyle, S., McClelland, L.E. *et al.* (2013) Quantitative narrative analysis software options compared: PC-ACE and CAQDAS (ATLAS.ti, MAXqda, and NVivo). *Qual Quant* 47, 3219–3247. doi:10.1007/s11135-012-9714-3

Niedbalski, J., & Ślęzak, I. (2016). Computer Assisted Qualitative Data Analysis Software. Using the NVivo and Atlas.ti in the Research Projects Based on the Methodology of Grounded Theory. *Computer Supported Qualitative Research Studies in Systems, Decision and Control*, 85-94. doi:10.1007/978-3-319-43271-7_8

Schlosser, D. F., Frasson, A. C., & Cantorani, J. R. (2019). Softwares livres para análise de dados qualitativos. *Revista Brasileira De Ensino De Ciência E Tecnologia, 12*(1). doi:10.3895/rbect.v12n1.9550

Schönfelder, W. (2011). CAQDAS and Qualitative Syllogism Logic—NVivo 8 and MAXQDA 10 Compared [91 paragraphs]. *Forum Qualitative Sozialforschung/Forum: Qualitative Social Research, 12*(1), Art. 21, http://nbn-resolving.de/urn:nbn:de:0114-fqs1101218.

Souza, M. A., Wall, M. L., Andrea C. D. M. C. T., Lowen, I. M., & Peres, A. M. (2018). O uso do software IRAMUTEQ na análise de dados em pesquisas qualitativas. *Revista Da Escola De Enfermagem Da USP,* 52(0). doi:10.1590/s1980-220x2017015003353

Trena, M.P.,& Jessica, N.L. (2016). ATLAS.ti for conversation and discourse analysis studies. *International Journal of Social Research Methodology*, *19*(4), 405-428. doi:*10.1080/13645579.2015.1021949*

Wiltshier, Fiona (2011). Researching with NVivo 8 [32 paragraphs]. *Forum QualitativeSozialforschung/ Forum: Qualitative Social Research,* 12 (1), Art. 23, http://nbn-resolving.de/urn:nbn:de:0114-fqs1101234

Woods, M., Macklin, R., & Lewis, G. K. (2015). Researcher reflexivity: Exploring the impacts of CAQDAS use. *International Journal of Social Research Methodology, 19*(4), 385-403. doi:10.1080/13645579.2015 .1023964

Chapter 17

Action Research in Medical Education

P F Kotur, Pushpa Kotur

ABSTRACT

Action Research (AR) is a systematic inquiry by the teachers in their respective work settings, to improve their practice. The dilemma and the challenge lies in applying the principles of Evidence Based Medicine (EBM), which is becoming increasingly applied for all scholarly activities performed by the teachers in medical colleges viz, teaching, research and administration. AR has gained much more significance in the context of the revised competency based MBBS medical curriculum rolled out by the National Medical Commission. There is an excellent opportunity as well as the challenge here, for the teachers to become agents of curriculum change by designing and implementing innovative techniques of instruction and assessment. This chapter describes the role of AR, its continuous cycle of planning a change, acting, and observing the consequences of the change, reflecting on the processes and replanning. Despite AR being collaborative, democratic, emancipatory, and practical in nature, it has some flaws such as subjectivity, vulnerability to pressure and time constraints.

Key Words: action research; evidence based medicine; qualitative research

ASSESS NEED

Medical education in India is struggling to cope up with the phenomenal expansion as well as the need to ensure quality of its graduates in shouldering health care of 132+ billion population. To achieve this gigantic task, research combined with faculty development becomes vital. The need for Medical Education Research (MER) has been felt more and more in recent years. Among various approaches which are commonly discussed in MER, the Action Research (AR) stands distinct because of its unique features. It is a systematic inquiry done by the teachers in their own work settings, to improve their practice. It is simple, affordable and authentic.

Many teachers think that research requires sophisticated design, huge data analysis and funding, which is something beyond their reach. They must realize that the environment where they are teaching is full of data, to conduct a high-quality action research, even with little knowledge in research methodology and data analysis (Craig, 2009). Unfortunately, most teachers are not familiar with the concept of action research, which is the focus of this chapter.

AR has gained all the more significance in the context of the revised competency based MBBS medical curriculum rolled out by the National Medical Commission. There is an excellent opportunity as well as the challenge here, for the teachers to become agents of curriculum change by designing and implementing innovative techniques of instruction and assessment.

The dilemma and the challenge lie in applying the principles of Evidence Based Medicine (EBM), and its correlates Evidence Based Medical Education (EBME) and Evidence Based Practice (EB) which are becoming increasingly applied for all scholarly activities performed by the teachers in medical colleges viz, teaching, research and administration (Todres et al, 2007).

BRIEF

- Meaning of Action Research (AR) and how is it different from other approaches
- Attributes of key features of AR
- Steps involved in conducting AR
- AR in the context of EBM and EBME
- Publication issues
- Critique of AR

CONTEXTUALIZE

Let us discuss a case scenario, in the context of a real educational dilemma faced by many of the Indian medical colleges, and possibly elsewhere too, during the Covid Pandemic.

Since 2019, a revised competency based MBBS curriculum was launched by the National Medical Commission (NMC). It is a product of nationwide expert consultation taking into consideration the present and future needs of the society. However, a question arises – do we have any evidence to prove that the medical graduate coming out of this new curriculum is likely to fair better than the one who has emerged out of traditional curriculum?

When the new curriculum was being launched the Covid 19 broke out. The Government and the Regulating bodies directed for the immediate closure of all the medical colleges across the country and to send all the students back home, as prophylactic measure against the spread of Covid 19. Further, all the colleges were also directed to adopt 'virtual mode of teaching and training' to avoid disruption of students' course of studies. The teachers resorted to online clinical training sessions. They had no clue whether students were learning or not, and if they were, how effective it was.

Reflect on this situation and think in what way this has implications for conducting action research. We will revisit this issue later in this chapter.

DESCRIBE

Educational Research (ER) versus Action Research (AR)

Harden (2000) described twelve different roles, spread over six areas of their day-to-day activity. The role as teacher, instructional designer, curriculum planner, resource material developer or even administrator offers exciting opportunities for him or her to get attracted towards research (Longstaffe et al., 1996; Ryan et al., 1996). Educational Research (ER) deals with the application of scientific methods and techniques to study and resolve educational problems. It primarily aims at improving the quality and efficiency of the teaching-learning process (Lodico, 2006). It serves four main purposes. First, it helps to develop new theories of teaching and learning. Second, it contributes to improve practice. Third, it can change a person from opinion-based teaching to evidence-based teaching. Fourthly, education research is a connecting link between education and the patient care. (Adkoli, 2020)

Action research (AR) isa term coined by Kurt Lewin in 1944. As the name implies, it is a type of research wherein the educators, while working in their work settings, encounter some problem or dilemma, conduct a systematic inquiry to find an answer to their problem. It has the potential to produce change quickly because the research is carried out by educators in their own work settings (Parsons and Brown, 2002). AR is aimed to bring about immediate and transformative changes through the processes of taking action and doing research simultaneously, using critical reflection. In nutshell, action research is – 'Research in Action'.

Is AR Quantitative or Qualitative?

Despite its wider acceptance, there is still debate on whether AR belongs to qualitative or quantitative research tradition (Ary, Jacobs, Razavieh & Sorensen, 2009). Some research scholars associate it with the qualitative tradition, while others assert that it relies more on quantitative inquiry (Burns, 2007). Because of its practical orientation, action research generally uses both quantitative and qualitative data (Lodico, 2006). Qualitative research helps teachers to addresses the complexity of the classroom environment, while quantitative research helps to observe the impact of the new curriculum but does not help them to perceive the causes of those happenings. The teachers through action research can systematically study problems within their educational setting and contribute not only in applying knowledge but also in generating new knowledge.

Attributes of AR

The main attributes of AR have been described by Lodico (Lodico, 2006).

1. AR is conducted in the teacher-researcher's own educational setting and the teacher takes an active part in the research
2. AR involves collaboration with other colleagues involved in the educational process.
3. AR focuses on taking action to change and improve educational practices.
4. AR is ongoing process and includes several waves of data collection, reflection, and action

In addition, other scholars have described some key features of AR. The success of AR depends on marshalling passion and building trust, wherein the teacher should act more as an active participant than an objective researcher (Burns, 2007). AR is a method of progressive problem solving which makes extensive use of real time scenarios and (Pine, 2008).

AR is value laden. It refuses neutrality and instead, finds ground for its inquiry in a setting where there are conflicting values or hierarchical differentials. It challenges traditional notions of power and values and investigates the problem by analyzing day-to-day realities (Craig, 2009).

The methodology of research is flexible, and tailor made to suit the demand of the situation. It involves a wide plethora of methods, tools and techniques which are found in the toolbox of educational researchers.

Most importantly, in AR, theory is prompted by practice, accompanied by observation, analysis, synthesis, reflection and evaluation. Reflexivity is said to be essential component of AR because it aims to interrogate and examine the benefits of actions implemented in the end (Craig, 2009). Action research is fluid and flexible in nature and hence one may expect some difficulty in following the steps serially (Herr, Anderson, & Herr, 2005).

The action research cycle described by Cooke & Cox (2005) provides a conceptual tool for conducting AR in any setting. (Figure 1). It consists of five stages, viz., identifying an area of focus; developing an action plan; Collecting data; analyzing and interpreting data; and reflecting. Some authors have described AR as a self- reflective *spiral* of planning a change, acting and observing the consequences of the change, reflecting on the processes which goes on continuously. In the entire research process, there could be multiple cycles and multiple foci of the study. (Koshy, 2005).

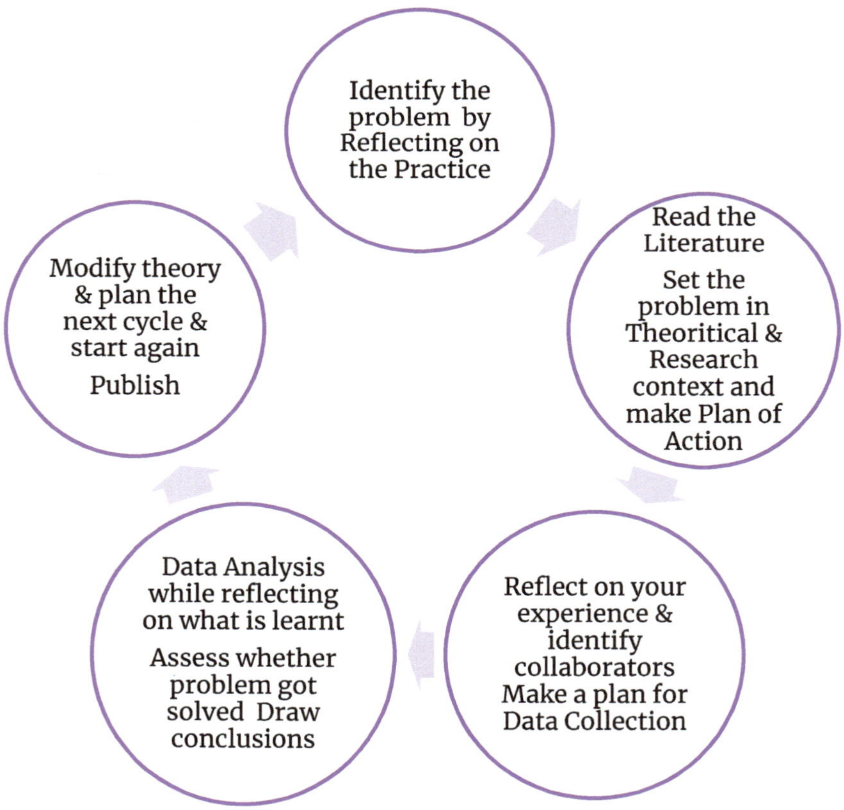

Figure 1: Action Research Cycle

Steps in conducting Action Research

We invite the attention of readers to consider the scenario described in the Contextualize section and appreciate the way, we have related the same with the following steps:

Step 1. Identifying the problem and formulating pertinent Question

Here in our case, the problem faced by the teachers is the difficulty in imparting and assessing 'virtual clinical training' to the students. If we convert this dilemma into an answerable question, the question shall be- How to impart and assess the clinical training to the students virtually (in the absence of patients or clinical material)? The question can be related to curricular issues, instructional strategy, or student assessment issues.

Step 2: Developing a plan of action:

Performing a thorough literature search, to find out the various methods suggested to teach and assess clinical skills virtually, is the next step of AR. Several methods such as using written case scenarios, use of Video clips (either self made or downloaded from the internet with due approval), clinical demonstrations using volunteers and usage of the virtual patients (a screen-based simulation) were explored to be to be possible solutions. In our set up, written case scenarios and use of Video clips (both self made and downloaded from the net) were used by our teachers. Assessment of clinical training through virtual mode, though far from being ideal, was done devising suitable tools (e.g., Google Forms) in the form of Questionnaires, Check lists etc. Each idea was implemented stepwise, keeping in mind the time required for the same.

Step 3: Collecting the data

Before the commencement of the clinical training, it was decided as what kind of data will be helpful for AR and how to collect it (depending upon the type of the clinical skill). Apart from the data to know whether the learning has happened, the practicality, student acceptance of the method was also obtained in the form of feedbacks. Meaningful data was collected from previous records and other daily records like attendance logs, Internal assessment marks of the students.

Step 4: Data analysis and conclusions

Simultaneous and frequent examination of the data during the collection process helped us to modify the action plan. The analysis of the data made our teachers to reflect on what actually was happening, guiding them to alter the teaching or assessing methodology. Tentative solutions for effective virtual clinical training were drawn from analysis. The results were discussed with other teachers in the monthly departmental faculty development meetings and after incorporating the valuable feedbacks from both the teachers and the students, the conclusions were drawn or the plan was refined.

Step 5: Modification of theory and repetition of the AR cycle

New cycle began again in light of the previous findings. New theory and modified plan of action, and collection of data again continued. A new question may be formulated addressing another problem. For example, the virtual clinical training can be commenced with the trained teachers and focus of AR can shift to measuring effectiveness of the virtual mode by collecting an altogether a different kind of data.

Step 6. Reporting of the results

While the ultimate goal of the AR is to promote effective change in the institution, the value of sharing the results with colleagues, other stakeholders and publishing it at least in an institutional or educational journal is equally important.

Translation of AR

The paradigm of 'Evidence Based Medicine', a five-step approach, is a time-tested tool for translating research in to practice (Gordon Guyatt 1992, Sackett, 2000). Extrapolating to AR, its findings will have to be critically appraised for rigor and validity before application (3rd Step of 5 step approach of EBM). In the process of AR, since the teacher is conducting the systematic enquiry, rigor and validity of AR can be questioned. In order to overcome this limitation, we suggest the need for a critical appraisal of AR by a peer (colleague), so that the research findings can be declared more trustworthy.

Thus, AR should selectively assimilate the practice of Evidence Based Medical Education (EBME) for Teaching, Evidence Based Medicine (EBM) for Patient Care and Evidence Based Management for administration respectively. This requires creation of awareness and the training of teachers as action researchers, as essential requirement within an institution (Longstaffe et al., 1996; Ryan et al., 1996). The capabilities of medical teachers both to conduct AR and also to critically appraise the same will go a long way in the progress of medical education.

Quality Evidence Synthesis (QES)

In AR, broad generalizations are made from specific or focused observations, that means AR is always inductive. Action researchers typically look at reality and try to develop a theory from the observations made and data collected from the class. AR places its emphasis on the local problems in a local setting. Its findings are to be evaluated in terms of local applicability, not universal validity. As in qualitative research, there is no hypothesis tested in AR and focus is on the understanding the phenomena, meanings, perceptions, concepts, thoughts and related experiences or feelings (Seers, 2012). An added advantage of AR can be that more number of teachers can be involved in research activity simultaneously. There is ongoing debate on whether or not quality assessment should be part of Quality Evidence Synthesis (QES) and if so, how to distinguish high quality studies from others. Quality, goodness, validity, trustworthiness, credibility, and workability have all been suggested as terms to describe criteria for good action research (Herr, Anderson, & Herr, 2005).

In a recent review by Cohen and Crabtree (2008) quality dimensions in existing appraisal instruments have been explored viz. researcher bias, validity, reliability, importance, clarity and coherence, ethics, and the use of appropriate and rigorous methods. The reviewers recommend the use three separate tools for 3 different purposes; critical appraisal skills program (CASP) tool for novice researchers as it is a popular and user-friendly, evaluation tool for qualitative studies (ETQS) for providing more detailed instructions on how to interpret criteria, and Joanna Briggs Institute (JBI) tool for its focus on congruity and being the most coherent (Hannes, 2010). There are several other critical appraisal tools available for determining the quality of AR. Mostly they are grounded in Qualitative research discussed elsewhere in this book.

Publication of Action Research

The common question that comes in the mind of a novice researcher is - what all can be included in the action research report so that it gets published? All the steps followed in the conduct of AR can be included sequentially, in the chronological order. Adopting the time tested IMRAD format if possible, can be an advantage.

Making use of the Lockwood's ladder of publishing can be of great help, which provides a framework by which emergent scholars can progress from modest report, shared with a colleagues in a safe environment, to authoritative peer- reviewed publication. (Emmanuelle, 2018)

Critique of Action Research

Despite AR being applied, emancipatory and practical, it may have following flaws as well.

Subjectivity: When left unchecked, results of AR may be laden with researcher's subjectivity.

Vulnerability to pressure. Researcher, by virtue of being a junior or subordinate in the organizational settings might be coerced to alter the findings by the seniors, to suit organizational objectives.

Time consuming: Because of AR's cyclical nature, there is a possibility that initial research question, depending upon the initial findings might get refined several times and thereby the refining of methodology taking time, making the entire research process time consuming. There is no clear time limit as when the research has to be stopped because technically, it stops only when the problem is resolved.

Knowledge generation: Sometimes the AR can be unpredictable and may fail to be included in referred journals. (Action Research-UK essays, 2017)

Some of the educators have disapproved ARas a true research saying that it's nothing more than the application of common sense. Notwithstanding this criticism, it definitely promotes application of scientific thinking and methods to solve real life problems and represents a great improvement over teacher's subjective judgements and decisions based upon traditional beliefs. (Wani, 2020)

Ethical issues in Action Research

Ethical dilemmas are intrinsic components of AR, precisely because of its collaborative nature and of the diverse motivations, perspectives, and institutional roles held by its participants. Since AR involves reflective contributions of many teacher-researchers, ethical issues are bound to arisewhen he/she engages in technical, practical or critical models of AR. Hence, there is a need to anticipate these ethical issues well before and be prepared to address them through honest dialogue with all the participants. (Banegas, Darío Luis, 2015) Teacher-researchers are teachers first and generally they respect the colleagues with whom they work, openly sharing information about their research. While they seek knowledge, they also care for the well-being of both students and professional colleagues (Monr, 1996). Many of the ethical issues of AR can be resolved by following the Golden Rule defined by Smith, of asking the following questions to ourselves viz. What are the likely consequences of this research? How well do they fit with my own values and priorities? If I were a participant, would I want this research to be done? What changes might I want to make me feel comfortable? (Smith, 1990)

Ethical issues in conducting action research are the same as those applicable for other types of research which have been discussed elsewhere in this book. However, since the researcher is 'insider' it is necessary to wear a 'neutral lens' for both the researcher and the ethics committee which can be challenging.

SUMMARIZE

The change over to Competency Based Medical Education (CBME), the surge of Covid 19 Pandemic and the urgent need for 'out of the box solutions' have created fertile soil for planting action research. We have elaborated on the meaning and key features of AR. We have outlined the steps of designing AR and discussed how AR can be aligned with the current trend of EBM. Deliberating on the strengths and weaknesses of AR, we have concluded that AR is an effective approach in the Indian context and it should be considered seriously by the researchers in health profession.

EVALUATE

After reading this chapter, take up the following assignment:

- Think of one educational problem which you face in your setting;
- Formulate a research question;
- Make an outline of steps which you would adopt to convert this in to an Action Research project.

ROAD AHEAD

Those who would like to pursue action research may consult the following open resources:

1. A Handbook for Exploratory Action Research (2018), (*http://bit.ly/handbook-EAR)*
2. ACTION RESEARCH Northeast and Islands Regional Educational Laboratory At Brown University by Eileen Ferranc*https://www.brown.edu/academics/education-alliance/sites/brown.edu.academics.education-alliance/files/publications/act_research.pdf*
3. Centre for Education Innovation. *http://cei.hkust.edu.hk/teaching-resources/action-research*
4. Action research - WHO | World Health Organizationhttps://www.who.int › alliance-hpsr › resources by L Gilson

The opportunities for action research come from local contexts of research. Be vocal on local. The Medical Education Units, Curriculum Committees can play mentoring role and form communities of practice.

The leadership should recognize the value of AR and make suitable policy to recognize and reward AR.

The avenues of publication at the local, national and international level should be explored. The medical education networks in India and abroad (SEARAME, AMEE, WFME etc.), many Universities of Health Sciences and centers of excellence also provide forums for sharing the reports of AR.

REFERENCES

Adkoli, B.V. (2020). Educational Research: Much Unexplored Pathway to Career Enhancement of Teachers in Health Sciences. *Annals of SBV* 9(1), 2–6.

Ary D., Jacobs, L.C., Razavieh, A., Sorenson, C.K. (2009) *Introduction to Research in Education*, Cengage Learning. ISBN.0495601225, 9780495601227

Banegas, D.I. & Luis, S. (2015). A look at ethical issues in action research in education. *Argentinian Journal of Applied Linguistics.* 3(1), 58-67.

Burns, D. (2007) *Systemic Action Research: A strategy for whole system change.* Bristol, UK: The Policy Press.

Cooke, B., & Wolfram Cox, J. (2005). *The Fundamentals of Action Research, Volume 1: The Early Years (Sage Benchmarks in Social Research Series).* Sage.

Craig, D. V. (2009). *Action research essentials* (1st Ed.). San Francisco, CA: Jossey-Bass. (Pp. 248).doi: *https://doi.org/10.33524/cjar.v13i2.40*

Ferrance, E. (2000). *Themes in education: Action research.* Providence, RI: Northeast and Islands Regional Educational Laboratory.

Kolk, M. *Embrace Action Research-The Action Research Cycle.* Creative Educator. https://www.thecreativeeducator.com

Guyatt, G., Cairns, J., Churchill, D., et al. (1992) Evidence-Based Medicine: A New Approach to Teaching the Practice of Medicine. *JAMA, 268*(17), 2420–2425. doi:10.1001/jama.1992.03490170092032

Harden, R.M., Crosby, J. (2000). AMEE Guide No 20: The good teacher is more than a lecturer – the twelve roles of the teacher. *Medical Teacher.* 22(4):334–34.

Hannes, K., Lockwood, C., & Pearson, A. (2010). A comparative analysis of three online appraisal instruments' ability to assess validity in qualitative research. *Qualitative health research*, *20*(12), 1736–1743. *https://doi.org/10.1177/1049732310378656*

Herr, K., & Anderson, G. L. (2005). *The action research dissertation: A guide for students and faculty.* SAGE Publications, Inc. *https://www.doi.org/10.4135/9781452226644*

Koshy, V. (2005). *Action Research for improving Practice.* Paul Chapman Publishing-SAGE Publications.

Longstaffe, J. A., Williams, P. J., Whittlestone, K. D., Hammond, P. M., & Edwards, J. (1996) *Establishing a support service for educational technology within a university. Association for Learning Technology Journal,* 4 (1). pp. 85-92.

Lodico, M.G., Spaulding, D.T. and Voegtle, K.H. (2006) *Methods in Educational Research: From Theory to Practice.* John Wiley, San Francisco.

Mohr, M. (1996) Ethics and standards for teacher research: drafts and decisions, in Research in Language and Learning: *Reports from a teacher research seminar.* Fairfax: Northern Virginia Writing Project, George Mason University.

Parsons, R.D., & Brown, K.S. (2002). *Teacher as Reflective Practitioner and Action Researcher.* Belmont, California: Wadsworth/Thomson Learning.

Pine, G. J. (2009). *Teacher action research: Building knowledge democracies.* SAGE Publications, Inc., *https://www.doi.org/10.4135/9781452275079*

Ryan, M., Wells, J., Freeman, A. & Hallam, G. (1996) Resource- based learning strategies: implications for students and institutions. *Association for Learning Technology Journal*, 4(1), 93-98. DOI: *10.1080/0968776960040114*

Sackett, D. L., Straus, S. E., Richardson, W. S., Rosenberg, W., Haynes, R. B. (2000). *Evidence-Based Medicine: How to Practice and Teach EBM.* (2nd ed) Edinburgh; New York: Churchill. Livingstone.

Seers K. (2012). Qualitative data analysis. *Evidence-based nursing*, *15*(1), 2. *https://doi.org/10.1136/ebnurs.2011.100352*. PMID: 22184739

Wani, S. R. (2020) *Educational Research-1.* M.A. Edu/Research Methodology/Educational Research.http://ddeku.edu.in

Smith, L. (1990) Ethics, field studies, and the paradigm crisis. In EgonG. Guba (Ed.) *The Paradigm Dialog*. Newbury Park, California: Sage Publications.

Todres, M., Stephenson, A., & Jones, R. (2007). Medical education research remains the poor relation. *BMJ (Clinical research ed.)*, *335*(7615), 333–335. *https://doi.org/10.1136/bmj.39253.544688.94*

Voulgre, E. (2018). Une lecture aujourd'hui des textes de 2002, 2003 et 2012. *Distances et médiations des savoirs*. doi: 10.4000/dms.2664

UK Essays. (2018). Criticism of Action Research. Retrieved from *https://www.ukessays.com/essays/education/research-methods-and-critique-action-research-in-education-education-essay.php?vref=1*

Key Points: Unique Attributes of Action Research

- Action Research is a process of simultaneous action taking and doing research, linked together by critical reflection by the teacher.
- Action Research enacts quickimprovements in an educational setting
- Action Research can convert a teacher from opinion-based teaching to evidence-based teaching
- Action Research can generate evidence for Competency based Curriculum
- Covid 19 Pandemic has opened unique opportunities for Action Research:
- Despite Action Research being applied, empowering, collaborative, democratic, emancipatory and practical in nature, some associated flaws viz. subjectivity, vulnerability to pressure by seniors, and time constraints have to be kept in mind.

Key Points: What is Not Action Research?

- Action Research is not what usually comes to any body's mind when we hear the word "research."
- Action Research is not a project where we learn more about a topic.
- Action Research is not problem-solving in the sense of trying to find out what is wrong, but rather a quest for knowledge about how to improve.
- Action Research is not about doing research on or about people or finding all available information on a topic looking for the correct. AR involves people working to improve their skills, techniques, and strategies.
- Action Research is not about learning why we do certain things, but rather how we can do things better.

(Eileen Ferrance, 2000)

Chapter 18

Mixed Methods Research In Public Health: From Theory to Practice

Krishnamurthy Jayanna, Satyanarayana Ramanaik, Manoj Kumar Pati, Arin Kar, Swaroop N, Tejaswini B D, Vinod Ramani

ABSTRACT

Mixed Methods study design is increasingly adopted in recent times by the public health researchers. The two critical components of mixed methods i.e., quantitative, and qualitative approaches are often discussed by domain experts in isolation, resulting in lack of practical application of these methods. The current chapter aims to address these gaps through blending theoretical knowledge in this domain with the practical experience of the authors. The chapter sheds light on scope, definitions, and practical considerations while planning, implementing, analyzing, and disseminating mixed methods research findings for programs and policy.

The mixed methods research draws upon the strengths of both qualitative and quantitative approaches. The methodology leverages effective engagement of patient and community for identifying health priorities. However, the designing of mixed methods research requires unique methodological skill sets The key challenge is to build a collaborative and cross-disciplinary team. When the perspectives of subjects are weaved into the research findings, the chances of engaging the community, health providers, systems authorities and policy makers are enhanced significantly. This facilitates effective implementation of programs and optimizes health outcomes.

Key Words: mixed-methods research; public health, health systems, community perspectives, quantitative research, qualitative research

ASSESS NEED

Mixed Methods study design is increasingly adopted in recent times by the public health researchers and programmers for finding solutions to the problems on the field (Tariq & Woodman, 2013). Public

Health discipline is tasked with determining the causes and solutions to complex challenges related to population health such as access, quality, coverage and inequity in health services and interventions. Once solutions are identified, they must be implemented effectively and efficiently to achieve the best possible outcomes at a population level. Then, these effective interventions need to be scaled up across geographies and should be sustained by the health systems (Aral & Blanchard, 2012). These three critical processes i.e., design, implementation and scale up, vary in complexity and sophistication depending on the nature of the problem. Program Science, Implementation Science and Implementation Research methods are increasingly adopted to solve these challenges (Aral & Blanchard, 2012; B M Ramesh, Halli, Jayanna, & Mohan HL, 2018; Medhanyie et al., 2019). These methods are critically reviewed and refined from time to time to suit the need. What is constant in all these approaches is the use of mixed methods at different stages of program design and implementation (Kar & Jayanna, 2021). The current chapter will focus on application of mixed methods approaches in a public health setting.

The chapter has high relevance to medical education & research community for two reasons. 1) Often the two mixed methods components, quantitative and qualitative are discussed by domain experts in isolation, and not in an integrated manner. This robs opportunities for trainees to internalize an integrated and practical application of the approach.2) The audience is often trained to lean toward one or the other but fail to find the rich connection and complementary roles of the two.

Traditionally the academic or the research community focuses on research and program evaluation, while the government, civil society and NGOs focus on implementation. The academicians though not fully aware of the field realities and complexities, are expected to find answers to the issues. The program implementers, managers and frontline workers who are on the field are expected to solve field level issues but are not equipped with scientific methods or skills to do so. In this backdrop, Program-Science is assuming importance, and program scientists who are equipped with skills and methods of both, are the need of the hour (Aral & Blanchard, 2012).

The current chapter is written by a team of experts, who are well-versed with program science and implementation research settings in low- and middle-income countries across a range of public health programs i.e., HIV, Maternal and Child Health, Adolescent Health, Non-communicable diseases, and Primary Health Care. While the chapter briefly outlines the theoretical aspects of mixed methods design, the main effort is to shed light on practical applications right through the planning, data collection and analysis. The chapter blends the theory with practical case studies that describe how the methodology was adopted in public health, and how the data informed programs and policy.

BRIEF

- Address needs of teaching faculty, doctoral and post-doctoral scholars interested in applying mixed methods research in public health
- Importance of mixed methods research and its relevance to solving complex public health challenges
- How to design, implement mixed methods, analyze, and disseminate results to influence programs and policy
- Case studies and practical application of mixed methods in the context of two national health programs: Maternal and Child Health and Non-communicable diseases.

CONTEXTUALIZE

Two scenarios provided below provide food for thought for visualizing the public health context where mixed methods research is relevant.

Case scenario 1. An high priority district in India continues to be affected by poor maternal and neonatal outcomes as a result of high rates of home deliveries in one of its blocks. Despite many health systems measures such as increasing delivery points, training of staff nurses and midwives, the situation hasn't changed. On further examination, several health behaviours of the population such as antenatal check-ups, immunisation rates are not optimal on account of local social and cultural norms, beliefs and practices of particular population living in the block.

Questions for self-reflections: *What is the best way to explore and understand the practices and local norms in the community? How does this data inform local communication strategies? Do these community based interventions complement health systems based interventions for optimizing district level performance?*

Case scenario 2. Growing burden of non-communicable diseases (NCD) in the country needs strengthening of primary health care systems so as to plan prevention, health promotion, treatment and care in a comprehensive way for the whole population. However, the medical officer of the primary health centre does not have data and the information of the population.

Questions for self-reflections: *What is the size of his population that already has one of the NCDs? How many are vulnerable for developing a NCD in future, as they have one or more of the risk factors? And finally where are they accessing care already? Should the PHC plan for it or not? Will population access care from PHC and what are possible health seeking behaviours and patterns?*

DESCRIBE

What is Mixed Methods Research?

The following explanations by experts and standard definitions give a comprehensive understanding of the term MMR to the reader.

Mixed methods research is a systematic integration of quantitative and qualitative methods in a single study for purposes of obtaining a fuller picture and deeper understanding of a phenomenon. Mixed methods can be integrated in such a way that qualitative and quantitative methods retain their original structures and procedures (pure form mixed methods). Alternatively, these two methods can be adapted, altered, or synthesized to fit the research and cost situations of the study (Chen, 2006).

In general, mixed methods research represents research that involves collecting, analyzing, and interpreting quantitative and qualitative data in a single study or in a series of studies that investigate the same underlying phenomenon (Leech & Onwuegbuzie, 2009)

'Mixed methods' is a term that is usually used to designate combining qualitative and quantitative research methods in the same research project. Few experts have preferred the term 'Multimethod Research' to indicate that different styles of research may be combined in the same research project. These need not be restricted to quantitative and qualitative; but may include, for example, qualitative participant observation with qualitative in-depth interviewing. Alternatively, it could include quantitative survey research with quantitative experimental research. And it may also include quantitative with qualitative styles (Hunter & Brewer, 2003).

Why is 'Mixed Methods Research' important?

Mixed methods research has many benefits in addressing complex public health challenges. In addition to gaining benefits from the inherent strengths of the two methods, combining them can address the limitations that are inherent in each method. By mixed methods research essentially we achieve five key things (Greene, Caracelli, & Graham, 1989).

1. **Triangulation** that seeks convergence, corroboration, correspondence of results from different methods. Ex: Using both quantitative survey data and the qualitative in-depth interviews to validate the underlying phenomenon or trait for a particular research question.
2. **Complementarity** that seeks elaboration, enhancement, illustration, clarification of the results from one method with the results from the other method. In other words, it refers how well two methods fit together and meet each other's needs. Ex: Elaborating the quantitative results by asking 'how' and 'why' questions through a qualitative study.
3. **Development** that seeks to use the results from one method to help develop or inform the other method especially during sampling, implementation, and measurement decisions. Ex: Developing quantitative survey tools by analyzing the themes emerged in a formative research which uses qualitative techniques.
4. **Initiation** that seeks the discovery of paradox and contradiction, new perspectives of frameworks, the recasting of questions or results from one method with questions or results from the other method and the last but not the least. Ex: Revising an interview guide for a qualitative study by carefully examining the survey results.
5. **Expansion** that seeks to extend the breadth and range of inquiry by using different methods for different inquiry components. Ex: asking follow-up questions in either of the methods.

How is mixed-method research carried out?

Mixing the method should be need based: The research design needs to be explicit about the intentional use of both quantitative and qualitative methods and how the combined strengths can answer the proposed research questions. Also, the selection of method should be informed by the nature of the problem one is studying (Creswell & Plano Clark, 2011). The rationale for using mixed methods needs to be elaborated in its design statement. For example, one data resource may not be enough, initial results need further explanations or a second method is needed to enhance the primary method (Creswell & Plano Clark, 2011).

Mixing may happen at different points of interface: Mixing ortriangulation is the key in any MMR and knowing its purpose, sequence, and the stages in which the integration or point of interface between the qualitative and quantitative methods would occur is very essential. Morse and Niehaus (2009) identified two possible points of integration: 1. ***Result point of integration and*** 2. ***Analytical point of integration*** (Morse, M, & Niehaus, 2009). They further noted, in the process of writing down the results of any first component, the result of the second component is added and integrated with the result point integration. Whereas in the analytical point of integration, a first analytical stage of a qualitative component is followed by a second analytical stage, in which the topics identified in the first analytical stage are quantified (Morse et al., 2009; Schoonenboom & Johnson, 2017).

Teddlie and Tashakkori 2009 (Teddlie, Charles, & A, 2009) identify four major stages of integration: 1. Conceptualization stage, 2. Methodological or data collection stage, 3. Analytical ordata analysis stage, and 4. Inferential and writing stage (Teddlie et al., 2009)

Despite these classifications, the decision on the sequencing and stages of point of integration could be taken based on the typology of MMR adopted. Also, as stated by O'Cathanin et al (2008) about the quality of mixed methods studies, it is important to report the type of integration, how it occurred in the context of the team working and who was involved in it, etc. in its study design.

The data collection could be together or at two different points in time: The timing of data collection is dependent on the type of mixed-method design. Four patterns are identified: 1. A parallel (both quantitative and qualitative together) data collection may take place in the ***convergent parallel design***. 2. the quantitative data collection and analysis will be carried out first and then the qualitative data collection and analysis will be conducted in ***explanatory sequential and transformative design***. 3. Qualitative data collection and analysis will be carried out first and then the quantitative data collection and analysis will be carried out in both ***exploratory sequential design and multiphase design***. 4. The collection and analysis of the second data set may occur before, during, and/or after the first data collection in ***embedded design*** (Creswell & Plano Clark, 2011; Morse et al., 2009; Schoonenboom & Johnson, 2017).

Collaborations between Quantitative and Qualitative Researchers: Quantitative is mainly a ***deductive method*** and ideal for measuring the pervasiveness of "known" phenomena and central patterns of association, including inferences of causality. Whereas the qualitative is an ***inductive method*** which allows for identification of previously unknown process, explanations of why and how phenomena occur (Pasick et al., 2009). The conceptual thinking and specific research skills required for data collection, analysis, and interpretation of findings in the two methods are different.

Data analysis and reporting considerations: The traditional approach to data analysis includes using statistical techniques for analyzing survey data and thematic analysis for interview data. ***Integrative strategy*** is another approach where-in qualitative data is quantitized or quantitative data is qualitized (Tariq & Woodman, 2013).

While reporting the outcomes of MMR, it is arduous to transparently delineate the level of data integration which in-turn results in the study design being disjointed (Kajamaa, Mattick, & de la Croix, 2020). ***Meta-inference*** conceptually refers to the interception of qualitative and quantitative strands, which needs to be precisely specified (Regnault, Willgoss, & Barbic, 2018). Researchers utilizing such designs should thus be mindful of the conflicting results and the challenges in interpreting them.

In general, finding an expert well versed with the nitty-gritty of both methods is quite challenging and it demands a multi-disciplinary team to conduct high-quality mixed method research (Jennifer Wisdom & Creswell, 2013).

Ethical considerations: Ethical considerations are an integral part of any MMR. In general, the ethical principles followed in MMR are common to other mono method research for example, ***making sure of no harm to participants, use of honest reporting, maintaining data quality measures***, etc. (Leia K. Cain, 2020). However, the use of new and innovative ways in design and different ways to approach data in MMR insists on the importance of more rigorous ethical considerations. Poth et al (2020) argue to intensify the ethical consideration in MMR considering its design which differs from mono research in terms of number of data collection and integration points, use of ***intensive data collection techniques, and participant expectations*** (Poth, 2020). Similarly, Hesse and Biber (2010) suggests to make sure of the ***validity and data quality*** at different stages: framing of design, methodological choice, sampling procedure, and the researcher's responsibilities towards participants. Collins et al (2013) highlights ***transparency*** as an imperative aspect in MMR.

Case studies and practical applications

Case Study 1: Maternal Neonatal and Child Health (Kangaroo Mother Care)

Background and problem: Despite having the policy to provide Kangaroo Mother Care (KMC) to babies with low birth weight (LBW) of less than 2500 gms, the estimated coverage of KMC globally was less than 5% (Chan, Labar, Wall, & Atun, 2016). KMC is defined as prolonged skin-to-skin contact of the baby with the mother or other caregiver for as long as possible during day and night, and exclusive breastfeeding or breast milk feeding. A 2016 Cochrane review shows that KMC can reduce neonatal deaths substantially by around 40% at the time of discharge from the hospital (Mazumder et al., 2019). Between 2016 and 2019, WHO supported by Bill and Melinda Gates Foundation, undertook implementation research in Ethiopia and India to improve coverage of Kangaroo Mother Care (KMC).

MMR design and methods: Implementation research is a useful iterative process that assesses or evaluates implementation strategies to understand what is working or not and also how and why it is going right or wrong (David H. Peters, 2013) World Health Organization. The project adopted a mixed-method approach where the **qualitative study** tried to understand the "why" and "how" practices affect the uptake of KMC in health facilities and community; and to identify potential solutions that can inform program design in improving coverage of KMC. Multiple in-depth interviews and focused group discussions were carried out with the stakeholders such as the health officials at the state and the district, medical officers, staff nurses, frontline health workers, mothers, fathers, and grandmothers of infants. The **quantitative study**was designed to estimate levels of existing practices affecting KMC, measure levels and trends of KMC practice in the hospital and at home and evaluate the intervention's influence in improving coverage of KMC to eight hours or more. This case study is from Koppal, a high priority district in Karnataka which was one of the study 7 sites across India and Ethiopia (Medhanyie et al., 2019)..

Results and implications: The ***qualitative studies*** informed that mothers were happy to learn and practice KMC but lacked clear message and support. Pediatricians perceived KMC as the skin-to-skin contact initiated soon after the delivery. It was also perceived as something that is *"known/ old practice"* and *"easy to do"* and not as an effective neo-natal care intervention. Staff nurses said that mothers were unclean and hence were not permitted to hold their low-birth-weight babies for fear of causing infections. Front line workers (FLW) shared challenges for continuing KMC at home because of beliefs like body heat not good for babies- "*body heat is not good for baby*", lack of support or privacy at home, and over-reliance on pre-lacteal feeds.

The project conducted continuing medical/nursing education (CME) for specialists and nurses. Regular visits by mentors (neonatologists and senior nurses) to the project sites to update doctors and handhold nurses were planned. Customized educational materials were printed for hospitals and FLWs. Training of FLWs included sessions on real-life problems and possible solutions; counsellors in hospitals were trained to motivate mothers on KMC. The qualitative evidence in the formative stages of the project helped to refine and finalize the messages, target groups for advocacy, intervention tools and methods. The ***quantitative data*** (concurrent monitoring) helped to monitor KMC uptake and practice in communities and hospitals and gave crucial information to review and improve programs. The pilot model that started in few villages and health facilities, was scaled up across the district. The government officials were engaged through the project planning and reviews. During the final year, the district wide project was evaluated to estimate the coverage. 87% of babies were initiated on KMC at the health facility and 53% practiced effective KMC at the facility and 36% practiced effective KMC at home after 7 days post-discharge. From as low as less than 5%, effective KMC went up to 53% in hospitals in a matter of two years, which revealed many important lessons to the policy and program managers. The lessons learnt and challenges were discussed with government officers and several best practices were integrated into the state action plans (Medhanyie et al., 2019)..

Case Study 2: Non-communicable diseases

Background and problem: The probability of an Indian, in the age groupof 30–70 years, dying at present from one of the four NCDs i.e. cardiovascular diseases (CVD), diabetes, cancer, and chronic respiratory disease is 26%. India has been called "the diabetes capital of the world," and it is estimated that 77 million Indians have the disease and "every fifth diabetic in the world is an Indian". It is projected to increase to 101 million by 2030 and 134 million by 2045. Evidence shows that the burden of NCDs and the prevalence of related risk factors are relatively higher in urban areasof India, and the prevalence is on the rise among the poor, making them particularly vulnerable tocatastrophic health expenditure, in addition to life-long morbidity and increased mortality. Gaps exist at multiple levels which hinder effective implementation of services for NCDs. Although tangible efforts have been made by the National and State government on NCD services, progress towards integration of care especially at primary care level has remain limited (Kar & Jayanna, 2021).

MMR design and methods: We used a mixed methods implementation research design to assess and address the gaps in an urban primary health centre (UPHC) catchment area covering around 58000 populations in Mysore city in Karnataka, India. We conducted a *population-wide screening* to detect prevalence of hypertension and diabetes in UPHC catchment area; a representative sample survey was also conducted to detect prevalence of risk factors in the population, understand out of pocket expenses and treatment adherence. *Facility audits* were undertaken to assess readiness to provide NCD care; we also conducted *qualitative research (focus group discussions (FGDs), and in-depth interviews (IDIs))* to understand client experiences and perceptions on NCD care, management, and lifestyle changes (Jayanna et al., 2019; Kar & Jayanna, 2021).

Results and implications: Around 35,000 adults over 18 years were screened of which about 12% and 19% had high blood sugar and high blood pressure respectively; 11% reported tobacco consumption; 6% high alcohol consumption; 40% inadequate physical activity and 81% inappropriate diet consumption. The ***facility audits*** revealed that public facilities lacked diagnostics and specialist services due to which most sought care in private facilities despite having to pay high out- of- pocket expenses. ***Qualitative studies*** revealed fear of side effects of mediations, myths and misconceptions that affected treatment adherence and lifestyle modification. It was found that majority of patients were not meeting treatment goals despite visits to healthcare facilities. Many challenges were encountered within the community, especially in relation to customized outreach, patient mobilization and communication, drug adherence, ensuring individualized patient care, counselling and lifestyle management. Empowering patients/families and enabling frontline workers to support and address health care needs of patients/families were major hurdles towards the continuum of care objective (Jayanna et al., 2019).

Based on the evidence generated by the MMR, urban health systems based implementation model was developed and is currently being implemented to address the gaps identified. This was one among the very few examples in the country where a comprehensive program for NCD was developed to address the entire care continuum (prevention, promotion, treatment, and care) in an integrated manner. The model is also informing thought process of how to strengthen comprehensive primary health care in India (Jayanna et al., 2019; Kar & Jayanna, 2021).

SUMMARIZE

Mixed methods research (MMR) draws upon the strengths of both qualitative and quantitative approaches for investigating the complex processes and systems in public health research. This method is the pertinent approach where diverse insights foster the investigation of complex research questions (Regnault et al., 2018). The lived experiences of individuals are captured in the MMR, which enables providing a patient or community perspective to the quantitative results of the study. This methodology leverages effective engagement of patient/community for identifying their priorities and improving the respective outcomes.

This design requires methodological skillsets for not just implementing best practices across the multiple methods, but also in articulating the quantitative and qualitative domains. This combination of skill sets enables generating different types of data and integrating them. The challenge is to build a collaborative and cross-disciplinary team for executing the complex mixed methods design and effectively manage the epistemological challenges *(Miller, Crabtree, Harrison, & Fennell, 2013)*. When the perspectives of subjects are weaved into the research findings, the chances of engaging community, health providers, system authorities and policy makers are enhanced which is critical for effective implementation and optimizing health outcomes. The implications of such findings are progressive when compared with findings based solely on statistical data.

EVALUATE

- What relevance do you see for 'Mixed Methods Research' in your context? Can you visualize a public health program that you are associated with?
- What are the different types of integrating quantitative and qualitative approaches in a MMR? When do you begin with quantitative and qualitative, and why?
- What are some practical considerations when you are analysing and reporting MMR data?
- What are the key obstacles to effectively conducting MMR? What are some steps you can visualize in your setting to overcome them?

ROAD AHEAD

To explore more of mixed methods, the following references are a good guide.

1. ***Combining the latest thinking in the field with practical, step-by-step guidance***

   The Third Edition of John W. Creswell and Vicki L. Plano Clark's Designing and Conducting Mixed Methods Research *is a good read that includes seven mixed methods designs with accompanying journal articles illustrating each design.*

   Available at: *https://us.sagepub.com/en-us/nam/designing-and-conducting-mixed-methods-research/book241842.* Accessed on 26-07-2021

2. ***For additional information on the major mixed methods design types***
   - Creswell, J. W., Plano Clark, V. L., Gutmann, M., & Hanson, W. (2003). Advanced mixed methods research designs. In A. Tashakkori & C. Teddlie (Eds.), Handbook of mixed methods in social and behavioral research (pp. 209–240). Thousand Oaks, CA: Sage.
   - Greene, J. C., Caracelli, V. J., & Graham, W. F. (1989). Toward a conceptual framework for mixed-method evaluation designs. Educational Evaluation and Policy Analysis, 11(3), 255–274.

3. ***More about Timing and Combining in MMR***
   - Caracelli, V. J., & Greene, J. C. (1993). Data analysis strategies for mixed-method evaluation designs. Educational Evaluation and Policy Analysis, 15(2), 195–207.
   - Morgan, D. L. (1998). Practical strategies for combining qualitative and quantitative methods: Applications to health research. Qualitative Health Research, 8(3), 362–376.
   - Morse, J. M. (1991). Approaches to qualitative-quantitative methodological triangulation. Nursing Research, 40, 120–123.
   - Tashakkori, A., & Teddlie, C. (1998). Mixed methodology: Combining qualitative and quantitative approaches. Thousand Oaks, CA: SageSpecial Interest Group on Mixed Methods Research

4. ***MMR Special Interest Group (SIG) from the American Educational Research Association***

   The SIG aims to support, encourage, and increase dialogue and idea exchange among educational researchers utilizing mixed methods and those interested in integrating qualitative and quantitative research approaches.

   Available at: *https://www.aera.net/SIG158/Mixed-Methods-Research-SIG-158* Accessed on 27-07-2021

REFERENCES

Aral, S. O., & Blanchard, J. F. (2012). The Program Science initiative: improving the planning, implementation and evaluation of HIV/STI prevention programs. Sex Transm Infect, 88(3), 157-159. doi:10.1136/sextrans-2011-050389

B M Ramesh, Halli, S., Jayanna, K., & Mohan HL. (2018). Maternal, Newborn and Child Health Programmes in India: A Programme Science Approach: Sage.

Chan, G. J., Labar, A. S., Wall, S., & Atun, R. (2016). Kangaroo mother care: a systematic review of barriers and enablers. Bulletin of the World Health Organization, 94(2), 130-141J. doi:10.2471/BLT.15.157818

Chen, H. (2006). A Theory-Driven Evaluation Perspective on Mixed Methods Research; Vol. 13, No. 1, 75-83

Creswell, J. W., & Plano Clark, V. L. (2011). Designing and conducting mixed methods research (2nd ed.). Thousand Oaks, CA: Sage Publications, Inc.

David H. Peters, N. T. T., Taghreed Adam. (2013). Implementation research in health: a practical guide; Accessed from https://apps.who.int/iris/bitstream/handle/10665/91758/9789241506212_eng.pdf;jsessionid=A3B1149E175A0766B7AD88B53CB86D2D?sequence=1. Retrieved from

Greene, J. C., Caracelli, V. J., & Graham, W. F. (1989). Toward a Conceptual Framework for Mixed-Method Evaluation Designs. Educational Evaluation and Policy Analysis, 11(3), 255-274. doi:10.2307/1163620

Hunter, A., & Brewer, J. (2003). Multimethod research in sociology. In T. C. Teddlie (Ed.), Handbook of mixed methods in social and behavioral research (pp. 577-594): Thousand Oaks, CA:Sage..

Jayanna, K., Swaroop, N., Kar, A., Ramanaik, S., Pati, M. K., Pujar, A.,... Mohan, H. L. (2019). Designing a comprehensive Non-Communicable Diseases (NCD) programme for hypertension and diabetes at primary health care level: evidence and experience from urban Karnataka, South India. BMC Public Health, 19(1), 409. doi:10.1186/s12889-019-6735-z

Jennifer Wisdom, & Creswell, J. W. (2013). Mixed Methods: Integrating Quantitative and Qualitative Data Collection and Analysis While Studying Patient-Centered Medical Home Models; https://pcmh.ahrq.gov/page/mixed-methods-integrating-quantitative-and-qualitative-data-collection-and-analysis-while#:~:text=Mixed%20Methods%20Studies,or%20sustained%20program%20of%20inquiry. Retrieved from

Kajamaa, A., Mattick, K., & de la Croix, A. (2020). How to ... do mixed-methods research. The Clinical Teacher, 17(3), 267-271. doi:https://doi.org/10.1111/tct.13145

Kar, A., & Jayanna, K. (2021). Using Mixed-Methods Approach in an Implementation Research Project to Design a Comprehensive Urban Primary Health Care Intervention for Management of Diabetes and Hypertension.

Leech, N. L., & Onwuegbuzie, A. J. (2009). A typology of mixed methods research designs. Quality & Quantity, 43(2), 265-275. doi:10.1007/s11135-007-9105-3

Leia K. Cain. (2020). Ethical Considerations in Mixed Methods Research; https://www.youtube.com/watch?v=O4mFApU4Xh4.

Mazumder, S., Taneja, S., Dube, B., Bhatia, K., Ghosh, R., Shekhar, M.,... Bhandari, N. (2019). Effect of community-initiated kangaroo mother care on survival of infants with low birthweight: a randomised controlled trial. The Lancet, 394(10210), 1724-1736. doi:10.1016/S0140-6736(19)32223-8

Medhanyie, A. A., Alemu, H., Asefa, A., Beyene, S. A., Gebregizabher, F. A., & Aziz, K. (2019). Kangaroo Mother Care implementation research to develop models for accelerating scale-up in India and Ethiopia: study protocol for an adequacy evaluation. 9(11), e025879. doi:10.1136/bmjopen-2018-025879

Miller, W. L., Crabtree, B. F., Harrison, M. I., & Fennell, M. L. (2013). Integrating mixed methods in health services and delivery system research. Health Serv Res, 48(6 Pt 2), 2125-2133. doi:10.1111/1475-6773.12123

Morse, M, J., & Niehaus, L. (2009). Mixed method design: Principles and procedures. Walnut Creek: Left Coast Press.

Pasick, R. J., Burke, N. J., Barker, J. C., Joseph, G., Bird, J. A., Otero-Sabogal, R.,... Guerra, C. (2009). Behavioral Theory in a Diverse Society: Like a Compass on Mars. Health Education & Behavior, 36(5_suppl), 11S-35S. doi:10.1177/1090198109338917

Poth, C. N. (2020). Little Quick Fix: Research Ethics; https://uk.sagepub.com/sites/default/files/upm-assets/115842_book_item_115842.pdf: Sage:.

Regnault, A., Willgoss, T., & Barbic, S. (2018). Towards the use of mixed methods inquiry as best practice in health outcomes research. Journal of Patient-Reported Outcomes, 2(1), 19. doi:10.1186/s41687-018-0043-8

Schoonenboom, J., & Johnson, R. B. (2017). How to Construct a Mixed Methods Research Design. Kolner Zeitschrift fur Soziologie und Sozialpsychologie, 69(Suppl 2), 107-131. doi:10.1007/s11577-017-0454-1

Tariq, S., & Woodman, J. (2013). Using mixed methods in health research. JRSM short reports, 4(6), 2042533313479197-2042533313479197. doi:10.1177/2042533313479197

Teddlie, Charles, & A, T. (2009). Foundations of mixed methods research: Integrating quantitative and qualitative approaches in the social and behavioral sciences. Los Angeles: Sage.

Chapter 19

Research Methods Applicable to The Medical Humanities

Upreet Dhaliwal, Satendra Singh

ABSTRACT

The application of the humanities in medical education should be evidence-based, relevant and grounded in the local context. To collect the evidence, it is important to use humanities research methods which are a key part of medical education research. They help gain insight into personal and societal factors that could impact the illness experience. Qualitative research methods can contribute to our understanding of the human condition - a critical prerequisite to helping learners become reflective, empathetic practitioners of patient-centered medicine. In this chapter, we first distinguish health humanities research from health humanities as a teaching-learning tool and then we go over five humanities research methods in detail: grounded theory, ethnography, phenomenology, narrative analysis and discourse analysis. We conclude that the method depends upon the research question and on what is the focus of the study.

Key Words: anthropology; cultural; grounded theory; humanistic competencies; humanities; literature; narrative inquiry.

ASSESS NEED

As biomedical researchers, we make use of mainly quantifiable data given the need for science to be objective. We are, as a result, conventionally trained to manipulate and measure well-defined variables and use statistical methods to support or refute our hypothesis. We frequently employ quantitative methods to measure changes in knowledge, attitudes, behavior and skills - and in the long term, changes in patient outcomes - after an educational intervention.

Within medical education, however, sometimes we wish to explore the values and experiences of the human stakeholders. In addition, now that the Phase 1 of the Competency-Based Curriculum for undergraduate medical education requires sessions on the medical humanities, we will need, over time, to study the impact of the humanities on the acquisition of humanistic competencies (Narrative competence, Critical thinking, Visual literacy, Advocacy, and Reflective capacity) in learners (Singh et al., 2020; Dennhardt et al., 2016). Values, experiences, and humanistic competencies are not measurable in numerical terms and we will be obligated to apply qualitative research methods.

To put it succinctly, we use quantitative analysis when we need to measure things and qualitative analysis when we want to understand phenomena. Studies may - and do - use a mix of quantitative and qualitative research methods for a well-rounded study. For example, some of us are familiar with employing questionnaires to capture both numerical and non-numerical data.

A book on research methods in medical education is incomplete without a discussion of those qualitative methods that are an integral part of humanities research. Use of such methods can contribute uniquely to improving our understanding of the human condition - a critical prerequisite to help learners become reflective, empathetic practitioners of patient-centered medicine (Ratka, 2018; Nazario, 2009; Pfeiffer et al., 2016). This chapter is about the specific qualitative research methods that are best geared towards capturing the humanistic attributes of stakeholders, and the human/socio-cultural factors contributing to the oppression due to illness.

BRIEF

- Humanities research methods are a key part of medical education research; they help gain an alternative insight and understanding of personal and societal factors that could impact the illness experience
- The application of the humanities in medical education should be evidence-based; the evidence should be collected through research methods that are relevant and are grounded in the local context
- Grounded theory, Ethnography, Phenomenology, Narrative analysis and Discourse analysis are methods borrowed from the humanities, but which are important ways to create evidence for the teaching and assessment of the health humanities in medical education.

CONTEXTUALIZE

The variety of ways in which qualitative data can be collected has been discussed in detail in preceding chapters. Suffice it to say that the data is primarily sourced from people and can be in the form of primary data (textual, visual, audio or video output of study participants) or secondary data in the form of existing text, images, audio or video recordings (Irwin, 2013; Klugman & Lamb, 2019).

The particular way to analyse the collected data will depend upon your research question. Let's take a look at the following scenario:

Scenario

You are in the middle of a devastating pandemic, and along with your medical students, you are trying to make sense of the chaos that has ensued. Your broad goal is to uncover the perceptions of people about the delivery of health care during the COVID-19 pandemic.

How would you proceed?

- **Approach One**: One group of students plans to use pandemic-related writing published by medical journals in the preceding months. They will examine the writing for patterns that may help with a conceptual understanding of how people navigate the healthcare delivery system. The analysis will provide an insight into the problems related to the pandemic; any theory generated as a result may help service planners find ways to improve healthcare delivery and prepare for future pandemics. This qualitative method is called **grounded theory** research as the outcomes are 'grounded' in the data.
- **Approach two:** Another group of students decide to visit a nearby leprosy colony repeatedly over a period of time and talk to residents about their experiences with health care during the pandemic. In response to lock down and social distancing norms, and by maintaining covid appropriate behaviour, they will conduct the visits in an open, outdoor space. This would be an **ethnographic** method of research which is conducted in participants' natural setting.
- **Approach three**: Yet another group decides to study events as they unfold in the Intensive Care Units of their institution again by maintaining covid appropriate behaviour. They choose to interview healthcare providers on site, and take videos (with permission), to capture perceptions of healthcare providers on the phenomenon of care delivery at point of care. This method is known as **phenomenology**.
- **Approach four**: A fourth group of students wish to examine personal incident narratives (verbal or written) of people (including from amongst themselves) who have experienced the COVID-19 illness directly themselves or in close family members. They will analyze the stories as a whole and look for patterns and clues that may point to the challenges faced by the narrators. This is the **narrative inquiry** method of qualitative research.
- **Approach five**: The last group of students choose to examine political leaders' statements on the pandemic published in leading newspapers to determine how language is used to influence public opinion about the healthcare scenario in the country. This is **discourse analysis**.

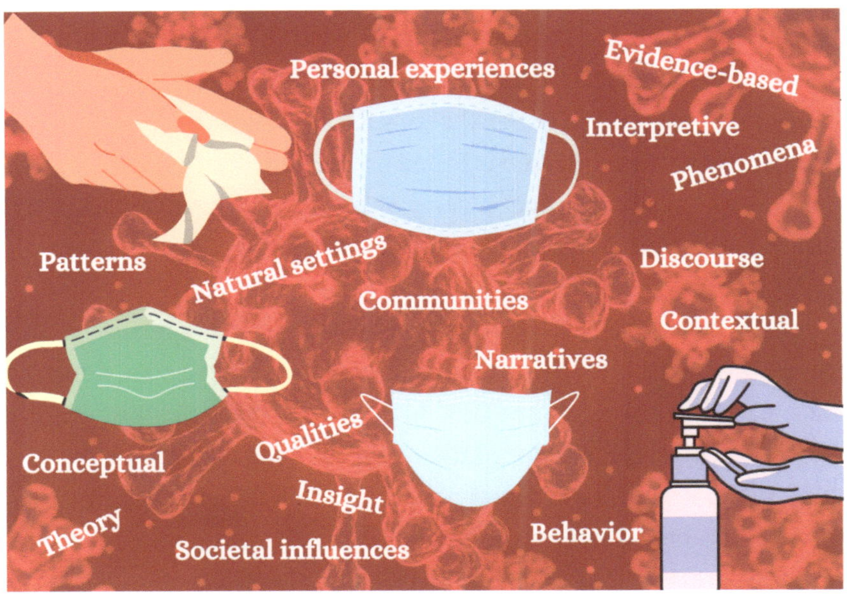

Figure 1: Terminology related to the scenario contextualised in this chapter

DESCRIBE

If the health humanities are about helping learners to reflect, to contextualise, to read between the lines, and to think critically so as to earnestly engage with the patient's illness experience, or to gain perspective on the caregiver's or provider's experience, then the methods we use must capture these attributes (Charon, 2017; Klugman, 2020; Callus, 2020).

Health humanities teaching versus research

Health humanities research may need to be distinguished from health humanities as a teaching-learning tool. When we use poetry in a classroom setting to introduce learners to the concept of empathy or of ethics, then poetry is a teaching tool or an intervention. At the end of the intervention, we could measure how many learners enjoyed the class and how the empathy scores changed after the intervention. Here, we have used a humanities tool (poetry) in an interventional study and have gathered quantitative data. Though the tool is from the repertoire of the humanities, the research method is not. On the other hand, we could ask the class to do a close reading of a single poem or a collection. They would go on to record significant words or phrases, and then consider the connotations and denotations of the words in the context of the poem so as to get a deeper understanding of how people communicate. Close reading with connotation and denotation is an important component of narrative analysis, which is a humanities research method (Pamboukian, 2019).

Here is another example: when we use a piece of fiction or ask students to write a creative piece, our goal could be to teach students to reflect and to critically analyse situations; that makes it a teaching method. However, when we examine the published literature for evidence of the human condition, and then we engage with the writing to understand how people experience illness in that specific context (the context may be of gender or economic disparities, or other differences), then it is a humanities research method (Kelly, 2013; Browne & Nash, 2016).

Qualitative research in the health humanities

Each of the approaches that we listed in the Contextualize section can help uncover new information that we may not think of otherwise. Nothing in the data can be predefined; qualitative researchers may be somewhat subjective as they will tend to make observations and interpret them through the perspective of their own lenses. The information collected is based on participants' perspectives as interpreted by the researchers, hence, is contextual and cannot be generalized to the larger population.

Let us now examine each of these approaches in greater detail.

A) **Grounded theory** (Charmaz & Thornberg, 2020)

This method is often used in sociology when the goal is to examine textual data in order to generate theory. By 'generate theory' is meant to generate a conceptual explanation of a process or an event when existing theories are unable to fully explain it. For example, if we consider the scenario we've given in the conceptualise section (pandemic-related writing published by medical journals), we may, upon data analysis, theorise that writings by people with disabilities (as opposed to writings by people without disabilities) expose many unique barriers that are specifically pandemic-related (like an inability to apply the face mask, or being subjected to inequitable triage decisions).

Grounded theory examines textual data line by line and looks for features of interest in the writing - each snippet of which is then coded inductively (versus deductive coding, vide infra, which is a component of content analysis). The hallmark of this method is that snippets are constantly compared with each other to look for patterns and the coding continues until theoretical saturation is reached, which means that no new codes are being generated. Codes may be descriptive single words or short phrases that are reflective of the feelings, actions or meanings implied by the narrator.

The other hallmark of this method is that data analysis and data collection go on simultaneously rather than starting the analysis only after all the data is collected. This is helpful because sometimes early coding may throw up surprises and suggest that some areas need greater exploration, and so the questions asked of the participants/text can be modified accordingly.

Inductive and deductive coding

Coding is used in most methods of qualitative analysis and will therefore be described in some detail here. In inductive coding, the codes are generated live as we progress with close reading of the data. Being a thorough, iterative process, it is time-consuming, but it allows an unbiased examination of the entire data without any preconceived ideas restricting thought. Deductive coding, on the other hand, is used when we already have a set of predefined codes, and we want to see how the data fits into those. Even during deductive coding, we should keep our options open and choose to assign inductive codes to text that seems to be important to the investigation even if it doesn't fit into any of the deductive codes. Deductive codes may be gleaned from our previous work or could be based on a review of the literature. When we use inductive coding, conversely, the review of literature is advisably done after the coding to avoid bias and to see how our themes correlate with what others have said on the subject.

We have often used both inductive and deductive coding to analyse the open-ended feedback from participants of our humanities workshops. For example, their reflective narratives were coded inductively, while their post-workshop reflections were examined for evidence of components of the ABCDE paradigm (appropriate analytical and attitudinal skills, ethical and professional behaviour, effective communication, respect for diversity, and empathy). The reasoning behind us using an inductive approach for the narratives was that they were submitted before we met for the workshop and it was impossible for us to know beforehand what they would reveal. The feedback, on the other hand, was obtained post-workshop, and we wished to examine if the workshop had been effective in introducing participants to the ABCDE attributes of physicians. A deductive approach ensured that our particular interest was captured through pre-decided codes.

Once coding is done, the codes are re-examined and the ones that are focussed and representative of the data are retained, while others are either merged or deleted. The focused codes are grouped together into a framework of categories that may be flat or have a hierarchical structure.

Flat framework of categories

Each code is given equal importance. This is simple to do when there are fewer codes, as in the example given above, where we used ABCDE as predetermined codes; however, for more complex analysis with multiple codes, a hierarchical structure may be more appropriate.

Hierarchical framework of categories

A hierarchical structure allows us to organize the codes into themes of varying importance and also helps to show how they relate to each other. There may be many tiers (Figure 2).

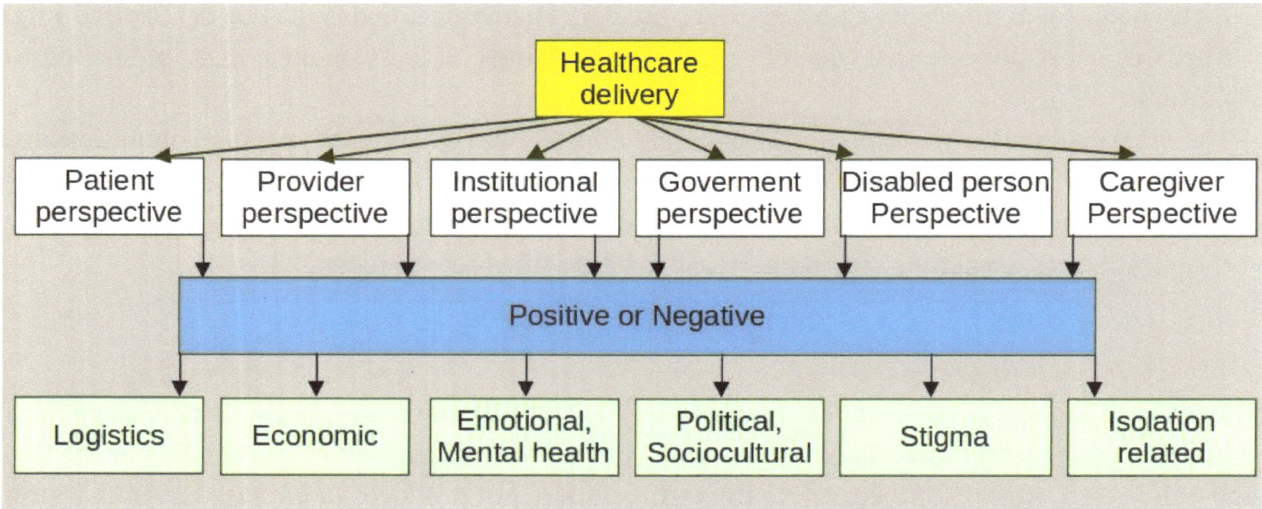

Figure 2: Hierarchical framework of categories generated during inductive coding of qualitative data

The figure shows possible codes that may arise out of the task we set out in the beginning of this section: an examination of pandemic-related writing published by medical journals around issues of healthcare delivery. The example shows many codes, but you may need fewer depending on the objective of the study. You could merge 'logistics' and 'economic' if you find that there is too little data to support either one of them. Similarly, 'stigma' and 'emotional, mental health' could be merged if needed.

Some tips on coding (Please also see chapter xxx: Qualitative Data Analysis of Interviews)

- Find a balance between having too many codes (becomes difficult to generate a coherent theory) and having only a handful (cannot learn anything new from the data).
- The code should not be so specific that it only applies to a few pieces of data, nor should it be so generic that every phrase fits into it.
- Avoid overlapping of codes - each should be different enough from the other so as not to confuse the coder.
- Constantly compare codes and categories to ensure that they are accurate and representative of the data and don't overlap.

The initial categories that we generate are tentative. The data is revisited to see if the categories are able to explain everything that is going on, and if the answer is yes, they are finalized and are interpreted to develop a theory that is 'grounded' in the data. This is the most frequently used methodology in medical education and medical humanities research and has consequently been described in relatively greater detail.

B. **Ethnography** (Hammersley & Atkinson, 2019; Varis, 2020)

Ethnography involves the direct observation of people in their natural settings or contexts. It is frequently used in anthropology to examine the influence of social and cultural beliefs and practices on people's behavior. Researchers need to immerse themselves in the setting and to engage with the participants to understand the situation from the inside. In the example given above with respect to the residents of a leprosy colony, students could use an ethnographic approach to study how the pandemic has affected healthcare delivery to this vulnerable section of society and how their own beliefs and attitudes towards healthcare have impacted/helped them in these troubled times. The outcome of this research would be an 'ethnography'. The ethnography could assist administrators and legislators in formulating policies that take into account socio-cultural factors that influence healthcare decisions, and could help in planning for equitable healthcare delivery to all vulnerable populations.

C. **Phenomenology** (Matua & Van Der Wal, 2015, Manen and Manen, 2021)

Phenomenology originated in philosophy and is about exploring the lived experience of participants. The process focuses on individual experiences around a phenomenon of interest, which may be a routine one, or an extraordinary one, like a pandemic. Phenomenology involves seeing or thinking about phenomena in a manner that is open-minded, perception-based, and serendipitous. In our example, we are interested in learning about the impact of the pandemic on healthcare delivery from the intensivist's perspective. Naturally, as is true for most humanities research, our own (the researcher's) perspective is added on to that of the participant, and it is common to clarify, in the final write up, in what way one's perspective may have influenced the results. An inductive analysis is conducted on the data - in our example, it will be done to uncover emotional, psychological, ethical, and professional implications of the pandemic. The outcome of the study might help administrators understand what kind of logistical support, and wellness/resilience interventions are needed so that service delivery at point of critical care can be optimised.

D **Narrative inquiry** (Woods, 2011; Shapiro, 2011)

This method of analysis is an examination of people's stories that directly relate to their experiences with real-life events like migration, an epidemic, or stigmatization for a communicable disease. The origin of this method lies in literary criticism. Narrative analysis, unlike other methods of qualitative data analysis, takes the story as a whole instead of coding it in bits and pieces. Thus, attention is paid not only to what has happened but also to the context of when and where it takes place, who the other people involved in the story are, and how they relate to each other. The chronology may or may not be linear, as is usual when the narrator is engrossed with making sense of impactful events.

Narratives usually do not display scientific objectivity but are moving accounts of struggle with emotional impact that make them engaging methods in medical humanities research. Several narratives around the same event can be examined to see if any patterns emerge.

The stages of narrative analysis (Greenhalgh et al, 2005):

It starts with a close reading of the text and an initial tentative coding. This is followed by a deeper reading to interpret the narrative and look for complex truths that may have been left unsaid. The findings are then verified through a review of the literature which also looks for alternative ways to explain or refute the findings. The final two steps are to write a representative account of whatever is learned, and to illustrate the account and provide evidence through the use of quotes from the narratives.

In the example we've chosen to work with, the personal incident narratives of people who have experienced illness due to COVID-19 may uncover important alternative ways to improve access to healthcare that may not otherwise be obvious. For example, their stories may disclose that resident welfare associations or groups of philanthropic private citizens may be roped in early for logistical support should the need arise again.

E. **Discourse analysis** (Mogashoa, 2014; Longhi, 2020)
This research method, commonly employed in linguistic and cultural studies, examines written or spoken material (including its non-verbal components) in the contexts in which the discourse takes place. Through discourse analysis, researchers seek to understand how language is used in real life situations; it focuses not so much on rules and syntax of language, but on the contextual meaning of the language used in the discourse. Attention is given to the purpose of the discourse, the assumptions and values communicated, and power equations between the speaker and the intended listener. The aim is to understand how language can expose social hierarchies and inequalities, or how it is used to achieve goals like trust-building, conflict resolution or rabble-rousing, among other things. Entire conversations (say, published interviews or videotaped ones) or texts (commentaries, newspaper articles) are examined for how the narrative has been built from beginning to end, the presumed intentions behind the euphemisms or metaphors used, how emphasis was created, how pauses were used, and how engagement was created.

The steps of a discourse analysis

- Once the research question is defined, the source of the discourse is identified (one source or a judicious mix of magazines, newspapers, interviews, political commentary, advertisements, manifestos etc). In our example, the students plan to use political statements published in newspapers.
- The next step is to gather and record relevant facts like when was the material published, who was the author and who was the intended audience, and what was the social and political context at the time.
- This would be a good time to conduct a literature review on the topic so that you have a theoretical framework ready on which to base your analysis. Thus, if you want to study the language used by politicians when referring to the pandemic, you might want to read up on the history and nature of political discourse in the country in general, and on the history of the relationship between the political parties and healthcare service providers and users.
- The analysis of the content is the next step where, as mentioned in the other methods above, we look for themes and patterns consistent with our research question, and explore the ideology, intentions, and attitudes conveyed by the wording and phrases used.
- The final step is to write out the results and to discuss it in the larger context while drawing conclusions that answer the research question.

Picking an appropriate research method

It depends on what your focus is: Is it the phenomenon you are trying to understand (Phenomenology)? Is it the political discourse around the phenomenon (Discourse Analysis)? If it is the people impacted by the phenomenon, are you interested in learning of their experiences through observing them in their natural settings (Ethnography) or would you rather study narrations of their first-hand experiences (Narrative Inquiry)? Is your interest in examining data so that you can generate a theory (Grounded Theory)?

SUMMARIZE

As medical education researchers, we will need, on occasion, to examine the values and experiences of the people we interact with. In readiness for that, we must familiarise ourselves with qualitative research methods which are frequently used in the humanities.

Which particular method we use depends on what question we plan to ask, and on the nature of the material we plan to examine. Methods like grounded theory, ethnography, phenomenology, narrative inquiry, and discourse analysis have an important role to play as we seek to create evidence in the fields of medical education and medical humanities.

EVALUATE

Have you used any of these methods in your research? If not, which of them would lend itself best to answering a question about medical education or the medical humanities that has been troubling you?

ROAD AHEAD

- The best way to learn more about these research methods is to read the references at the end of the chapter and then to embark on the journey as soon as possible.
- Plan out a research project that uses one of these qualitative methods and share the results with the larger community of medical educators who might be looking for ways to integrate these methods into their work and could benefit from your experience.

REFERENCES

Browne, K., & Nash, C. J. (2016). Queer methods and methodologies: An introduction. In *Queer Methods and Methodologies* (pp. 1-24). Routledge.

Callus, A. M. (2020). The Contribution of Disability Studies to the New Humanities. Word and Text, *A Journal of Literary Studies and Linguistics*, 10(1), 70-90.

Charmaz, K., & Thornberg, R. (2020). The pursuit of quality in grounded theory. *Qualitative Research in Psychology*, 1-23.

Charon, R. (2017). To see the suffering. *Academic medicine: journal of the Association of American Medical Colleges*, 92(12), 1668.

Dennhardt, S., Apramian, T., Lingard, L., Torabi, N., & Arntfield, S. (2016). Rethinking research in the medical humanities: a scoping review and narrative synthesis of quantitative outcome studies. *Medical Education*, 50(3), 285-299.

Greenhalgh, T., Russell, J., & Swinglehurst, D. (2005). Narrative methods in quality improvement research. *Quality & safety in health care*, 14(6), 443–449. https://doi.org/10.1136/qshc.2005.014712

Hammersley, M., & Atkinson, P. (2019). Ethnography: Principles in practice. Routledge.

Irwin, S. (2013). Qualitative secondary data analysis: Ethics, epistemology and context. *Progress in development studies*, 13(4), 295-306.

Kelly, C. (2013). Building bridges with accessible care: Disability studies, feminist care scholarship, and beyond. *Hypatia*, 28(4), 784-800.

Klugman, C. M. (2020). What is a Bioethics of the Oppressed in the Age of COVID-19?. *The American Journal of Bioethics*, 20(10), 29-31.

Klugman, C. M., & Lamb, E. G. (Eds.). (2019). Research methods in health humanities. Oxford University Press.

Longhi, J. (2020). Proposals for a discourse analysis practice integrated into digital humanities: theoretical issues, practical applications, and methodological consequences. *Languages*, 5(1), 5.

Matua, G. A., & Van Der Wal, D. M. (2015). Differentiating between descriptive and interpretive phenomenological research approaches. *Nurse researcher*, 22(6).

Mogashoa, T. (2014). Understanding critical discourse analysis in qualitative research. *International Journal of Humanities Social Sciences and Education*, 1(7), 104-113.

Nazario, R. J. (2009). Medical humanities as tools for the teaching of patient centered care. *Journal of Hospital Medicine: An Official Publication of the Society of Hospital Medicine*, 4(8), 512-514.

Pamboukian, S. A. (2019). Denotation and Connotation. *Research Methods in Health Humanities*, 15.

Pfeiffer, S., Chen, Y., & Tsai, D. (2016). Progress integrating medical humanities into medical education: a global overview. Current opinion in psychiatry, 29(5), 298-301.

Ratka, A. (2018). Empathy and the development of affective skills. *American Journal of pharmaceutical education*, 82(10).

Shapiro, J. (2011). Illness narratives: reliability, authenticity and the empathic witness.

Singh, S., Dhaliwal, U., & Singh, N. (2020). Developing Humanistic Competencies Within the Competency-Based Curriculum. *Indian Paediatrics*, 57(11), 1060-1066.

van Manen, M., & van Manen, M. (2021). Doing Phenomenological Research and Writing. *Qualitative health research*, 31(6), 1069–1082. https://doi.org/10.1177/10497323211003058

Varis, P. (2020). Ethnography. *In The Routledge Handbook of English Language and Digital Humanities* (pp. 185-201). Routledge.

Woods, A. (2011). The limits of narrative: provocations for the medical humanities. *Medical humanities*, 37(2), 73-78.

Chapter 20

Integrative Medicine & Health Research: Methods, Case Studies and Research Priorities

Krishnamurthy Jayanna, Gangadharan GG, Sai Baba M

ABSTRACT

Integrative Medicine Research (IMR) refers to a *systematic and scientific integration of the Modern and Traditional* systems of Medicine to achieve best possible outcomes of health and wellbeing for the clients. Lack of adequate communication between the disciplines, lack of clarity in execution of integrated protocols has affected research and clinical practice. IMR aims to effectively integrate subjective and the objective dimensions of health and wellbeing to enhance quality of life. This is particularly relevant in today's scenario where interventions that lead to increase in longevity of life are not necessarily improving quality of life and wellbeing.

The current chapter targets the medical education fraternity from modern and traditional medicine backgrounds, and provides clarity, direction and practical guidance in planning and conducting IMR. The chapter also provides case studies and best practices in the space of Ayurveda research, and finally sheds light on relevance of appropriate communication and knowledge translation in this space.

The authors conclude that the successful conduct of IMR requires conducive ecosystem, coming together of multidisciplinary experts jointly led by the clinicians from modern and traditional systems with the backing of a clear vision, roadmap and funding. Research methods can vary from simple exploration to observational studies (case series, case reports) to experimental trials within hospitals to observe clinical impact, as well as health systems and public health research to observe population level impact. Often the research methods and instruments in one discipline may not be applicable to other disciplines, which should be duly considered. Appropriate attention to ethical considerations and consent procedures while conducting research, and systematized knowledge translation with the stake holders will go a long way in strengthening IMR.

Key Words: integrative health, complementary and alternative medicine, integrative medicine, research methods, research priorities.

ASSESS NEED

'Integrative Medicine', 'Complementary & Alternative Medicine' (CAM) are the terms used interchangeably in relation to how traditional systems of medicine relate to mainstream or conventional medicine. Lack of clarity of these terms among the stakeholders and the community has hindered research on the ground and policy formulation (Agarwal, 2018; Nayak, 2012) particularly in basic sciences. Some work in this direction is already going on and outcomes are awaited with bated breath. For instance the 'ASIIA (A Science Initiative In Ayurveda (Zollman & Vickers, 1999). While the need for more options to promote holistic health and wellbeing are clearly felt by both care providers and the public, and is also well articulated in the policies, the 'know-do' gap, inadequate capacities and systems to carry out multi-disciplinary & integrative medicine research have affected progress in research and knowledge uptake. (Singh, 2010; Bansal, 2020). This was witnessed most recently in the COVID-19 pandemic context (Seifert et al., 2020).

Over the last 150 years, the average lifespan of population globally has increased from under 30 years to over 70 years (Max Roser, Esteban Ortiz-Ospina and Hannah Ritchie, 2019). The most common killers then used to be communicable diseases which are now replaced by the non-communicable diseases. Despite advances in clinical and public health infrastructure in the space of modern medicine that have led to this transition and improvements in longevity, the quality of life and wellbeing continues to be sub-optimal (Megari, 2013) with a large number of people living with chronic diseases that can adversely affect their quality of life. The aim of the present paper is to study quality of life and especially Health-related quality of life (HRQoL. The non-communicable diseases are characterized by lifestyle changes; chronic nature of medical conditions which at best can be controlled and managed, but not cured; require constant attention to health behaviors, risk factors and treatment compliance which put people to lot of stress and anxiety, affecting their wellbeing and quality of life (Pati et al., 2020; Varni et al., 2007). Sustainable Development Goal 3 refers to both 'Health' and 'Wellbeing' but modern medicine has challenges in addressing the wellbeing and quality of life which have personal and subjective connotations(Robert et al., 2005) (Bansal, 2020). This aspect of subjectivity also poses a challenge for research and clinical practice in this space.

In the recent years, Complementary Medicine Research and Integrative Medicine Research are emerging as solutions to explore how the conventional and non-conventional systems of medicine may come together to address both the objective and subjective measures of health and wellbeing (Complementary, Alternative, or Integrative Health: What's In a Name?, n.d.). Alternate approaches when integrated scientifically with modern medicine can not only promote holistic health and wellbeing but can also be cost-effective and preventative in nature (Anand et al., 2017), thus offering many benefits at individual and public health level. India has been the home of traditional systems of healing such as Ayurveda, Yoga and others which are increasingly researched in the past few decades. The current policy environment both globally and locally is more favorable for multi-disciplinary research in the space of Integrative Medicine. However, the research capacities to conduct Integrative Medicine Research, and the institutional mechanisms and training systems to support clinicians and researchers are not quite there to fill this growing void. Efforts are proactively undertaken globally to address this gap (NCCIH Strategic Plan FY 2021–2025, n.d.). Medical Education systems both in the schools of Modern Medicine as well as AYUSH need to be strengthened in this direction (Bansal, 2020).

In this backdrop, the current chapter is written keep the target audience as faculty and postgraduates of Allopathy, AYUSH and other health science disciplines to address the following needs:

1. Clarify terminologies, scope and relevance of complementary, alternative, and integrative medicine.
2. Provide direction to designing and implementing integrative medicine research
3. Illustrate case studies and best practices in this space considering the current health situation in the world
4. Highlight relevance of appropriate communication and knowledge translation in the space of integrative medicine research
5. Outline ideas to trigger Integrative Medicine Research within the universities and institutions

BRIEF

- Standard definitions, scope, relevance of Complementary, Alternative and Integrative medicine
- How to design and implement integrative medicine research
- Emerging priorities and best practices in Integrative Medicine Research
- Communicating or Translating knowledge of research in this space.
- Outline ideas to trigger IMR within universities and institutions

CONTEXTUALIZE

A key hurdle to the fulfilment of the 'Sustainable Health and Wellbeing' is the lack of synergistic and holistic approach to patient care. Efforts are divided between the health and wellbeing dimensions, between the objective and subjective verticals there by depriving opportunities to understand synergistic effects of interventions that address both (Krishnamurthy Jayanna, 2021). For ex: growing body of knowledge in meditation and yoga research is indicating physiological improvements in functioning of several body systems – circulatory, cardiovascular, neuro-endocrinal, etc. in addition to improvements in wellbeing and quality of life. Modern medicine has established evidence in optimizing clinical effects for several disease conditions. *How can they be integrated for enhancing patient outcomes comprehensively?*

Non-communicable diseases are a growing concern today (Jayanna et al., 2019). How does modern medicine, Ayurveda and the other AYUSH practices come together to mitigate the problem? Where do we begin and how do we proceed in planning integrative medicine research to derive benefits at individual and population level?

Ayurveda is an age-old school of healing and offers curative and preventative remedies to many conditions that are prevalent today. *What are some of the case studies and success stories in Ayurveda research that offers lessons for building integrative research agenda today?*

These are some questions that provide a context and build the content for the subsequent sections of the chapter.

DESCRIBE

This section will shed light on key terminologies commonly used in this space. Further it alludes to practical considerations in designing and conduct integrative research, and some sensitivities involved in science communication and knowledge translation in this domain. The section lists few ideas and suggestions for universities and institutions to initiate IMR in the context of National Education Policy (NEP) 2020. Toward the end, few case studies and success stories of Ayurveda research are provided as relevant examples of IMR in today's scenario.

Definitions and Terminologies

Complementary Medicine refers to a context where a *non-mainstream medicine is practiced along with mainstream medicine*; Alternate Medicine, where *non-mainstream medicine substitutes mainstream medicine*, whereas Integrative Medicine refers to a *systematic and scientific integration of the two* to achieve best possible outcomes in health and wellbeing for its clients (Complementary, Alternative, or Integrative Health: What's In a Name?, n.d.). In the same line, the authors use the term '*Integrative Health research*' to extrapolate the idea to the health of the populations (instead of clients) with adequate focus on prevention and health promotion (Jayanna, 2020). This is particularly relevant today as the research is highly skewed toward curative research without necessarily addressing the lifestyle, prevention and health promotion aspects related to both communicable and non-communicable diseases.

Multidisciplinary scope and Ecosystem Preparedness

Integrative Health or Integrative Medicine Research (IMR) calls for a systems level effort with a focus on holistic or wholesome care of not just the patients, but their families as well. Working as a team with the common goal of highest outcomes for clients is the focus here; and the outcomes are not limited to 'clinical cure or relief of symptoms' but also accommodates aspects of 'wellbeing' and 'quality of life'(Nayak, 2012) particularly in basic sciences. Some work in this direction is already going on and outcomes are awaited with bated breath. For instance the 'ASIIA (A Science Initiative In Ayurveda (Nguyen et al., 2019) miscommunication is a leading cause of patient harm and is associated with reduced patient satisfaction, health literacy, treatment compliance and quality of life. In conventional healthcare settings, the differences in professional hierarchy, training, communication styles and culture are recognised communication barriers. Less is known about interprofessional communication (IPC. Hospital administration and systems must promote conducive working atmosphere for specialists from different back grounds. The care should extend to families and community that the hospital caters to. Essentially it requires a multi-disciplinary approach involving clinicians and specialists from Modern medicine and AYUSH backgrounds, Nursing and Physiotherapy, Public Health, Counselling, Wellness and Wellbeing, Hospital Administration, etc. Indian Council of Medical Research in its strategic plan and agenda 2030 document gives impetus to strengthening infrastructure and interdisciplinary research capacities in this space through a network of centers, collaborations with AYUSH agencies and guideline formulation in carrying out integrative medicine research (Swaminathan, 2017)

Vision, Orientation and Capacity Building

A high-level vision and commitment from the hospital and health authorities to generate best possible outcomes for their clients, families and society through multi-disciplinary and integrative approaches is the starting point. Conscious effort toward orientation and training of teams in undertaking multidisciplinary research, regular multidisciplinary research meetings and journal clubs, conferences and seminars will go a long way in building competencies, and in opening the mindsets and appropriate attitudes required in his space.

In hospital settings during postgraduate clinical training, PG dissertations and collaborative research between modern and AYUSH postgraduates may be encouraged. In addition, integrative medicine fellowships, electives and workshops on integrative medicine research are ways and means of expanding capacities in this domain. Several of these best practices are already in vogue in the west and it is time these are stepped up within the country which has been a home to many traditional systems of medicine and healing. Integrative Medicine Health Incubators within the universities and institutions can be yet another platform to trigger momentum and interest in young minds (Anand et al., 2017).

Designing, Conducting and Communicating IMR: Examples and Practical Considerations

The research methods can vary from simple exploration and observational studies to experimental designs. Mixed methods study design integrating quantitative and qualitative approaches have been adopted commonly which generates rich information from multiple perspectives (Bishop & Holmes, 2013)80 of which met criteria for applying the quality appraisal tool. The most popular formal mixed methods design was triangulation (used by 74% of studies. The study objectives and the available funding will inform the scope and rigor of the research design. While planning research studies, due consideration should be given to available evidence and efforts should be made to build on the existing knowledge base. All clinical studies should be registered at the clinical trials registry of Government of India (CTRI) prior to the commencement of data collection.

A good beginning for aspirants can be to integrate non-pharmacological interventions advocated by the traditional disciplines (Yoga, Meditation, Ayurveda) with current evidence-based management of Diabetes Mellitus (type 2) or Hypertension (Hagins et al., 2013). Ayurveda has specific recommendations on diets and lifestyle modification which are not researched adequately (Chandola, 2012) and their effects on lifestyle modification and there by disease control will be worthwhile to explore. Monitoring the blood glucose and blood pressure levels before and after the integration can give good indication of effects of these interventions.

In the contexts of pre-hypertension and pre-diabetes where the mainstream recommendations are completely non-pharmacological and lifestyle oriented, experimental trials may be adopted to delineate the actual impact of traditional interventions. A randomized control trial can establish additional incremental effects of yoga and meditation on the control of blood glucose and blood pressure in comparison to the subjects that are exposed only to the routine management and lifestyle modification, but without yoga and meditation. In addition to the clinical outcomes, we can also study the impact on subjective wellbeing and quality of life. Studies do indicate their positive impact on management of stress and anxiety, and promotion of healthy behaviors which are very relevant in chronic medical conditions (Satyapriya et al., 2009) India, were randomized to practicing yoga and deep relaxation or standard prenatal exercises 1-hour daily. The results for the 45 participants per group who completed the study were evaluated by repeated measures analysis of variance.\nRESULTS: Perceived stress decreased by 31.57% in the yoga group and increased by 6.60% in the control group (P=0.001.

In settings where current modalities of treatment are not effective (terminal management of certain cancer conditions) or in case of new challenges (such as COVID-19), exploration of alternative remedies such as AYUSH should be boldly explored, with due attention to the rigor of scientific exploration. Case series or case reports can precede experimental studies. In terminal cases of cancers where the clients and families go through high distress with substantial loss of quality of life, more open exploration of integrative medicine to mitigate the suffering can be explored.

Health systems research and Public Health research are yet another area with wide scope and ramifications for population health and wellbeing. In India, health and wellness centers are emerging as platforms at primary care level to improve disease prevention and health promotion efforts (Pati et al., 2020). Several pilots have been attempted to integrate Yoga and Meditation at these centers, to improve population control of non-communicable diseases and to promote healthy lifestyles. Large scale research programs while measuring population-based outcomes will go a long way in adding new knowledge in this space (Jayanna, 2020).

While the traditional disciplines are required to be researched adequately, due considerations should be given to scenarios that are not compatible to a particular research design or a method for philosophical and discipline specific reasons. For example, Ayurveda and Yoga disciplines rely on the subjective component of individual such as body-mind constitution (Prakruti) as well as the role of mind in disease causation. These theories of causation are non-linear and complex and pose a challenge for research through the lens of modern science that rely on biological markers at a physical and physiological level. Experts suggest that the research methods in integrative space should be flexible and customized to support the theories and objectives of the discipline (Sankar Sylapan et al., 2020; Singh, 2010) a unique passive form of meditation. We carried out a pilot study recruiting male heartfulness meditators (proficient n = 24, with 6–28 years of meditation experience; novice n = 24, 5 to 16 months of experience. These issues should be overcome through consultations and dialogue between the researchers and clinicians of different disciplines, paving way for newer advances in research methods as well.

The role of clear communication to the clients, their informed consent with regards to research participation, appropriate approvals from institutional ethics review board are critical in effective conduct of high quality IMR. Systematic planning of data gathering and transparency in making the data available for public consumption and validation by other experts will go a long way in building credibility of IMR. Communication and dissemination of research findings, both positive and negative, through high impact peer reviewed journals, joint conferences targeting clinicians of modern and traditional disciplines, multidisciplinary health researchers, policy makers will help to advance research in this space further. Policy makers, health systems and local hospital systems should come forward with dedicated investment to support IMR in an uninterrupted and ongoing manner.

Education and Science Communication of Integrative Medicine Research: Perspectives and Considerations

Education plays a vital role in laying the foundation for shaping minds for responsible actions. The progress made by utilizing the advancements in Science and Technology has solved several problems humanity is facing and will continue to solve many in future. Ancient Indian Knowledge system had the wisdom to take care of physical, mental, social, emotional, and spiritual wellbeing (Jayanna, 2020; Sai Baba, 2021). There is a need to bring awareness about ancient Indian knowledge systems, communicate the essence in a language that is simple and impactful that paves way for integration. Particularly, the communication should be targeted to the medical education systems and clinical practitioners to dispel the myths and concerns and equip them to deal with the current needs constructively (Fischhoff & Scheufele, 2013). The requirement is to look for easily adoptable and large-scale implementable nuggets of ancient Indian knowledge systems, be it yoga or meditative and spiritual practices. With the Industrial Revolution, the whole world, including India embraced urbanization, and focused on western methods of education and medicine; the ancient systems and institutions providing education and health became weaker.

The world has seen many epidemics and pandemics like Zika, Ebola, H1N1(Swine flu), AIDS, Asian Flu, Spanish Flu, Polio, etc. For a few, solutions were found and got contained or almost eradicated (polio). The impact of COVID and its long-term consequences on people's health is yet to be understood (Mahase, 2020). While vaccines could be introduced, not much progress is made in terms of finding drugs for a cure for the affected. Some combination drugs finding a cure, though not 100% effective, are giving relief to the affected. A glimmer of hope is the anti-Covid-19 drug 2-deoxy-D-glucose (2-DG) developed by DRDO, India (DRDO, 2021). Initial trials have indicated that the molecule used in the drug helps COVID affected patients recover faster, and their dependency on supplemental oxygen is also reduced. The property of only accumulating in virally infected cells has made this drug unique. The COVID pandemic brings into sharp focus the importance of investing in social policies protecting the most vulnerable. Science must remain open and continue to find solutions, and the scope for integrative medicine research is vast.

There are many diseases that humanity is yet to find a cure, posing a challenge to the researchers in the field of medicine. Many people are forced to learn to live with diseases like Asthma, Hearing loss, Diabetes, Dengue, Rabies, Hepatitis B, Herpes simplex. Some are life-threatening, like HIV/AIDS, Leukaemia. Some like bipolar disorder and Schizophrenia disrupt the life of the patient and family members. Diseases like Parkinson's, Dementia and Alzheimer's are life-limiting and pose a challenge to handle. With life expectancy increasing all over the world and the elderly population increasing, providing care for the elderly has become a challenge. Lifestyle diseases are threatening to cripple the world.

The response of individuals is different to different medicines and treatments paving way for personalized medicine today. Ayurveda always advocated customized and personalized approach recognizing the uniqueness of each being. Allopathy has its chain of side effects connected with every prescribed medication. Healthcare systems like Ayurveda, Yoga and Naturopathy, Unani, Siddha, and Homoeopathy (AYUSH) have been given impetus in India realizing the need for reviving the profound knowledge of ancient systems of medicine and ensuring the optimal development and propagation of the AYUSH systems of healthcare (Tillu, 2018; Sai Baba, 2021). AYUSH systems of medicine focus on changing the human body to respond better and making the entire body-mind system intact. The allopathic system focuses on rigorous measurement of the success of any drug and treatment. *It seems ironical and unfair to measure the efficacy of one medicine system in terms of what is established for another system.*

Wellbeing is essential, and all the progress of science and technology is toward enhancing the quality of life. Providing affordable and holistic health care is the challenge societies are struggling to achieve. Integrative Medicine or Health research is the need of the hour and policies, investments and infrastructure should be conducive to encourage high quality research in the years to come to realize the goals of sustainable health and wellbeing.

Role of Health Science Universities and Institutions in the context of NEP 2020

National Education Policy 2020 provides impetus to universities and higher educational institutions in the direction of multidisciplinary research and education. Here is a list of suggestions to initiate IMR within the institutions and universities:

- Create **Stewardship for Integrative Medicine - Multidisciplinary research** at Institutional level
- Create **Integrative Medicine Incubation Centers** to promote innovations and multidisciplinary research
- Develop **Electives, Certificate courses and Fellowship programs** in Integrative or Complementary & Alternative Medicine
- Initiate **Doctoral programs** in Integrative Medicine
- Support **Cross-disciplinary PG dissertation projects** supported by institutional seed funding

Case studies in Ayurveda Research

Ayurveda can be integrated in different ways for achieving better patient outcomes in Integrative medicine practice. Ayurveda therapies and medication when used concomitantly with Western medicine help reduce the dependence on the Western medicine, many of which are associated with severe side effects when used long-term. They also help to enhance the effectiveness of other medicine or therapies. In this section, we briefly discuss few case studies wherein integrating 2 or more systems of medicine has profoundly benefited patients with chronic illnesses. It has also given evidence regarding safety such a combination.

***Ulcerative colitis** a chronic, debilitating inflammatory bowel disease is usually managed with anti-inflammatories, corticosteroids, biologicals and surgery, in severe cases (Kucharzik et al., 2020). These treatments are associated with side effects including treatment resistance and risk of malignancies and other organ damage. Oral administration of extract of Holarrhenaantidysenterica (1 g thrice daily), decoction of Ficus glomerata (40 ml twice daily), powder combination of Cyperus rotundus, Mesua ferrea, and Symplocosracemosa (1 g each thrice daily) and recto-colonic administration of 100 ml Ficus glomerata decoction significantly reduced the symptoms of Ulcerative colitis including frequency of bowel movements, bleeding in stools, and abdominal pain. Hemoglobin increased, erythrocyte sedimentation rate (ESR) decreased, red blood cells (RBCs), pus cells and occult blood in stool were reduced. Patients were receiving conventional medication as well. However, by the end of the Ayurveda treatment, Intake of aminosalicylates was reduced by 82.86%, corticosteroids gradually by 25% and finally stopped (Patel et al., 2010) general debility and with abnormal structural pathology in the descending colon, particularly sigmoid colon. In modern medical science, there is no permanent curative and safe treatment for this disease. This study can be helpful for reducing the need of steroids and surgical processes in the patients of ulcerative colitis. A clinical study of 43 patients of ulcerative colitis has been conducted at the O.P.D. (outdoor patient department.*

*Osteopenia is a precursor to **Osteoporosis** and fractures and is very prevalent in women around and beyond menopause. Management with Hormone replacement therapy (HRT), selective estrogen receptive modulators (SERMs) and Bisphosphonates are effective but associated with side effects (Qaseem et al., 2017). A traditional Ayurveda preparation Panchatiktaghrita given along with calcium and vitamin D3 supplements for 1 year, significantly improved Bone mineral density (BMD) and bone-specific biomarkers, namely serum vitamin D3, osteocalcin, and TRAP-5b when compared with calcium and vitamin D3* *supplements alone. The Ayurveda formulation contains plants, such as Azadirachta indica (Nimba), Trichosanthes dioica (Patola), Solanum xanthocarpum (Kantakari), Tinospora cordifolia (Guduchi), and Adhatodavasica (Vasa). These herbs are katu (pungent) and tikta (bitter) in taste that are helpful in slowing down the degeneration processes. The herbs are processed in ghee and administered with milk, all adding to its therapeutic effectiveness. The bone-stabilizing effects of the formulation reduced the risk of major osteoporotic fractures and improved the quality-of-life scores (Munshi et al., 2019).*

Integrative management is the need of the hour in ***Cancer care****. Ayurveda is routinely sought after for minimizing the side effects of cancer chemo and radiotherapy and also for prevention of recurrence. A study comparing the effect of adjuvant Ayurveda treatment, started during and after chemotherapy (CT) has shown promising results in reducing CT induced toxicity and improving quality of life. Ayurveda herbo-mineral preparations MauktikyuktaKamdudha (MKD), MauktikyuktaPravalPanchamruta (MPP) and Suvarnabhasmadi formulation (SBD) were administered along with six cycles of CT. The CT drugs were based on the type of malignancy. One group received only the CT and the second group received Ayurveda preparations, with sub-groups receiving MKD and MPP along with CT, MKD and MPP after CT and MKD, MPP and SBD after CT. It was observed that all the Ayurveda sub-group patients had significantly reduced nausea, loss of appetite, constipation, and fatigue. There was significant improvement in the Karnofsky score for assessment of general well-being and activities of daily life and global score of the Quality of Living Questionnaire, which incorporates symptomatic criteria, general condition, functional ability, and disease-related symptoms (Deshmukh et al., 2014).*

*Recently, a "****Nano-Ayurvedic Medicine****", a proprietary combination of gold nanoparticles and phytochemicals from mango was piloted as an adjuvant to CT in a small group of 6 breast carcinoma patients. All the patients (n=3) treated with the Ayurveda adjuvant showed 100% disease control rate (DCR) or clinical benefit rate (CBR) (Khoobchandani et al., 2020) herein, full details: (i.*

Pain and the need for use of analgesics reduced considerably by administration of solid lipid Boswellia serrata particles (SLBSP) and standardized Boswellia serrata gum extract (BSE) in knee osteoarthritis. SLBSP was superior to BSE (Kulkarni et al., 2020). Ayurveda medications given alone and in combination with Methotrexate had similar benefits in ***Rheumatoid arthritis*** *patients. This study is of high importance as for the very first time CAM has been compared with allopathic medicine with all the trappings of a placebo-controlled, double blind, randomized trial. Placebos were developed to mimic the 148 Ayurveda formulations used in the study. The physician was allowed to draw from this list of 148 formulations to individualize the treatment in the Ayurveda group (Furst et al., 2011) methotrexate (MTX.*

A comprehensive Ayurveda regimen consisting of calorically unrestricted Ayurvedic diet, yoga, meditation, breathing; and Ayurvedic herbs significantly improved arterial pulse wave velocity, reduced BMI, total cholesterol, LDL cholesterol, and triglycerides and reduced or eliminated the need for antihypertensive medications in a majority of ***Coronary Heart Disease*** *patients (DuBroff et al., 2015). Five to ten sessions of Abhyanga (massage) with Ayurveda oils significantly reduced the need to use antispastic drugs, helped achieve standing with minimal assistance sooner, and gave better locomotion at discharge to Stroke patients, when given in conjunction with Physiotherapy. The Modified Ashworth Score improved supporting the hypothesis that interneuron overactivity was impacted by the Abhyanga (Sankaran et al., 2019).*

SUMMARIZE

- Integrative Medicine Research refers to a *systematic and scientific integration of the Modern and Traditional Medicine* to achieve best possible outcomes of health and wellbeing. IMR effectively integrates subjective with the objective dimensions of health and wellbeing, andcan significantly impact quality of life. This is particularly relevant in today's scenario where improvements in longevity of life is associated with changing disease profile and poor quality of life in chronic disease conditions.
- Successful conduct of IMR requires conducive ecosystem, vision and funding, coming together of multidisciplinary experts across Modern Medicine, AYUSH, Nursing, Counselling, Public Health, Technology and Hospital Administration. Research methods can vary from simple exploration to observational studies (case series, case reports) to experimental trials as well as health systems research, with due consideration to building on the existing evidence available. Often the research methods and instruments in one discipline may not be applicable to other disciplines, which should be duly considered. The sole purpose of IMR is to advance health, wellbeing and quality of life that should promote advances in integrative medicine as well as research methods.
- Appropriate attention to ethical aspects, consent procedures while conducting research and appropriate dissemination with a focus on clinical practitioners from multiple disciplines, policy makers and health systems will go a long way in building credibility of IMR.
- It is critical to focus on the young minds and shape their attitudes and perspectives toward IMR through appropriate institutional level policies, ecosystem preparedness and capacity building programs. Fellowships in Complementary and Alternative Medicine and IMR, electives and workshops, cross-disciplinary PG dissertations and PhD programs, integrative medicine health incubators will go a long way.

EVALUATE

- What do you understand of the terms 'Complementary Medicine', 'Alternative Medicine', and 'Integrative Medicine'?
- What are the key obstacles for effective implementation of Integrative Medicine Research? What are different types of integrative medicine research one can undertake?
- What hospital systems and larger policy and health systems preparedness will facilitate integrative medicine research?
- What are some low hanging fruits to begin integrative medicine research? Where do you think you can start in your setting? Who is a strong collaborator with whom you can take up a research work in your area of work?
- What aspects of science communication needs special consideration when it comes to general public and health policy makers

ROAD AHEAD

For more clarity and understanding of integrative health, its relevance in current times and policy ramifications:

- Nayak, J. (2012). Ayurveda research: Ontological challenges. *Journal of Ayurveda and Integrative Medicine*, 3(1), 17–20. https://doi.org/10.4103/0975-9476.93942

- *Complementary, Alternative, or Integrative Health: What's In a Name?* (n.d.). https://www.Nccih.Nih.Gov. Retrieved July 19, 2021, from https://www.nccih.nih.gov/health/complementary-alternative-or-integrative-health-whats-in-a-name
- Bansal, P. (2020). Medical Education in India: History, current scenario and future perspectives in an Integrative Health System context. *NITI AAYOG, Govt of India*, 25.
- Jayanna, K. (2020). *Science and Practice of Integrative Health and Wellbeing Lifestyle.*
- Tillu, G. (2018). AYUSH research for New India: Vision and strategies. *Journal of Ayurveda and Integrative Medicine*, 9(3), 240–244. https://doi.org/10.1016/j.jaim.2018.06.001

For more on good case studies, research methods and designs in relation to integrative medicine research,

- Bishop, F. L., & Holmes, M. M. (2013). Mixed Methods in CAM Research: A Systematic Review of Studies Published in 2012. *Evidence-Based Complementary and Alternative Medicine*, *2013*, 1–12. *https://doi.org/10.1155/2013/187365*
- Furst, D. E., Venkatraman, M. M., McGann, M., Manohar, P. R., Booth-LaForce, C., Sarin, R., Sekar, P. G., Raveendran, K. G., Mahapatra, A., Gopinath, J., & Kumar, P. R. K. (2011). Double-blind, randomized, controlled, pilot study comparing classic ayurvedic medicine, methotrexate, and their combination in rheumatoid arthritis. *Journal of Clinical Rheumatology: Practical Reports on Rheumatic & Musculoskeletal Diseases*, 17(4), 185–192. *https://doi.org/10.1097/RHU.0b013e31821c0310*
- Kulkarni, P. D., Damle, N. D., Singh, S., Yadav, K. S., Ghante, M. R., Bhaskar, V. H., Hingorani, L., & Gota, V. S. (2020). Double-blind trial of solid lipid Boswellia serrata particles (SLBSP) vs. Standardized Boswellia serrata gum extract (BSE) for osteoarthritis of knee. *Drug Metabolism and Personalized Therapy*, 35(2),/j/dmdi.2020.35.issue-2/dmpt-2020-0104/dmpt-2020-0104.xml. https://doi.org/10.1515/dmpt-2020-0104
- Hagins, M., States, R., Selfe, T., & Innes, K. (2013). Effectiveness of Yoga for Hypertension: Systematic Review and Meta-Analysis. *Evidence-Based Complementary and Alternative Medicine*, *2013*, 1–13. *https://doi.org/10.1155/2013/649836*
- Singh, R. (2010). Exploring issues in the development of Ayurvedic research methodology. *Journal of Ayurveda and Integrative Medicine*, *1*(2), 91. *https://doi.org/10.4103/0975-9476.65067*

For more science communication about ancient knowledge systems

- Fischhoff, B., & Scheufele, D. A. (2013). The science of science communication. *Proceedings of the National Academy of Sciences*, *110*(Supplement_3), 14031–14032. *https://doi.org/10.1073/pnas.1312080110*
- Nguyen, J., Smith, L., Hunter, J., & Harnett, J. E. (2019). Conventional and Complementary Medicine Health Care Practitioners' Perspectives on Interprofessional Communication: A Qualitative Rapid Review. *Medicina*, 55(10), 650. *https://doi.org/10.3390/medicina55100650*
- Sai Baba, M. (2021). *Communicating Ancient Indian Knowledge Systems* (pp. 5–14). NIAS/NSE/U/SP/05/2021.*https://niascom.in/tooonlogs*

Good journals and programs on IMR and CAM

- *http://www.jaim.in*
- *https://www.hindawi.com/journals/ecam/*
- *https://www.cancer.gov/about-cancer/treatment/cam*
- *https://www.sciencedirect.com/journal/european-journal-of-integrative-medicine*

- *https://nunm.edu*
- *https://journals.sagepub.com/home/chp*
- *https://www.sciencedirect.com/journal/advances-in-integrative-medicine*

REFERENCES

Agarwal, V. (2018). Complementary and Alternative Medicine Provider Knowledge Discourse on Holistic Health. Frontiers in Communication, 3, 15. https://doi.org/10.3389/fcomm.2018.00015

Anand, A., Tyagi, R., & Kaur, P. (2017). Incubating Integrative Medicine in India through PMO's Atal Incubator Scheme of Niti Aayog. Annals of Neurosciences, 24(3), 131–133. https://doi.org/10.1159/000477149

Bansal, P. (2020). Medical Education in India: History, current scenario and future perspectives in an Integrative Health System context. NITI AAYOG, Govt of India, 25.

Bishop, F. L., & Holmes, M. M. (2013). Mixed Methods in CAM Research: A Systematic Review of Studies Published in 2012. Evidence-Based Complementary and Alternative Medicine, 2013, 1–12. https://doi.org/10.1155/2013/187365

Chandola, H. (2012). Lifestyle disorders: Ayurveda with lots of potential for prevention. AYU (An International Quarterly Journal of Research in Ayurveda), 33(3), 327. https://doi.org/10.4103/0974-8520.108814

Complementary, Alternative, or Integrative Health: What's In a Name? (n.d.). https://www.Nccih.Nih.Gov. Retrieved July 19, 2021, from https://www.nccih.nih.gov/health/complementary-alternative-or-integrative-health-whats-in-a-name

Deshmukh, V., Kulkarni, A., Bhargava, S., Patil, T., Ramdasi, V., Gangal, S., Godse, V., Datar, S., Gujar, S., & Sardeshmukh, S. (2014). Effectiveness of combinations of Ayurvedic drugs in alleviating drug toxicity and improving quality of life of cancer patients treated with chemotherapy. Supportive Care in Cancer: Official Journal of the Multinational Association of Supportive Care in Cancer, 22(11), 3007–3015. https://doi.org/10.1007/s00520-014-2294-0

DRDO. (2021). DCGI approves anti-COVID drug developed by DRDO for emergency use. https://pib.gov.in/PressReleasePage.aspx?PRID=1717007

DuBroff, R., Lad, V., & Murray-Krezan, C. (2015). A Prospective Trial of Ayurveda for Coronary Heart Disease: A Pilot Study. Alternative Therapies in Health and Medicine, 21(5), 52–62.

Fischhoff, B., & Scheufele, D. A. (2013). The science of science communication. Proceedings of the National Academy of Sciences, 110(Supplement_3), 14031–14032. https://doi.org/10.1073/pnas.1312080110

Furst, D. E., Venkatraman, M. M., McGann, M., Manohar, P. R., Booth-LaForce, C., Sarin, R., Sekar, P. G., Raveendran, K. G., Mahapatra, A., Gopinath, J., & Kumar, P. R. K. (2011). Double-blind, randomized, controlled, pilot study comparing classic ayurvedic medicine, methotrexate, and their combination in rheumatoid arthritis. Journal of Clinical Rheumatology: Practical Reports on Rheumatic & Musculoskeletal Diseases, 17(4), 185–192. https://doi.org/10.1097/RHU.0b013e31821c0310

Hagins, M., States, R., Selfe, T., & Innes, K. (2013). Effectiveness of Yoga for Hypertension: Systematic Review and Meta-Analysis. Evidence-Based Complementary and Alternative Medicine, 2013, 1–13. https://doi.org/10.1155/2013/649836

Jayanna, K. (2020). Science and Practice of Integrative Health and Wellbeing Lifestyle. www.Cihw.In. https://www.cihw.in/book-release

Jayanna, K., Swaroop, N., Kar, A., Ramanaik, S., Pati, M. K., Pujar, A., Rai, P., Chitrapu, S., Patil, G., Aggarwal, P., Saksena, S., Madegowda, H., Rekha, S., & Mohan, H. L. (2019). Designing a comprehensive Non-Communicable Diseases (NCD) programme for hypertension and diabetes at primary health care level: Evidence and experience from urban Karnataka, South India. BMC Public Health, 19(1), 409. https://doi.org/10.1186/s12889-019-6735-z

Khoobchandani, M., Katti, K. K., Karikachery, A. R., Thipe, V. C., Srisrimal, D., Dhurvas Mohandoss, D. K., Darshakumar, R. D., Joshi, C. M., & Katti, K. V. (2020). New Approaches in Breast Cancer Therapy Through Green Nanotechnology and Nano-Ayurvedic Medicine—Pre-Clinical and Pilot Human Clinical Investigations. International Journal of Nanomedicine, 15, 181–197. https://doi.org/10.2147/IJN.S219042

Krishnamurthy Jayanna. (2021). 2019_KJ_Med_Abstract_Ref.pdf. 178425 Bytes. https://doi.org/10.6084/M9.FIGSHARE.14483292

Kucharzik, T., Koletzko, S., Kannengießer, K., & Dignaß, A. (2020). Ulcerative Colitis—Diagnostic and Therapeutic Algorithms. Deutsches Aerzteblatt Online. https://doi.org/10.3238/arztebl.2020.0564

Kulkarni, P. D., Damle, N. D., Singh, S., Yadav, K. S., Ghante, M. R., Bhaskar, V. H., Hingorani, L., & Gota, V. S. (2020). Double-blind trial of solid lipid Boswellia serrata particles (SLBSP) vs. Standardized Boswellia serrata gum extract (BSE) for osteoarthritis of knee. Drug Metabolism and Personalized Therapy, 35(2),/j/dmdi.2020.35.issue-2/dmpt-2020-0104/dmpt-2020-0104.xml. https://doi.org/10.1515/dmpt-2020-0104

Mahase, E. (2020). Covid-19: What do we know about "long covid"? BMJ, m2815. https://doi.org/10.1136/bmj.m2815

Max Roser, Esteban Ortiz-Ospina and Hannah Ritchie. (2019). Life Expectancy [https://ourworldindata.org]. https://ourworldindata.org/life-expectancy#

Megari, K. (2013). Quality of Life in Chronic Disease Patients. Health Psychology Research, 1(3), e27. https://doi.org/10.4081/hpr.2013.e27

Munshi, R. P., Kumbhar, D. A., Panchal, F. H., & Varthakavi, P. (2019). Assessing the Effectiveness of Panchatikta Ghrita, a Classical Ayurvedic Formulation as Add-on Therapy to Vitamin D3 and Calcium Supplements in Patients with Osteopenia: A Randomized, Open-Labeled, Comparative, Controlled Clinical Study. Journal of Alternative and Complementary Medicine (New York, N.Y.), 25(10), 1044–1053. https://doi.org/10.1089/acm.2019.0124

Nayak, J. (2012). Ayurveda research: Ontological challenges. Journal of Ayurveda and Integrative Medicine, 3(1), 17–20. https://doi.org/10.4103/0975-9476.93942

NCCIH Strategic Plan FY 2021–2025. (n.d.). https://www.Nccih.Nih.Gov. Retrieved July 19, 2021, from https://www.nccih.nih.gov/about/nccih-strategic-plan-2021-2025

Nguyen, J., Smith, L., Hunter, J., & Harnett, J. E. (2019). Conventional and Complementary Medicine Health Care Practitioners' Perspectives on Interprofessional Communication: A Qualitative Rapid Review. Medicina, 55(10), 650. https://doi.org/10.3390/medicina55100650

Patel, M. V., Patel, K. B., & Gupta, S. N. (2010). Effects of Ayurvedic treatment on forty-three patients of ulcerative colitis. Ayu, 31(4), 478–481. https://doi.org/10.4103/0974-8520.82046

Pati, M. K., Swaroop, N., Kar, A., Aggarwal, P., Jayanna, K., & Van Damme, W. (2020). A narrative review of gaps in the provision of integrated care for noncommunicable diseases in India. Public Health Reviews, 41(1), 8. https://doi.org/10.1186/s40985-020-00128-3

Qaseem, A., Forciea, M. A., McLean, R. M., Denberg, T. D., & Clinical Guidelines Committee of the American College of Physicians. (2017). Treatment of Low Bone Density or Osteoporosis to Prevent Fractures in Men and Women: A Clinical Practice Guideline Update From the American College of Physicians. Annals of Internal Medicine, 166(11), 818–839. https://doi.org/10.7326/M15-1361

Robert, K. W., Parris, T. M., & Leiserowitz, A. A. (2005). What is Sustainable Development? Goals, Indicators, Values, and Practice. Environment: Science and Policy for Sustainable Development, 47(3), 8–21. https://doi.org/10.1080/00139157.2005.10524444

Sai Baba, M. (2021). Communicating Ancient Indian Knowledge Systems (pp. 5–14). NIAS/NSE/U/SP/05/2021.

Sankar Sylapan, B., Nair, A. K., Jayanna, K., Mallipeddi, S., Sathyanarayana, S., & Kutty, B. M. (2020). Meditation, well-being and cognition in heartfulness meditators – A pilot study. Consciousness and Cognition, 86, 103032. https://doi.org/10.1016/j.concog.2020.103032

Sankaran, R., Kamath, R., Nambiar, V., & Kumar, A. (2019). A prospective study on the effects of Ayurvedic massage in post-stroke patients. Journal of Ayurveda and Integrative Medicine, 10(2), 126–130. https://doi.org/10.1016/j.jaim.2018.02.137

Satyapriya, M., Nagendra, H. R., Nagarathna, R., & Padmalatha, V. (2009). Effect of integrated yoga on stress and heart rate variability in pregnant women. International Journal of Gynaecology and Obstetrics: The Official Organ of the International Federation of Gynaecology and Obstetrics, 104(3), 218–222. https://doi.org/10.1016/j.ijgo.2008.11.013

Seifert, G., Jeitler, M., Stange, R., Michalsen, A., Cramer, H., Brinkhaus, B., Esch, T., Kerckhoff, A., Paul, A., Teut, M., Ghadjar, P., Langhorst, J., Häupl, T., Murthy, V., & Kessler, C. S. (2020). The Relevance of Complementary and Integrative Medicine in the COVID-19 Pandemic: A Qualitative Review of the Literature. Frontiers in Medicine, 7, 587749. https://doi.org/10.3389/fmed.2020.587749

Singh, R. (2010). Exploring issues in the development of Ayurvedic research methodology. Journal of Ayurveda and Integrative Medicine, 1(2), 91. https://doi.org/10.4103/0975-9476.65067

Swaminathan, S. (2017). ICMR Strategic Plan & Agenda 2030: Transforming Health of Indian People through Responsive Research. ICMR, Government of India. https://main.icmr.nic.in/sites/default/files/Books/ICMR_Strategic_plan.pdf

Tillu, G. (2018). AYUSH research for New India: Vision and strategies. Journal of Ayurveda and Integrative Medicine, 9(3), 240–244. https://doi.org/10.1016/j.jaim.2018.06.001

Varni, J. W., Limbers, C. A., & Burwinkle, T. M. (2007). Impaired health-related quality of life in children and adolescents with chronic conditions: A comparative analysis of 10 disease clusters and 33 disease categories/severities utilizing the PedsQLTM 4.0 Generic Core Scales. Health and Quality of Life Outcomes, 5(1), 43. https://doi.org/10.1186/1477-7525-5-43

Zollman, C., & Vickers, A. (1999). ABC of complementary medicine: What is complementary medicine? BMJ, 319(7211), 693–696. https://doi.org/10.1136/bmj.319.7211.693

Section III

Publication

Chapter 21

Publication Ethics

Shanthi Ananthakrishnan, Ananthakrishnan N.

ABSTRACT

Publication ethics refers to rules and guidelines to be followed and practiced when publishing a research work. This is necessary to maintain professional and academic honesty which is essential when the information is shared with a larger audience who may incorporate some of the conclusions and recommendations in their practice. The code of conduct for publication was laid down by the committee on publication ethics (COPE), founded in 1997, to prevent misconduct in publication. The chapter highlights various types of misconducts associated with publication which include falsifying and manipulating data, plagiarism, duplicate publishing, salami slicing, self-citation, simultaneous publication, conflicts of interest and authorship issues. Attention is drawn to the guidelines framed by The International committee of medical journal editors (ICMJE).

The authors have given a comprehensive checklist which can be used by the research workers to ensure that there is no academic dishonesty of any sort during publication. Any unethical practice noticed by the editors or brought to their attention can lead to serious consequences ranging from tendering an apology to imprisonment.

Key Words: publication ethics; academic dishonesty; authorship; plagiarism.

ASSESS NEED

Out of the many waves of change which are engulfing medical education, one with an immense magnitude is the importance given to medical research. Medical students, though minimally sensitised to research, are not aware of the importance or steps in submission and publication of their research work as a platform to share the knowledge arising out of research activities, however small the contribution might be considered. Just as there are ethical guidelines for conducting research, there are guidelines for sharing the results of the work to a wider audience on printed or electronic media. Breaching the guidelines will amount to academic dishonesty and may lead to retraction of the published work. Hence researchers need to be aware of the issues involved and ensure that the manuscript proposed to be submitted for publications meets all current ethical guidelines. This chapter will discuss the proper and ethical way of publishing research.

BRIEF

- Define publication ethics.
- List and explain various types of unethical practices in publication.
- Create awareness of consequences of unethical publication.
- Provide Checklist for authors to avoid unethical issues.
- Provide links to useful URLs for this purpose.

CONTEXTUALISE

Presented below are some of the glaring examples of unethical publication practices and their consequence:

1. Alfredo Fusco (Italy), a cancer researcher at the University of Naples has, since 2012, been under criminal investigation for fraud, including manipulation of images in his published studies. As of 2020, Fusco has had 22 of his publications retracted, and an additional four papers corrected (Fusco, 2018).
2. A request by an author to correct one of his papers in 2015, led to an investigation by the journal which led to 19 of his papers being retracted for falsification (Retraction Watch, 2016).
3. Edward Awh and graduate student David Anderson (US), formerly from the University of Oregon, retracted nine of their publications due to data fabrication (Retraction Watch, 2016).
4. A former postdoc at the National Institutes of Health committed misconduct in a study of hepatitis by falsely claiming that data from a single trial subject were actually from more than a dozen different people (Retraction Watch, 2013).

The knowledge of publication ethics, therefore, is mandatory for all young authors to avoid such unpleasant consequences.

DESCRIBE

What is publication ethics?

It is a set of rules or guidelines to be followed while publishing, to enable the researchers to share genuine authentic data without any fabrication and simultaneously giving due credit to all those and only those concerned with the scientific or scholarly research work. Both the publishers and authors need to follow some basic core practices to win the trust and confidence of the readers. The term "Publication Ethics" has been attributed in Psychology Dictionary to one Dr. Halvorson who noticed a remarkable similarity of his earlier work in another article published later (Pam, 2013). The same author has gone on to define publication ethics as "Publication ethics are rules of conduct generally agreed upon when publishing results of scientific research or other scholarly work. Generally, it is a standard that protects intellectual property and forbids the re-publication of another's work without proper credit. It also forbids the use of plagiarism of another's efforts". Data and information published as original must, in fact, be original. There are so many incidents and anecdotes of malpractices such as stealing another person's work etc., which have brought disgrace both to the publishers and the authors.

In 1997, a group of editors who had experienced publication malpractice had a meeting and their deliberations led to the formation of The Committee on Publication Ethics (COPE) to prevent misconducts in publication. The committee was officially registered in the UK in 2007 and is funded by subscription by its members composed of publishers, journal editors and others involved in academic publication (About COPE – Core Practices 2017). Guidelines have been laid to define and deal with publication misconduct (Kutz, 2019).

Types of unethical practices in publication (Sengupta and Honavar, 2017)

Data manipulation and Research Fraud

This refers to research where the original data is altered and fraudulent results or conclusions are published. This is particularly seen in clinical studies. On suspicion, the reviewers can ask for the original datasheet from the researchers. The researchers are generally advised to keep intact the original datasheet for at the least 5 - 10 years after publication of the work for verification, in case there is dispute as to the veracity of the data.

Plagiarism

This term refers to one researcher using the work of another researcher without any consent or acknowledgement of the latter's contribution. In other words, it amounts to a 'theft' of intellectual property of one researcher by another. This is a very common form of fraudulent practice observed in practice. There are several types of plagiarism: (Bowdoin)

- ✓ **Clear plagiarism**: Here, large portions of the text or data including tables, figures are copied verbatim by the researcher and incorporated into his/her own work.
- ✓ **Minor plagiarism**: This refers to copying only short phrases or sentences without any misappropriation of data.
- ✓ **Accidental plagiarism**: When a researcher misquotes the source of information or fails to cite their sources, it is called accidental plagiarism. This is usually unintentional. Using similar phrases or groups of words is also accidental and not intentional.
- ✓ **Mosaic plagiarism**: When phrases are quoted from another work without using quotation marks, or text is used with synonyms without altering the general structure in parts of the manuscript, it is called patchy or mosaic plagiarism.
- ✓ **Self-plagiarism**: This describes a situation where the researcher incorporates the contents wholly or in part of his/her own work published earlier into his/her new work. Authors might feel that using their own work might be ethical. From a scientific point of view this amounts to reusing a previously used material to pass off as a new work and is academically dishonest.

  Examples of a few types of self-plagiarism are:

  - Duplicating the publication in another journal without informing the publisher or the reader.
  - Publishing a large study as a number of smaller studies to increase the number of publications by that author

There are several software packages for checking plagiarism. Some of the popular ones are "Plagaware", "Urkund", and "iThenticate". The authors should check for plagiarism using one of the recognised software before sending the manuscript for publication.

Many journals carry out a rigorous plagiarism check before publishing a manuscript. COPE provides guidelines to check plagiarism when detected either in the review phase or after publication (Ithenticate, 2011). Authors, before submitting a manuscript, should ensure a thorough check for plagiarism using good commercially available software. The report of these software usually shows the text with highlighted areas which are similar to what is found in other references. It is the responsibility of authors to ensure that they pay particular attention to these highlighted areas and rewrite them, cite sources, or delete them before the paper is submitted. Plagiarism is a legal offence in India with prescribed punishment which may be fine or even imprisonment (NRI Legal Services).

Simultaneous submission

When an author submits his manuscript simultaneously to more than one journal at the same time to increase the chances of publication, it is called simultaneous publication. Many journals obtain an undertaking from the author that the manuscript has not been sent to any other journal. The authors should wait for a decision from the editor before sending it to another journal. If there is an inordinate delay in getting a reply from the editor, the corresponding author with the consent of his/her co-authors can withdraw the submission officially and resubmit it to another journal. Presenting a research work in an academic meet or having an abstract published in the conference proceedings does not preclude it from submission for publication in a journal as a full paper.

Duplicate Publication

When an author uses the same hypothesis, data, discussion points and conclusions from a previous study and publishes it as a new study it is duplication. It is different from self-plagiarism in that the same phrases, images, tables are not used. The authors might change the title, change the order of authors, or bring in hidden evidence not used in the previous publication. Authors generally use non-English journals for duplication.

Salami slicing

This is another form of duplication wherein the same author from a single study, with the same set of data, the same research question and methodology analyse the subgroups separately or just extends the follow up period and present it as different result in a new paper.

Self-citation

When an author cites his/her own work which is out of context with the current research topic, it is called self-citation. Citation is important for senior researchers as it is the basis for increasing their I and H-indices which are important for career advancement. However, citations of one's own work which are relevant to the current research are permissible.

Authorship issues, (ICJME, Bavdekar, 2012)

The International committee of medical journal editors (ICMJE) has laid down criteria for authorship of publications. Authorship is important to a researcher because it has academic and to some extent financial implications. The authors are responsible for the content of publication and have to take accountability for their work. Since, in many a case, the role of co-authors in the research work is not evident, several journals now insist that the contributions of each author towards the research work be disclosed at the time of submission of the manuscript.

Criteria for authorship

The ICMJE recommends that authorship be based on four criteria. These mandate that the author should have made substantial contribution to:

1. The design of the study, acquisition of data, analysis and interpretation.

AND

2. Preparing the draft of the manuscript or revising it critically and intellectually contributing

AND

3. Approving the final version of the manuscript

AND

4. The author should besides take accountability for all aspects of the work in and ensuring that questions related to the accuracy or integrity of any part of the work are appropriately investigated and resolved.

In addition, the author should also identify co-authors responsible for different parts of the work. The order of authors is determined by the extent of their contribution. It is better to resolve the issues of authorship at the beginning of the study itself. It is possible to change the order of authorship after acceptance or even after publication, provided, the co-authors agree, and submit a signed no objection form to the editor individually.

The corresponding author takes the responsibility of communicating with the journal during manuscript submission, peer review and publication process. He/she is responsible for answering the queries raised during peer review and provide clarification or details that are asked for. He/she should also be available after publication to sort out issues that might arise later. Although the corresponding author is responsible for all issues related to publication, it is advisable to share the correspondence with co-authors also.

Non-Author contributors

Others involved in the research project, but who do not fulfil the above said criteria are referred to as non-author contributors. Personnel involved in funding the research work, general supervision of the research work, administrative support, technical support, typing the manuscript, language editing, proof reading etc are considered non author contributors. Though they do not qualify for authorship, they can be acknowledged by the authors mentioning specific nature of their contribution.

Ghost Authors

They are the authors who have made substantial contribution to the work but are not given authorship. They are usually paid authors or professional writers (Lacasse and Leo, 2010, Chabner, 2009). They should not be included as authors but may be acknowledged. The other significant type of ghost authorship is to suppress the name of junior contributors, usually postgraduate students, who have contributed substantially to the paper (Bavdekar, 2012). Several steps have been suggested for curbing the undesirable practice of ghost writing (Lacasse and Leo, 2010, Chabner, 2009)

a. Journals should clearly state their approach to ghost writing in the instructions to authors.
b. Make authors declare the participation of a ghost writer and their role in the preparation of the manuscript.
c. Identify the person or the agency which provided ghost writing services at the end of the manuscript.

Gift Authors: Authorship is given to persons from the affiliated Institute although they have not contributed to the research work. Gift authorship is generally given to a person form the institute in which the research work was carried out and to the Heads of the Institutions or departments where the research work was carried out. It is an unethical practice to include them as authors if they do not fulfil the ICMJE guidelines.

Guest Authors: This authorship is given to a person(s) whose inclusion might improve the chances of publication of the manuscript. This again is an unethical publication practice. It is done in a belief that, having a senior or a well-known academician as one of the co-authors will influence the weightage given to the paper by the reviewers, editors or readers and increase the chance of acceptance.

Conflict of Interest or Competing interest (COI)

This refers to the fact that the author may have in conducting the research which might directly or indirectly affect the outcome of the research work. Having such conflicting interests is not considered unethical, but failing to disclose it, is. Once the COI is disclosed, the readers can judge the work with discretion.

COI can be direct or indirect. Direct COI is when the author receives employment, owns stocks, or patents of the product investigated in the research. Indirect COI is when the author receives grant to conduct the study, honoraria or paid lectures to popularise the product.

Retraction (COPE, 2019)

This refers to the act of withdrawing an article after publication form the journal. The decision to withdraw is made by the editors. A notification regarding retraction must be given to the data base and on acceptance of retraction, the article with the authors' names will have the word "Retracted" before it's title. Sometimes the article can be totally removed from the data base. The reasons for retraction must be disclosed by the editors. The general reasons are any flaw or academic dishonesty brought to the notice of the editors after publication. Retraction will be done as soon as the editors are convinced about the unethical issues related to the article. In some situations where the editors are convinced about the validity of the findings of the research work and the dispute is about authorship or conflict of interest the article might not be retracted.

Consequences of breach

What will be the consequence if any of these unethical practices is discovered? COPE has laid down guidelines for solving this misconduct. The editorial board should contact the authors and inform them about the discovery of the misconduct. If the authors accept their fault and apologise, the paper is rejected and the Head of the Institute is informed. If the paper has already been published, the authors must confess to their guilt which will be published as an erratum in the journal. If the misconduct is severe and proved, the editor has the right to retract the paper. The authors can be blacklisted by the journal and the information is shared with COPE so that the same is disseminated to other journals. If the authors deny their misconduct, the editor can take appropriate action as per COPE guidelines. They can also be questioned by the local ethical authorities.

Authors should be guided by a checklist to ensure that they have fulfilled all the required norms before submission of the manuscript to a journal.

SUMMARIZE

Publication ethics refers to the rules and guidelines that are to be followed and practiced when publishing a research work. Academic honesty is essential when the information is to be shared with a larger audience who may incorporate some of the findings and conclusions in their practice. The code of conduct during publication was laid down by the committee on publication ethics (COPE) founded in 1997 to prevent misconducts in publication.

Misconducts associated with publication are falsifying and manipulating the data, plagiarism, duplicate publishing, salami slicing, self-citation, simultaneous publication, conflicts of interest and authorship issues. Authorship issues include, gift authorship, ghost authorship, guest authorship and non-authorship contribution. Ethical guidelines in giving authorship to an author are laid down by, the International committee of medical journal editors (ICMJE).

Research workers are advised to use a checklist to avoid academic dishonesty of any sort during publication. Any unethical practice noticed by the editors or brought to their attention can lead to consequences ranging from tendering an apology to imprisonment.

EVALUATE

1. What is self-plagiarism?
2. What is the difference between gift and guest authorship?
3. What do you understand by conflicts of interest?

Based on the information contained in this chapter make a list of five points which you will consider while writing your next research paper in medical education

ROAD AHEAD

Checklist for Authors regarding Publication Ethics before submission (Modified from Sengupta and Honavar, 2017, Reference Number 8). Consulting and conforming to the items on this checklist would go a long way to avoid ethical pitfalls in publishing.

Approval for research:

1. Approval from regulatory agencies, if required.
2. Mandatory registration of all clinical trials with number.
3. Proper informed consent procedure which is recorded in the manuscript.

Data:

1. Accurate.
2. Verifiable.
3. Available for review, if required.

Plagiarism

1. Is any part of the work copied from others?
2. Has copyright permission been obtained where required?
3. Has plagiarism check been carried out and corrective measures taken?

Submission

1. Has duplicate submissions been avoided?
2. Has salami slicing been avoided?
3. Has self-citation been employed only where appropriate?

Authorship issues

1. Have authorship been provided to all those who fulfil the norms of COPE and proper sequence?
2. Has Ghost, Guest and Gift authorship been avoided?
3. Have all authors seen and agreed to the final version of the publication?

Conflict of interest

1. Has conflict of interest issues been discussed clearly with all co-authors and declared in uncertain terms in the paper wherever there is a conflict of interest?

Acknowledgments

1. Has the contribution of all those who have helped in the study, but who do not qualify to be authors, been acknowledged?

USEFUL URLs FOR PROSPECTIVE AUTHORS

COPE-*https://publicationethics.org/core-practices*

ICMJE-*http://www.icmje.org/recommendations/browse/roles-and-responsibilities/defining-the-role-of-authors-and-contributors.html*

REFERENCES

Bavdekar SB. (2012). Authorship issues. Lung India, 29:76-80. DOI: *10.4103/0970-2113.92371*

Boudoin. The Common types of Plagiarism.*https://www.bowdoin.edu/dean-of-students/judicial-board/academic-honesty-and-plagiarism/common-types-of-plagiarism.html. Accessed July17, 2021*

ChabnerBA.(2009).Ghostwritersinthesky.Oncologist,14:199-200.DOI:10.1634/theoncologist.2009-0031

Committee on Publication Ethics (COPE) (2019). Version 2.*https://publicationethics.org/files/cope-retraction-guidelines-v2.pdf*. Accessed July 20, 2021.

COPE (2007). COPE – Core Practices, (2017). *https://publicationethics.org/core-practices*. Accessed July 7, 2021.

International Committee of Medical Journal Editors, ICJME (2021). Roles and Responsibilities of Authors, Contributors, Reviewers, Editors, Publishers and Owners.*http://www.icmje.org/recommendations/browse/roles-and-responsibilities/defining-the-role-of-authors-and-contributors.html. Accessed July 18, 2021*

Ithenticate. (2011). White paper – The Ethics of Self-plagiarism. *https://www.ithenticate.com/hs-fs/hub/92785/file-5414624-pdf/media/ith-selfplagiarism-whitepaper.pdf. Accessed July 15, 2021*

Kutz K. (2019). What is COPE – (The committee on publication Ethics),

https://www.econtentpro.com/blog/what-is-cope-the-committee-on-publication-ethics/69. Accessed July 5, 2021

Lacasse JR, Leo J. (2010). Ghost writing at elite academic medical centres in the United States. PLoS Med, 7: 1 1000230. DOI: 10.1371/journal.pmed.1000230.

NRI Legal Services. Laws relating to plagiarism in India.*https://www.nrilegalservices.com/laws-relating-to-plagiarism-in-india/. Accessed July 14, 2021*

Pam N. (2013). Publication Ethics. PsychologyDictinary.org. *https://psychologydictionary.org/publication-ethics/*. Accessed July 5, 2021

Sengupta S, Honavar HG. (2017). Publication Ethics. Indian Journal of Ophthalmology, 65: 429-432. DOI: 10.4103/ijo.IJO_483_17.

Retraction watch (2013). Former NIH scientist falsified images in hepatitis study. *https://retractionwatch.com/2013/12/*. Accessed on July 24th, 2021.

Retraction watch (2016). How a researcher's request to correct one paper turned to 19 retractions. *https://retractionwatch.com/2016/11/*. Accessed on July 24th, 2021.

Retraction watch (2016). Two more retractions bring total to 9 for neuroscience duo. *https://retractionwatch.com/2016/04/19/two-more-retractions-bring-total-to-9-for-neuroscience-duo/*. Accessed on 24th July 2021.

Retraction watch (2018). Alfredo Frusco facing misconduct charges in Italy, up to 21 retractions. *https://retractionwatch.com/2018/12/24/alfredo-fusco-facing-misconduct-charges-in-italy-up-to-21-retractions/*Accessed on 24th July, 2021.

Chapter 22

Reference Management

Chinmay Shah, Sanjay Bedi

ABSTRACT

Every research whether it would be it in the domain of social sciences or of health sciences starts with review of literature and ends acknowledging these references. This process till date was done manually. Understanding this concept this is a tedious process which takes up a substantial part of the researcher's time.

The advent of software has brought about a revolutionary change in the way we do our reference management. Importing and storing references, changing the referencing format, locating missing references have been made much easier and less time consuming. In this chapter we will discuss the need for reference management, explain the basic principles of software use in reference management and compare the different tools that are available to the researcher

Key Words: review, information retrieval, reference management, publication

ASSESS NEED

In previous chapters you have seen how to do literature search, how to do research and how to write research article. Now comes most important part of research writing or thesis writing i.e. reference management. Reference management has gain due importance and it used widely in present time of plagiarism. University Grant Commission, all Journal are checking your research project for plagiarism check so if you have not cited your reference properly, your work will go above acceptable range of plagiarism. A Decade before reference management concept was not much known and researcher were writing reference on card & were keeping it in box. Secondly when you are defending your thesis or supporting your result with appropriate theory, proper referencing increase the authenticity and trust on project presented to reader.

In many of thesis work it is observed that due to workload and hasty preparation, we see mismatch between references cited and reference mentioned at the end of thesis. This is because of insufficient knowledge regarding reference management. For any research project, investigator collect large amounts of data from various source i.e. book, journal, periodicals, online database, website etc. Different sources require different format for writing it in reference section and to keep track of all these can be tiresome. Writing literature reviews require large amount of time during the manuscript writing, reference management help to simplify this entire task so that researchers can focus on scientific aspects of the research process.

BRIEF

- What is reference
- Why Reference to be done
- What is reference Management Software
- Why to use reference Management Software
- How to do reference management
- Tools, software available for reference management
- How to cite reference in publication

CONTEXTUALIZE

Pranav is doing Ph.D. in Health Professions Education (HPE), His topic of Ph.D. is gender equality in HPE. He has done review of literature and collected information from various 128 sources including Past Ph. D Thesis, Books, General Article, News, Blogs unpublished literature, offline thesis from library. He has started preparing his thesis and now looking at resources stored in drive of desktop, meanwhile he is also getting few new resources related to result he has got from his study. He now wants to quote from different source but

- He is not sure which resource is placed in which folder of computer
- Which resources are new and which are old
- In few of the resources he has duplicate information so he is unsure which information is correct
- He wants to cite reference as per APA Style in-text as well as in reference section as and when he progresses in writing
- He also wants to make sure that he is not giving two reference number to same article
- He also wants to update his resource data as and when new resource material is available
- He wants to access all his resource data from different location with different devise so that he can continue to work even if he is not in office

Let us see in following section that how reference manager will help him

DESCRIBE

Reference is, what we cite and refer to in our thesis or research paper to indicate source of original document/method/data, which can be from book, chapter in book, Journal, thesis, published or unpublished communication with author, monogram, website, blog, news paper, image etc. we should choose reference based on relevance, latest year of publication or access, number required by appropriate authority or Journal.

In present era of technology, we must cite reference as:

- It gives credit to authors of original works
- It adds credibility to our work as it reflects that we are working on valid base
- It helps us to show the continuation of previous work

There are more than thousands of reference styles, but broadly we can classify as:

- In '**Numbered style**', the in-text citation is a number, and the bibliography is a sequentially numbered list of references at the end of the text which provides full details of the corresponding in-text citation. Vancouver style is an example of numbered style and is commonly used in the field of Medicine.
- In '**Author-Date style**', in-text citation generally includes author(s)' surname/last name along with date of publication in round brackets and bibliography is listed at the end of the document, in alphabetical order of first author's surname/last name. Examples of author-date style include the Harvard style and APA (American Psychological Association) style.
- In '**Footnote style**', in-text citations are in the form of superscripted numbers and details of the reference are provided as footnotes at the end of the page. In addition, a complete list of references is provided at the end of the document, in alphabetical order of first author's surname/last name. Chicago style is an example of Footnote style.

Each university or journal subscribes to one of these styles, with litter personal variations.

Many of time we commit error in reference management due to lack of organisation, improper file name, unclassified collection, downloading same reference from different resources, vanishing of downloaded article due to hardware issue or change in working environment of devices. This all error can be taken care by reference management.

Reference management is a **systematic process** of organizing the searched literature in an easily searchable, retrievable, and citable fashion.

A reference manager (also known as citation manager or bibliographic management software) is software which allows research scholar to manage reference collected in different format (PDF, PostScript, HTML, XML, RTF, RIS) from different sources (PubMed, Google Scholar, Web of Science, Manual, other reference manager, Scopus) and also help in citation.

Reference Management basically deals with three type of activity searching, storing and writing of article. Common task performed by reference management can be listed as follow:

- Storing of search result i.e. reference into web account as well as on our computer
- Storing reference in different folder and tag it with topic, date, author, project etc
- Arrange reference according to date of publication, author, journal etc
- Retrieval of reference information from online bibliographic databases
- Automated management of PDF files
- Open Access for easier access to full-text content
- Web-based reference management for easier collaboration and use across multiple devices from multiple location
- Culling resources to collect information, idea etc from different places automatically from online databases
- Creating bibliographies.
- Changing the reference system for resubmission

- Inserting Numbered sequential/Numbered alphabetical/Author/date
- insert in-text citations into a document as you type. This will also generate a reference list or bibliography at the end of your document, based on those citations.
- Help to manually add print only resources
- share your references with others in different format and also allow to create collaborative libraries of references

All above action can be broadly put in to following heading,

- Collection/importing
- Managing/Storing
- Citing
- Sharing

Collection/importing

Most of reference magenta software have website, desktop application for installation in computer and web browser which help in collecting/importing software from different sources. Reference can be collected from resources/database where we usually search our Scholarly literature i.e. PubMed, Google Scholar, Web of Science, Scopus. We can also import reference from other reference manager in prescribe format or we can manually add reference using "add reference" option in reference manager.

It is best to collect/import reference when we are doing literature search, this can be done in either one step or two steps depending on type of reference manager you use. In one step method, reference will be directly stored to reference management website using web browser while in two step method we need to download it first and then import to desktop application. In both cases we need to synchronize website and desktop application once we finish literature search so that it's available everywhere. In most of the software you can collect/import more than one reference at a time.

You can collect reference form most of the database but method of collection will differ depending on database you are choosing. The image given below is showing how to collect reference using web importer from Google scholar.

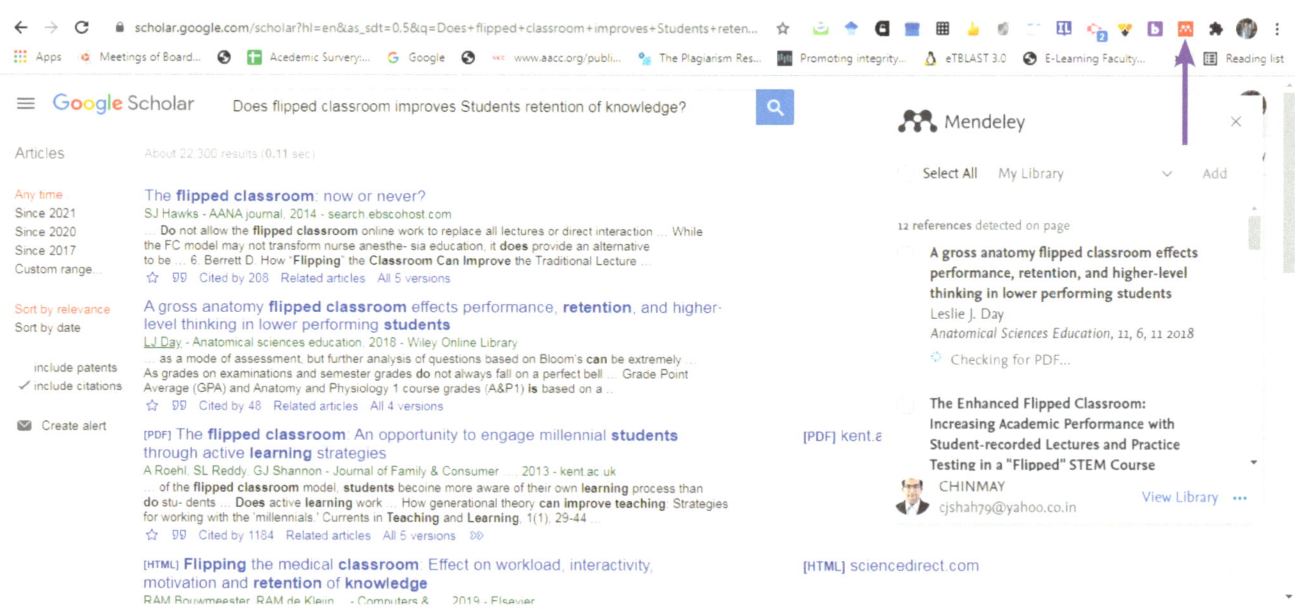

Figure 1: Showing webimporter of Mendeley

You can see web importer as well as function of saving one or more articles directly from Google scholar.

During collection/importing of software please check that you have complete information about the reference i.e. Title, author, date, volume, issue, page number and other publication details, once should also look for Abstract & the full text PDF (if it is available). In present era most of the article will have DOI Number so do not forget to mention it. If anything is missing, enter it manually.

Managing/Storing

Principle of managing/storing/organizing reference in software is more or less same but operability of software will be different depending on software customization and feature availability.

Reference can be grouped in Endnote, can be put in folder/subfolder in case of Mendeley while it can be labeled in paperpile. This is one way we can organize our reference as per project we are working on. Sometimes you may find same reference imported from different website, in such case you can use "find duplicate" function of reference manager to remove duplicate after viewing file with maximum information.

As you can see in image below you can organize your reference based on author/year/title/source/ date of adding reference. You can mark it as favorite, read or unread. Similarly, you can find it in all reference, recently added, recently read, your own publication and favorite reference. You can also use search option to do direct search of reference. You can also tag the bibliography or can apply filters to bibliography.

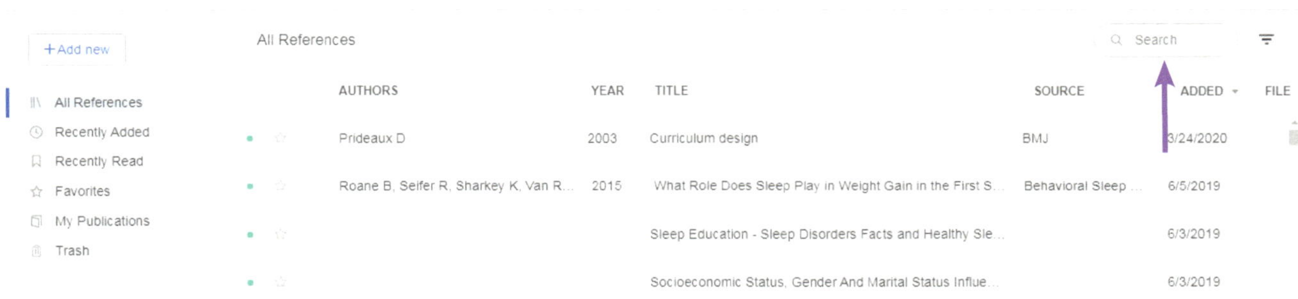

Figure 2: Showing Filter searching reference in reference manager

Further you may need to add data manually, almost all reference manager allow addition of reference from chapter, book, case, computer program, conference proceeding, encyclopedia, journal, report, television broadcast, online broadcast, thesis, webpage and other category. You need to ensure that you do all required entry for further process.

Caution: once you add reference manually you must press synchronize button to synchronize between desktop, web and mobile application of reference manager. Synchronization will pull down any changes made on all devices. It's a good idea to synchronize regularly to ensure that your documents and annotations are saved in the cloud.

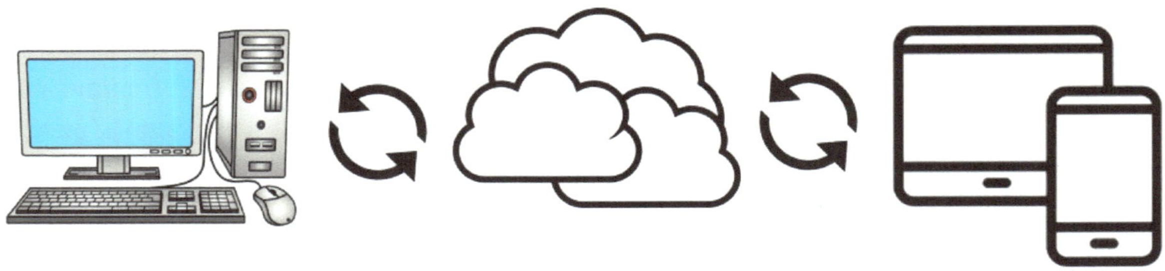

Figure 3: Showing synchronisation between different devices

Citing/creating bibliography

Once you have your references collected, you can use reference management software to generate lists of references and to insert citations from your library as you write. This page looks at setting up the right referencing style and how to cite references in your work.

In all reference manager there is option of insert citation/insert reference from library created by you in the reference manager using word Plugin. When you use this function, reference will be inserted in your word file and will look little different from your other text & you will find it as hyperlink text which is connected with your reference library so if you update your reference in your library it will be automatically updated in your word file.

Some of the reference manager may have extra feature of cite while you write option & some will allow you to copy reference from library and insert it in to word document, but this may take more time than routine.

Once you finish writing your document along with citing reference at appropriate places, use option of creating annotated bibliography to complete your thesis or paper with all reference mentioned in the reference styled chosen by you.

The biggest advantage of using reference manager during preparing of manuscript or thesis is, if you delete or insert new reference after preparing your complete document, it will automatically change sequencing of reference after that so there is no need to rewrite/cite reference again. Secondly if you are changing journal and need new citation style, with single click it will be changed in whole document.

Please keep in mind that when you are sharing or submitting document, create a plain text copy that is no longer connected with your reference manager so that it will not get change or affected by reference manager used by recipient of word document.

Sharing

Once you are done with your research project and want to publish it, your work is visible to other and they might contact you other investigator might contact you for getting reference you quoted in the paper/ thesis.

Reference manager also help you in this by using their built-in function of share reference. Alternately you can export reference in specific format (RIS or BibTeX format) and then mail to other investigator who can import in their software.

Reference Management software

There are many types of reference manager available in market (BOX Below).

Box 1: Commonly Available reference manager

- EndNote
- Mendeley
- Zotero
- RefWorks
- Papers
- JabRef
- CiteULike
- Outlook
- Microsoft word
- Google Doc
- Citavi
- ReadCube
- Paperpile
- Sciwheel
- EasyBib.com

From the large number of available reference managers, we have chosen few of them to discuss in detail. You can choose depending on pros and cons of different reference manager.

Zotero

- Zotero is a free reference management tool developed as a project developed at Carnegie Mellon and supported by a small team at George Mason University.
- It is a free, easy-to-use tool to help you collect, organize, cite, and share your research sources.

Mendeley

- Mendeley, an Elsevier company headquartered in London, offers their eponymous reference management software suite,
- It includes Mendeley Reference Manager, Web Importer, the Citation Plugin add-on, available in Premium package. It has a desktop and web program for managing and sharing research papers, discovering research data and collaborating online.

EndNote

- Clarivate Analytics headquartered in Philadelphia offers EndNote, a reference library and management software.
- You can Find, use and share research with EndNote. It's for more than bibliographies. Sync your EndNote library across your desktop, iPad and online. Work on your research from anywhere.

Read Cube Papers

- Papers offers a cross-platform suite of reference management & discovery tools which can dramatically improve the way researchers find, access, organize, read, annotate, share, and cite research literature.

P	**Paperpile** • Clean and simple and reference management for the web. Sync your library to all your devices and read and annotate like on paper on your iPad, iPhone, or Android device. Cite your papers in Google Docs and Microsoft Word.
citavi Organize your knowledge.	**Citavi** • Citavi is a software program that helps you organize your research projects and manage your time. Keep track of all the sources you read and their contents. • Analyze PDF articles with annotation tools and save ideas for future projects. Create outlines for drafts and write reports, articles, or books – faster and more efficiently than you ever thought possible. Citavi is the only academic productivity tool this comprehensive and the only program that supports the entire research process.
	RefWorks • RefWorks is an online research management, writing and collaboration tool that is designed to help researchers easily gather, manage, store and share all types of information, as well as generate citations and bibliographies
W	**Microsoft word** • With updated Microsoft word, it has features like creating list of reference, citing it and creating bibliographic database based on it
Google docs	**Google Docs** • This is an online tool help to cite and creating bibliography, it also has facility of one click change in style of reference citation.

An extensive list and comparison of available reference management software can be found on Wikipedia. Image below shows comparison of important reference manager.

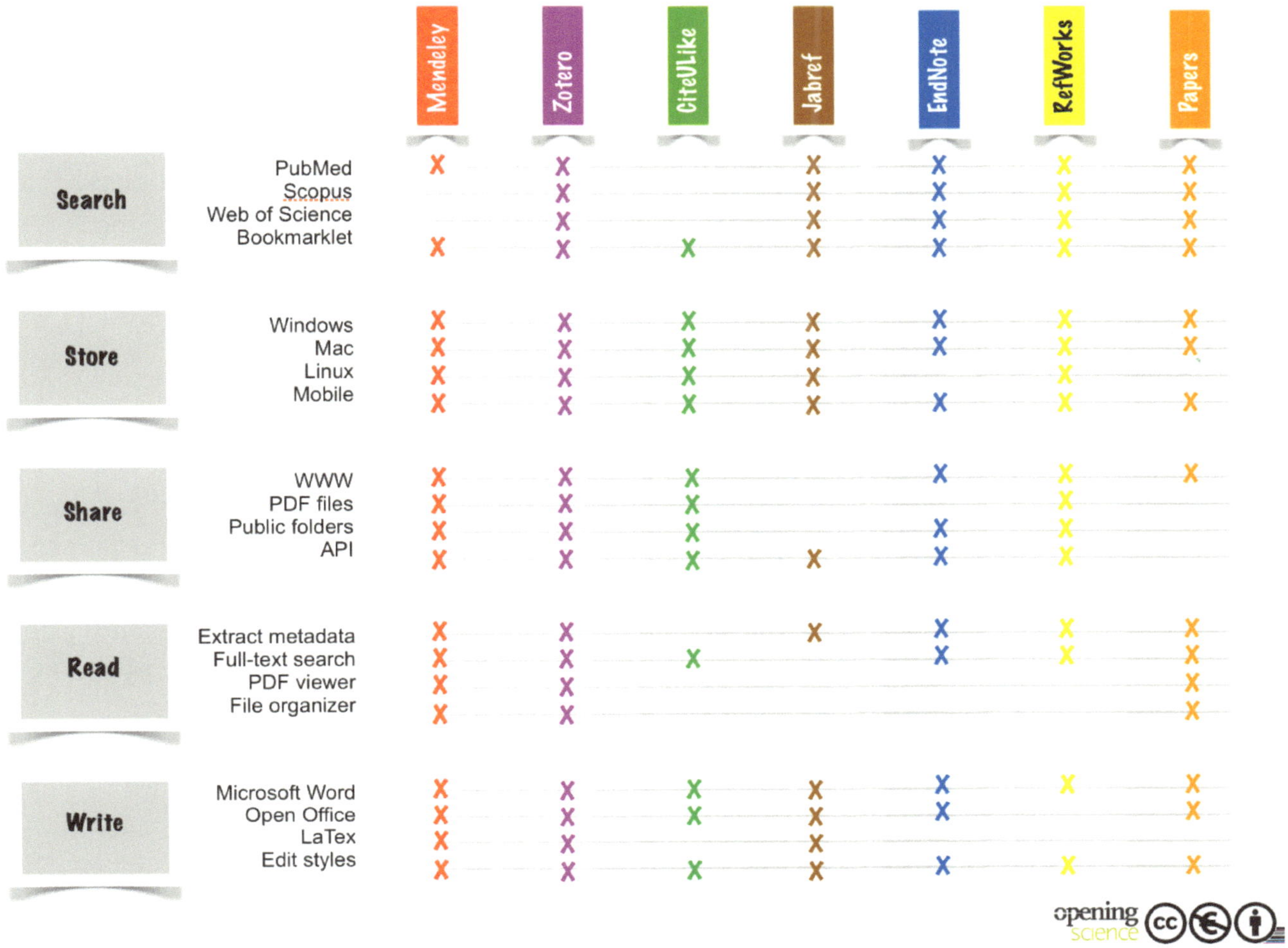

		Mendeley	Zotero	CiteULike	Jabref	EndNote	RefWorks	Papers
Search	PubMed	X	X		X	X	X	X
	Scopus		X		X	X	X	X
	Web of Science		X		X	X	X	X
	Bookmarklet	X	X	X	X	X	X	X
Store	Windows	X	X	X	X	X	X	X
	Mac	X	X	X	X	X	X	X
	Linux	X	X	X	X		X	
	Mobile	X	X	X	X	X	X	X
Share	WWW	X	X	X		X	X	X
	PDF files	X	X	X			X	
	Public folders	X	X	X		X	X	
	API	X	X	X	X	X	X	
Read	Extract metadata	X	X		X	X	X	X
	Full-text search	X	X	X		X	X	X
	PDF viewer	X	X					X
	File organizer	X	X					X
Write	Microsoft Word	X	X	X	X	X	X	X
	Open Office	X	X	X	X	X		X
	LaTex	X	X		X			
	Edit styles	X	X	X	X	X	X	X

Figure 4: Feature comparison of popular reference managers. Adapted from (M. Fenner 2010)1.

Which software should I use?[2]

Please keep in mind following question before choosing your reference manager

1. Do you want to work online or offline?
2. Is paying for use of a package an option for you?
3. Will the package always be free?
   - Mendeley is free to use, and it is free to download the desktop app.
   - Zotero is free to use, and it is free to download the desktop app.
4. Which operating system will you be using?
   - Windows/Apple Mac (MacOS).
5. Which word-processor are you going to use?
6. Do you want to collaborate with other people to build bibliographies and/or share libraries?
7. Which databases do you expect to use for searching?
8. Which reference style are you expected to use, or do you wish to use?
9. Can you create or edit reference styles?
10. Does the software allow you to edit the data fields (those relating to elements of your references/ citations)?

Writing for publication

If you are writing for publication, publishers usually require you to use their nominated [RM] referencing style. In the case of journals, this is usually the journal's own style. Reference management software encompasses many thousands of referencing styles and so it is likely that packages will contain the style you are required to use, as well as the more well-known styles such as APA, Chicago, Harvard and Vancouver. It is also easy to import a style into a package. If it is not available, for example, the OSCOLA footnotes style which law students and legal researchers use. Alternatively, you may be able to create a new style by editing an existing one and saving it separately. As previously mentioned, there are a number of advantages for using an RM, which include the following:

Inserting references

As previously mentioned, RMs typically insert coded citation information that refers back to the author's locally saved library. Depending on the specifications of a journal's guidelines, these references may require the use of brackets [1], parentheses (1), superscripted text1, bracketed or parenthesized superscripted text[1],(2), or commas to separate the author's name and date of publication ("Hantla 2013" vs. "Hantla, 2013"). All of these formatting differences can be automatically adjusted by setting up specifications in the RM.

Creating bibliographies

Depending on how you are accustomed to writing for your field, you may reserve inserting citations until after you have finished drafting the paper and keep a large bibliography in a separate file. Doing this often requires the use of notes and placeholders in the text that run the risk of being submitting with the article to the journal editor, which can make your work appear careless. Using an RM to manage the order in which citations appear in your bibliography can greatly reduce the amount of time you spend drafting an article, leaving more time for data collection and experimentation.

Changing the reference system for resubmission

As is often the case, when an author is rejected from one journal, he/she must begin the manuscript preparation process for a new journal. Sometimes, this requires a reorganization of the paper, but most of the time, the authors are required to reformat the paper's references and bibliography according to a new set of standards (typically found under the "Guidelines for Authors" section of the journal's website). These specifications come in one of at least three different styles:

SUMMARIZE

Reference Manager is very crucial and important technological support available to researcher. It will reduce burden of research of managing reference collected from different source. Reference manger not only help us to collect, store and cite reference, if used effectively it will also work as reference library of future research.

EVALUATE

For research project "effect of flipped classroom on students retention of knowledge" perform following exercise:

1. Choose reference Manager or choice, download it and **set up** it for online browser, plugin as well as desktop version
2. Search reference in Google Scholar or pubmed and collect it using browser plugin.
3. Now try exporting some reference in different formate available on that software
4. Save PDF of article whenever available
5. Check completeness of each reference
6. Check for the duplicate and remove incomplete reference
7. Create Folder/Group as per the need
8. Open Microsoft word and now start using word plug-in
9. Select one of the reference style and do citation in text, do citation of around 10 reference
10. Create bibliography of cited reference
11. Save document for submission
12. Look at share option in the software and share it with your friend
13. Try to export as well as import reference from other source
14. Try to do manual entry of book and journal

ROAD AHEAD

1. **Detail comparison of all reference management software**
   - *https://en.wikipedia.org/wiki/Comparison_of_reference_management_software*
2. **The following are useful comparisons of reference management software:**
   - *Imperial College London: Reference Management Software comparison*
     Comparison of EndNote, EndNote Online, Mendeley, Zotero and RefWorks based on nine criteria (some only locally relevant).
   - *Oxford Bodleian Libraries: Comparison of Reference Management Software*

   Comparison of EndNote, EndNote Online, Mendeley, Zotero and RefWorks based on four criteria.
3. **Online guide is available in following link:**
   - *EndNote: Further help*
   - *Mendeley: Further help*
   - *Zotero*
   - *EndNote Training*: Book into the Library's EndNote Sessions
   - *Mendeley training*: Book into the Library's Mendeley training
   - *Zotero training*: The Library runs training for Zotero from time to time
4. **Transferring records and libraries between different reference management programs**
   - *https://docs.google.com/document/d/1OuIqnAiDgTtlkRiITWlZU6Xlu8JCds7C1bvjn_VKuPU/edit#*

Acknowledgements: We acknowledge Vasumathi Sriganesh, MLIS – CEO of Qmad foundation for imparting knowledge of reference management in us and creating it is interesting for future study

REFERENCES

Fenner, M., Scheliga, K., & Bartling, S. (2014). Reference management. In Opening Science (pp. 125-137). Springer, Cham

Which software should I use? (n.d.). https://Library-Guides.Ucl.Ac.Uk/Reference-Management-Software/Which-Software. Retrieved September 20, 2021, from https://library-guides.ucl.ac.uk/reference-management-software/which-software

Chapter 23

Can we Trust Systematic Reviews in Medical Education?

How to write good reviews to impact practice and research

Madalena Patricio, Sucheta Dandekar

ABSTRACT

Medical education was facing one of its most challenging moments due to the complexity of developments with implications in health care, when the COVID-19 pandemic situation emerged, which resulted in the most dramatic changes in medical education, forcing schools to abandon face-to-face teaching, during the night.

These challenges require schools and teachers to make difficult decisions. Therefore, a shift from 'opinion-based' to 'evidence-based' is crucial, but evidence is difficult to find for the busy teacher. This becomes even more imperative because social responsibility is required from medical schools that are now under scrutiny, which implies providing evidence to justify their curricula.

The question now is to explore whether we can have something reliable in medical education, equivalent to what COCHRANE is doing for clinical medicine. BEME (Best Evidence Medical Education) COLLABORATION, introduced in 1999, is the answer while offering secondary research, which involves a comprehensive search of all potentially relevant studies using reproducible criteria, transparent selection of studies, research design, synthesized data and interpreted results. BEME, with more than sixty published systematic reviews, is at the forefront of evidence-informed practice in medical and health professional education (www.bemecollaboration.org).

This chapter will take you through the basis of educational evidence compared to clinical evidence, the impact of BEME on practice and research, how to write and submit a BEME Systematic Review and what BEME authors can expect from BEME and AMEE (Association for Medical Education in Europe). It hopes to be a guideline for authors to write good systematic reviews, which, therefore, will have an impact on practice and research.

Key Words: BEME, best evidence medical education, evidence-based teaching

ASSESS NEED

Systematic reviews are a critical component of evidence-informed policy making not only in health but also in many other domains (O'Connor et al. 2019). A high-quality systematic review is described as the most reliable source of evidence to guide clinical practice. The purpose of a systematic review is to deliver a meticulous summary of all the available primary research in response to a research question. Systematic reviews search, appraise and collate all relevant empirical evidence in order to provide a complete interpretation of research results. It is a form of analysis that medical researchers carry out to synthesize all the available evidence on a particular question. (O'Connor et al. 2019).

The BEME (Best Evidence Medical and Health Professional Education) Collaboration is an international group of individuals, universities and professional organisations, established in 1999 by Harden et al., as an effort to move from the use of anecdotal information in medical education to the use of evidence synthesis through systematic review, mirroring the revolution seen in healthcare.

After its founding, much of BEME's energy was put into a 'proof of concept' (Gordon & Patricio, 2016) to demonstrate that the synthesis and review techniques that were becoming a mainstay of evidence-based medicine could be applied within the health education arena. In line with the work of the Cochrane Collaboration 2015 (*www.cochrane.org*), the BEME methodology involves a comprehensive search of all potentially relevant studies, the use of explicit, reproducible criteria in the selection of studies for review, appraisal of research designs, data synthesised and results interpreted (Patricio and Carneiro, 2012).

Searching for evidence to inform best practices in medical education is a complex and very demanding undertaking. Therefore, the objective of this chapter is to contribute to a better understanding of why BEME is important, how much it is trustworthy and to inform on the process of writing and submitting a BEME Systematic Review.

BRIEF

- Medical education is facing complex challenges, implying schools and teachers' decisions
- Schools and teachers' decisions must be evidence-based, but is this possible?
- Evidence in clinical medicine (COCHRANE) versus evidence in medical education (BEME)
- BEME as a feasible and trustworthy answer for moving to 'Evidence-based Teaching'
- Writing and submitting a BEME Systematic Review (SR)
- BEME impact.

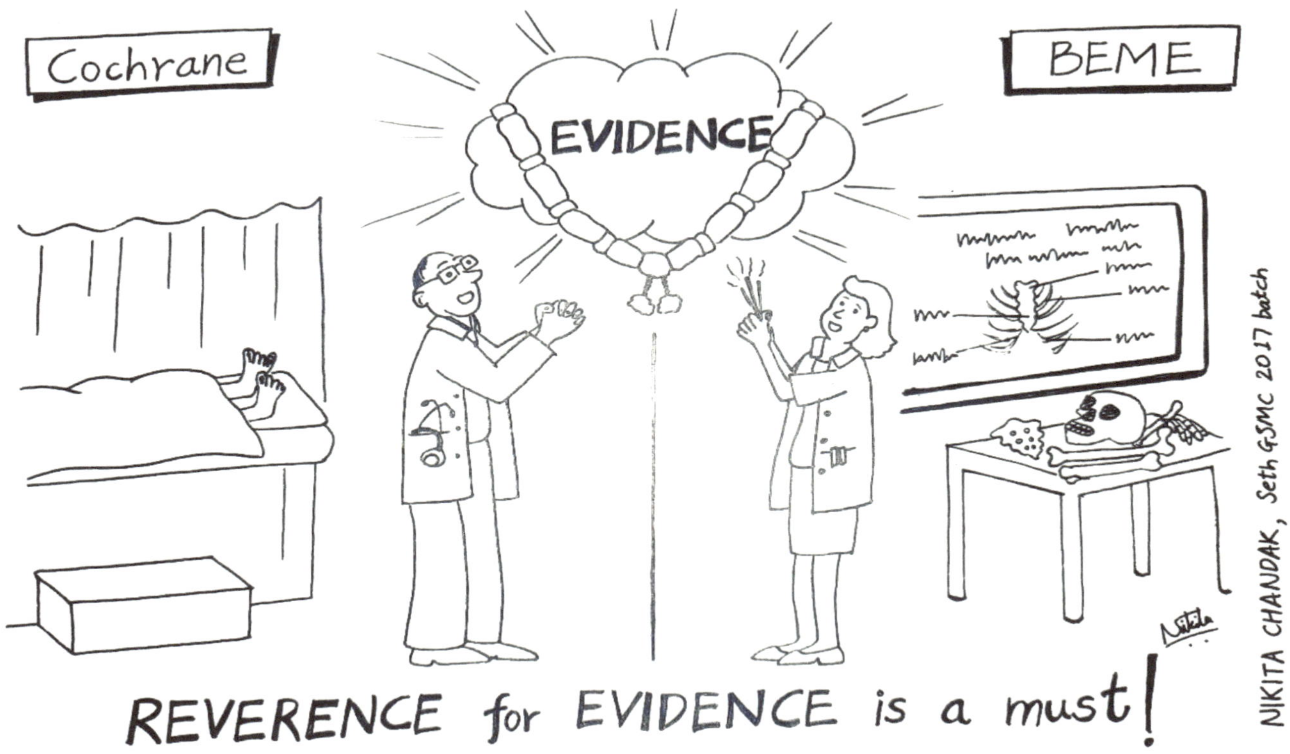

CONTEXTUALIZE

The question '*What's a good Doctor and how do you make one*', on the cover and in September 2002 British Medical Journal editorial (Hurwitz B & Vass A. 2002), sums up the question that medical schools have been asking themselves during the last two decades as they seek to find what works best in medical education, questioning whether their teachers are making the best decisions concerning the needed changes to be implemented.

The problem is that in medical education we continue to witness intense debates on the best methods for teaching and assessing students and there is no such thing because there is no 'one best' method in education. This is why there was a need for 'evidence-based' - a movement started to be recognized by Harden et al., who stated in 1999, 'there is a need to move from opinion-based education to evidence-based education'.

BEME, the Best Evidence Medical and Health Professional Education (*www.bemecollaboration.org*) is the implementation, by teachers in their practice, of methods and approaches to education based on the best evidence available' (Harden et al. 1999).

This move to '*evidence-based education*' is also crucial because more social accountability is currently required by medical schools who are now under scrutiny, not only from faculty but also from the public, needing evidence to justify their decisions. Therefore, the question remains, if evidence is possible in education.

DESCRIBE

Medical Education is facing dramatic changes implying difficult decisions which require a move to evidence-based teaching

Medical education is facing one of its most challenging times due to the complexity of undergoing developments with implications in health care.

Globalization, the explosion of medical knowledge and new technologies, patients' new requisites, new rights and new expectations, the new generations of students arriving at universities requiring new teaching methods and the need for social accountability of medical schools, are just some examples already in place, when the COVID-19 pandemic situation arose, implying the most dramatic changes in medical education, forcing schools to abandon face-to-face teaching, overnight.

These multiple challenges require schools and teachers to make rather difficult decisions. The problem is that the medical education community continues to witness intense debates on the '*best method*' for teaching and assessing students when there is no such thing because there is not a '*single best method*' in education applicable to all situations around the world.

This is why there is a need for education to move from '*opinion-based*' to '*evidence-based*' to identify '*what works, for whom and in what circumstances* 'as stated by Harden et al., back in 1999, when proposing the implementation of the BEME (Best Evidence Medical Education) Collaboration.

Searching for evidence to inform best practices in medical education is a complex and very demanding undertaking. As in clinical medicine (Sackett DL. 1997), information overload is one of the main problems when looking for evidence in medical education. This is recognized by many authors for more than two decades namely by Frazer & Dunstan 2010; Smith R 2010; Azer et al. 2016 just to give some examples. Smith (2010) in a paper entitled 'Strategies for coping with information overload', imagining himself asking God as he arrives in Heaven '*Will we ever solve the problem of information overload? Sure, He´ll answer, but not in my lifetime ...*'

The question now is to explore if we can have in medical education something equivalent to what COCHRANE Collaboration - *an international group dedicated to Evidence-based Medicine, which is based on the application of the scientific method to all medical practice* - is doing in clinical medicine. This leads us to the question 'can we trust BEME as much as we trust COCHRANE *in medicine?*'

Is evidence possible in education?

To answer this question, a study was implemented (Patricio & Carneiro, 2012), at the Faculty of Medicine of the University of Lisbon (FMUL), to examine the basis of educational evidence compared to clinical evidence as well as the different nature of the science behind each approach. 'Which are the major similarities and differences between a COCHRANE and a BEME Systematic Review?' were the research questions. BEME reviews in medical education and COCHRANE reviews in clinical medicine were compared based on reviews undertaken at the CEMBE (Center for the Study of Evidence-Based Medicine) at the FMUL.

Common steps were identified in both approaches:

- Asking a relevant question
- Researching/selecting primary studies
- Carrying out critical coding and evaluation
- Synthesising evidence
- Identifying implications for practice

While the major differences, were:

- Research questions are more complex in BEME reviews than in COCHRANE
- In BEME there are no standard guidelines for all studies
- Synthesis in COCHRANE gives a point of estimate when in BEME it only shows '*what works, for whom, in what circumstances*'
- In COCHRANE, a statement can be made when in BEME it may be just a general recommendation.

In conclusion, both approaches seem to be similar in terms of methodology. The differences between them are perhaps more a matter of degree than the existence of fundamental differences.

The need to define causality in education

In medical education as in clinical medicine, a hierarchy of evidence should support decision-making but evidence alone is never sufficient for sound practice (Patricio & Carneiro, 2012). This is why it is important to define causality in medicine and education, to understand the difficulty of undertaking a systematic review in education. The causal relationships in medicine and health care in general are of central importance, because answers to several types of clinical questions depend on the assessment of whether a cause and effect relationship truly exists (Haynes et al. 2006). A factor is a cause of an event if its operation increases the frequency of that event (Elwood, 2017). This is true for clinical medicine and medical education but, in education (and all social sciences), you need to pay attention to other variables namely to the strong effect of the 'confounding variables', which are external factors that correlate with the outcome but are not directly causal as described in the figure below.

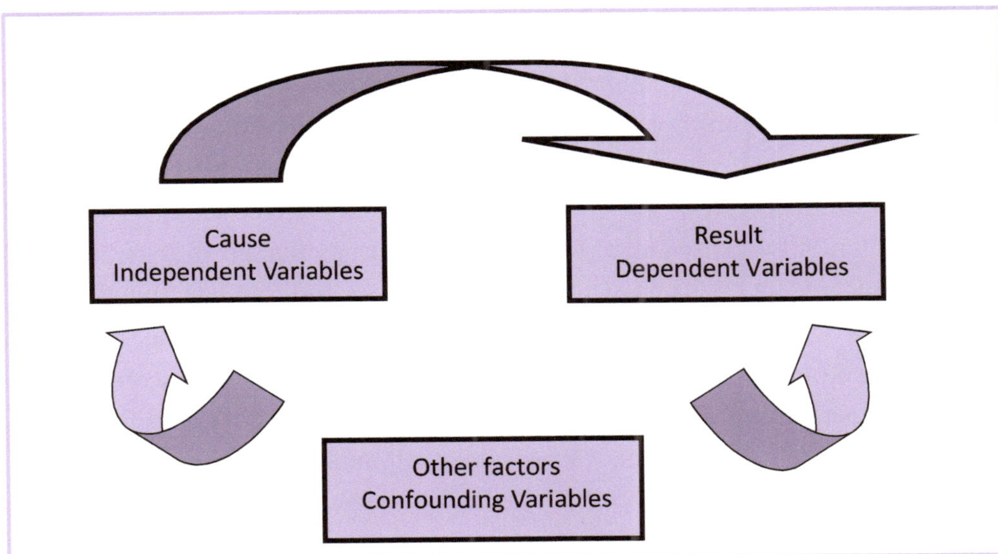

Figure 1: Confounding variables

This is extremely important when analyzing study results in education. Let us give an example: if in clinical medicine a benefit is found in an experimental study to test the efficacy of aspirin in a specific disease, then there should be no doubt that the intervention (an aspirin pill with a predefined size: 100 mg, 325 mg, etc.) is the same for all patients, so it can be easily replicated.

However, if positive results are found in medical education, in an experimental study to identify the impact of a specific method implemented by a specific teacher, the transferability of results to practice is more difficult, because it is impossible to dissociate the effects of the confounding variables – namely, the teacher charisma, enthusiasm, capacity for motivating students, etc., from the intervention itself.

BEME and 'Evidence-based Teaching'

In many circumstances, when previous teaching solutions are not effective to address the complex challenges, medical education is facing or when medical schools wish to introduce new developmental changes, BEME, whose goal is to provide and make available the latest findings of scientifically-grounded educational research, can be the answer enabling teachers and administrators to take informed decisions.

To achieve this goal, BEME identifies the best evidence available to support evidence-based decisions rather than opinion-based ones, offers opportunities for training and development in relation to the implementation of evidence-informed teaching and translates research findings into practice.

As evidence in education is possible and BEME is trustworthy, we share below some examples of BEME Guides giving answers to support teaching daily practice.

- *Should we use simulation in my teaching and what are the 10 measures I can take to make it more effective?*
  Yes, we should, and the features are; providing feedback, repetitive practice, curriculum integration, range of difficulty level, multiple learning strategies, capture clinical variation, controlled environment, individualized learning, defined outcomes and ensuring of simulator validity.

- *Should we use a multiple mini-interview (MMI) or a traditional method for selecting students for undergraduate health programmes?*
  The answer is that MMIs used for selection to undergraduate health programmes appear to have reasonable feasibility, acceptability, validity and reliability. Reliability is optimized by including 7-12 stations, each with one examiner. The schools must identify the attributes they value and blueprint them to the interviews. The evidence is stronger for face validity, with more research needed to explore content validity and predictive validity. In published studies, MMIs do not appear biased against applicants on the basis of age, gender or socio-economic status. However, applicants of certain ethnic and social backgrounds did not fare as well in a very small number of published studies. Performance on MMIs does not correlate strongly with other measures of non-cognitive attributes, such as personality inventories and measures of emotional intelligence. The answer is given by BEME Guide 37, '*Evidence regarding the utility of multiple mini-interview (MMI) for selection for undergraduate health programmes: a BEME systematic review*' by Rees et al. 2016.

- *What developments/changes in medical education have been deployed as a response to COVID 19, what is their impact? What lessons have been learned?*
  The introduced changes are: a rapid shift to synchronous and asynchronous remote learning occurred that is likely to persist beyond the pandemic, and attention must be paid to learner engagement, structure and organization in the future. Early developments supported alternatives to clinical placements or continued clinical exposure using telehealth, personal protective equipment (PPE), and physical distancing. A few articles of exceptional quality, most notably a digital learning package

to support well-being (Blake et al. 2020) were identified that can serve as models to guide future educational developments and reporting. Gaps in the literature were identified with additional studies needed in the areas of assessment, admissions and selection to post-graduate training, and faculty development. While there was often a lack of practical detail to support the educational community in enactment of novel interventions and limited evaluation data, the range of options deployed offers much guidance for the medical education community. The answers are given in BEME Guide 63, 'Developments in medical education in response to the COVID-19 pandemic: A rapid BEME systematic review' (Gordon et al. 2020) and also in BEME Guide 64 *'An update on Developments in medical education in response to the COVID-19 pandemic: A rapid BEME systematic review' (Daniel et al. 2021)*. It is important to highlight that they were the last two BEME Guides published at the time this chapter was written, to answer the main questioning of the medical education agenda.

The above 'questions and answers' are just 3 examples from around 160 research questions available from the 64 Systematic Reviews published so far. (*www.bemecollaboration.org/Published+Reviews/)*

Writing a BEME systematic review

A systematic review is a secondary research process, based on primary studies. It attempts to collect all existing evidence on a specific topic in order to answer specific research question(s). They offer a number of benefits, namely providing an overview of the evidence, helping to identify gaps in the field, highlighting concerns in studies and providing guidelines for practice and future research. Writing a good BEME systematic review, as said above, is a demanding process especially due to the strong effect of the confounding variables. Some requisites are crucial for a successful BEME systematic review:

- At the beginning, a relevant educational problem needs to be identified. Then, research question(s) should be established, which need to be feasible and relevant. They can be framed using PICO criteria - **P**opulation, **I**ntervention, **C**ontrol, and **O**utcomes (Liberati et al. 2009; Page et al 2020) and should be used to help establish your search strategy (Sackett, 1997)
- At the end, the research questions need to be answered and implications to practice and research must be stated.
- It must be a coherent process from the educational problem until the transferability of results into practice and research. Therefore, the methods, data synthesis, discussion and the conclusions need to be aligned. Systematic reviews that end up concluding only that more research is needed are no longer acceptable

Submitting a BEME systematic review

There are two ways of submitting a systematic review:

- *The Traditional BEME Review Process* which consists of 4 stages
  - ✓ Stage 1: Topic registration (2-4 weeks)
  - ✓ Stage 2: Protocol development and review (6 months maximum)
  - ✓ Stage 3: Review development (~1 year)
  - ✓ Stage 4: Final adjudication of the review and Publication (1-2 months).

All stages are crucial, but the protocol is probably the one requiring special attention because a good protocol almost assures the success of the review and the decision on protocol allows the authors to progress further. Detailed information on BEME stages is outlined at BEME website (*https://bemecollaboration.org/Steps+in+the+Review+Process/*).

The protocol is peer reviewed by an assigned BEME International Collaborating Centre (BICC) and, following any requested revisions, is posted on the BEME website. It must clearly:

- Identify what type of review is planned (narrative review, scoping review, systematic, realist review, etc.)
- Identify what the practical contribution to knowledge will be once the review is complete
- Argue that there is a sound link between the research question(s) and the secondary research methodology that will be used to identify answers to the question(s).
- Give a clear definition of the key concepts in the review question(s) or show how these will be arrived at (*https://bemecollaboration.org/Step+4+Protocol+Preparation/*)
- *The Alternative Review Process*

High quality systematic reviews may become a BEME review without progressing through stages 1-4. This pathway is good for groups who already have significant expertise in reviews and do not require the support offered by BICCs and the BEME Review Committee to be successful. The advantages to authors include the recognition of the review as meeting BEME's high standards, and the extended abstract/manuscript word limits which are reserved for BEME reviews.

BEME peer-review process is supportive

It is important to clarify what authors can expect from BEME whose peer review process is supportive, unlike what happens in other peer-reviewed journals: BEME is highly committed to support authors throughout the handling process for a successful systematic review as well as providing an editorial service, while keeping high quality standards of exigency. During the process of writing a systematic review, the authors are supported by a BICC, which is appointed by the BEME Review Committee to supervise the authors. Supervision is given from protocol stage until the submission of final manuscript. The list of current BICCs is available at *https://www.bemecollaboration.org/BICCs/*

A second example of BEME support is the fact that the two checklists used by BEME reviewers to assess the protocols (*https://bemecollaboration.org/Step+4+Protocol+Preparation/*) or the final manuscripts (*https://bemecollaboration.org/Step6CompletedReview/*) are made available to authors immediately after acceptance of their topic registration. From them, the authors can check their protocol of final manuscript against the BEME criteria used by reviewers.

To understand what authors can expect from AMEE is also important: after registration and protocol are accepted, AMEE is committed to publish the review. Publication depends on the successful achievement of all steps of the handling process. BEME Reviews are published in two formats: BEME Spotlight and a paper in Medical Teacher once final manuscript is accepted. It will be listed in the content pages of the journal and indexed in *Index Medicus.*

BEME impact

For almost two decades BEME has been contributing with great impact to Evidence-based Teaching. Considering 2019, the year immediately prior to the COVID-19 pandemic situation arose, when BEME celebrated its 20th anniversary, we verified that:

- *Three BEME Guides are among the four papers with the most citations in Medical Education Journals, namely:*
    - A BEME systematic review of the effects of inter- professional education: BEME Guide 39, by Reeves et al., 2016.
    - A systematic review of faculty development initiatives designed to enhance teaching effectiveness. A 10-year update: BEME Guide 40, by Steinert et al.
    - Evidence regarding the utility of multiple mini-interview (MMI) for selection to undergraduate health programs. BEME Guide 37, by Rees et al., 2016.
- *Two BEME Systematic Reviews are among the top ten papers most downloaded from Medical Education Journals:*
    - A Best Evidence in Medical Education systematic review to determine the most effective teaching methods that develop reflection in medical students: BEME Guide No. 51 by Jane Uygur et al., 2019
    - A Best Evidence Medical Education (BEME) systematic review of: What works best for health professions students using mobile (hand-held) devices for educational support on clinical placements? BEME Guide No. 52, by Gillian et al., 2019.

These benchmarks are important because there is no benefit in making systematic reviews available if schools, teachers, students and other stakeholders do not see the need. This is why we need 'YOU', the readers of this chapter to join BEME Collaboration to help the dissemination of the BEME culture.

Each school around the world has a crucial role to play to develop the BEME culture of evidence. Let us share some examples of school contributions made in the countries of the authors of this chapter:

- In India, many researchers are now using systematic reviews to consolidate evidence-based strategies. Not only are the systematic reviews related to the subject disciplines but also the reviews related to health professions education are gaining momentum. This is indeed a very encouraging time for evidence base medical education. The reviews are being registered in International Prospective Register of Systematic Reviews (PROSPERO). We have many BEME contributors of Indian origin. Two BEME reviews deserve a mention – '*Predictive values of measurements obtained in medical schools and future performance in medical practice.* BEME guide 5' (Hamdy et al. 2006) and '*The effect of educational games on medical students' learning outcomes: a systematic review.* BEME guide 14' (Akl, 2009), which include Indian authors from New Delhi and Coimbatore. We hope that this will provide enough incentive for all of you to explore this new world of Best Evidence in Medical Education!
- In Portugal, medical schools are progressively basing their decisions on evidence. The CEMBE (Center for the Study of Evidence-Based Medicine) at the FMUL published one study 'Systematic reviews of evidence in medical education and clinical medicine: *Is the nature of evidence similar*? (Patricio M, Carneiro AV. 2012) and a Systematic Review '*Is the OSCE a feasible tool to assess competencies in undergraduate medical education*? (Patricio et al. 2013). An update of the last review was submitted to BEME.

If joining BEME interests you, please contact us (*beme@amee.org*).

You are most welcome!

SUMMARIZE

We have seen that medical education is facing dramatic developments, with COVID 19 in top of them. These developments imply medical schools and teachers to make difficult decisions. This is why a move to Evidence-based Teaching is needed to support those decisions. To find evidence is difficult namely for the busy teacher and BEME Collaboration may be the answer, while impacting in practice and research. We also have seen that BEME is feasible and trustworthy and how to write and submit a BEME Systematic review.

With more than 60 systematic reviews currently published and 20 under processing, BEME is starting to be recognized as the leader in secondary research whose main challenges in the near future concern to offer more training to the public, to the BICC reviewers and authors and above all increase the dissemination of the Evidence-based teaching culture.

EVALUATE

Before concluding, we leave some questions below as a self-assessment opportunity:

- How do you justify the need to move to 'Evidence-based Teaching'
- Which are the three fundamental requisites for a good systematic review?
- If all 'stages' are important when writing a BEME systematic review, which is the most critical one?
- Which are the two processes to submit a BEME systematic review?
- Why is the BEME peer-review process different from peer-review in other journals?
- How is BEME supporting the authors? Please give two examples.

It would be great to have your feedback on this chapter. Please let us know: What is the main message you got from this chapter and what else, should we have done to improve this chapter?

Your comments and suggestions are most welcome (*beme@amee.org*).

ROAD AHEAD

- Try to generate new topics based on existing knowledge, trends, gaps observed and medical education needs/problems
- Select a methodology that suits your research question(s)
- Adapt your findings to your local context and translate them into practical recommendations
- Arrive at a conclusion that would be appropriate for stakeholders, policymakers and scientific community.
- Do not forget that a hierarchy of evidence should support decision-making but evidence alone is never sufficient for sound practice
- Above all, it is crucial to contribute to the move from education based in opinion to education based in evidence

REFERENCES

Akl EA, Pretorius RW, Sackett K, Erdley S, Bhoopathi PS, Alfarah Z, and Schünemann HJ (2009). The effect of educational games on medical students' learning outcomes: a systematic review. BEME Guide No 14. Medical Teacher 32, 1, 16-27

Blake H, Bermingham F, Johnson G, Tabner A. (2020). Mitigating the psychological impact of COVID-19 on healthcare workers: a digital learning package. Int J Environ Res Public Health. 17(9):2997.

Daniel M, Gordon M, Patricio M, Hider A, Pawlik C, Bhagdev R, Ahmad S, Alston S, Park S, Pawlikowska T, Rees E, Doyle AJ, Pammi M, Thammasitboon S, Haas M, Peterson W, Lew M, Khamees D, Spadafore M, Clarke N, Stojan J. (2021). An update on developments in medical education in response to the COVID-19 pandemic: A BEME scoping review: BEME Guide No. 64, Medical Teacher.

Gillian Maudsley, David Taylor, Omnia Allam, Jayne Garner, Tudor Calinici & Ken Linkman (2019) A Best Evidence Medical Education (BEME) systematic review of: What works best for health professions students using mobile (hand-held) devices for educational support on clinical placements? BEME Guide No. 52, Medical Teacher, 41:2, 125-140.

Gordon M, Patricio M, Horne L, Muston A, Alston SR, Pammi M, Thammasitboon S, Park S, Pawlikowska T, Rees EL, Doyle AJ, Daniel M. (2020). Developments in medical education in response to the COVID-19 pandemic: A rapid BEME systematic review: BEME Guide No. 63, Medical Teacher, 42:11, 1202-1215.

Hamdy H, Prasad K, Anderson MB, Scherpbier A, Williams R, Zwierstra R and Cuddihy H (2006). BEME Guide No 5, BEME systematic review: Predictive values of measurements obtained in medical schools and future performance in medical practice. BEME Guide no 5. Medical Teacher 28(2):103-116.

Harden RM, Grant J, Buckley G, Hart IR. (1999). BEME Guide No. 1: Best Evidence Medical Education. Med Teach 21(6):553–562.

Hurwitz B & Vass A. (2002). What's a good doctor and how do you make one? Editorial BMJ vol. 325: 711.

Haynes RB, Sackett DL, Guyatt GH, Tugwell P. (2006). Clinical epidemiology. How to do clinical practice research 3d ed. Philadelphia: Lippincott Williams & Wilkins. BMJ 2002;325:g

Issenberg SB, McGaghie W, Petrusa E, Gordon DL, Scalese RJ. (2005). Features and uses of high-fidelity medical simulations that lead to effective learning: a BEME systematic review. *Medical Teacher,* 27, 10 - 28.

Liberati A, Altman DG, Tetzlaff J, Mulrow C, Gøtzsche PC, Ioannidis JPA, Clarke, Devereaux PJ, Kleijnen J, Moher D. (2009). The PRISMA statement for reporting systematic reviews and meta-analyses of studies that evaluate healthcare interventions: explanation and elaboration. BMJ; 21, 339:b2700

O'Connor AM, Tsafnat G, Thomas J, Glasziou P, Gilbert SB, Hutton B. (2019). A question of trust: can we build an evidence base to gain trust in systematic review automation technologies? Syst Rev 18; 8(1) 143.

Page MJ, McKenzie JE, Bossuyt PM, Boutron I, Hoffmann TC, Mulrow CD, et al. The PRISMA (2020) statement: an updated guideline for reporting systematic reviews. BMJ 2021; 372:n71.

Patricio M, Carneiro AV. (2012). Systematic reviews of evidence in medical education and clinical medicine: Is the nature of evidence similar? Medical teacher; 34(6): 474–482.

Patricio M, Juliao F, Filipa F, Carneiro AV. (2012) Is the OSCE a feasible tool to assess competencies in undergraduate medical education? Medical teacher 2013; 35(6): 503–514.

Rees EL, Hawarden AW, Dent G, Hays R, Bates J, Hassell AB. (2016). Evidence regarding the utility of multiple mini-interview (MMI) for selection to undergraduate health programs: A BEME systematic review: BEME Guide No. 37. Med Teach. May; 38(5):443-55.

Reeves S. Fletcher S, Barr H, Birch I, Boet S, Davies N, McFadyenA, Rivera J, Kitto S. (2016) A BEME systematic review of the effects of interprofessional education (update). BEME Guide No 39. Medical Teacher 38.7.

Sackett DL. (1997). Evidence-based medicine. Seminars in Perinatology. Volume 21, (1):3-5.

Steinert Y, Mann K, Anderson B, Barnett BM, Centeno A, Naismith L, Prideaux D, Spencer J, Tullo E, Viggiano T, Ward H, Dolmans D. (2016). A systematic review of faculty development initiatives designed to enhance teaching effectiveness: A 10-year update: BEME Guide No. 40, Medical Teacher, 38:8, 769-786.

Uygur J, Stuart E, De Paor M, Wallace E, Duffy Seamus, O'Shea M, Smith S, Pawlikowska T. (2019). A Best Evidence in Medical Education systematic review to determine the most effective teaching methods that develop reflection in medical students: BEME Guide No. 51, Medical Teacher, 41:1, 3-16.

Chapter 24

How to Enhance the Acceptance of Your Manuscript?

Ballambattu Vishnu Bhat, Sambandam Ravikumar

ABSTRACT

Scientific research has become an integral part of our academic activities. Once the research is completed, the findings should be published in an indexed journal so that others will get the benefit of the findings. Rejection of a manuscript is not a pleasant experience for the author. There could be several reasons for the rejection of a manuscript. Not selecting the appropriate journal, lack of novelty, improper methodology, poor writing, inadequate use of tables, graphs and figures, and incomplete referencing can all lead to rejection. If the author takes care of these issues before submitting the manuscript, chances of acceptance will be higher. In this article, we analysed some of the issues and suggested methods for avoiding rejection.

Key Words: desk manuscript acceptance, manuscript rejection, medical education journal, plagiarism, indexed journal, impact factor.

ASSESS NEED

Successful publication of papers in a peer-reviewed journal is very important for all academicians because it will contribute to their promotion, professional recognition and research grants. In the current scenario, publication is important not only for career advancement but also for the economic survival of departments in the medical institution. Other outcomes of publications include credibility to the researcher, advancement of the science leading to improvement in practice, and quality of health care. One of the key areas for recognition and accreditation by the regulators is research productivity measured by the number of successful publications by the faculty members. In addition, other attributes of publications such as citation, h-index and the impact factor of the journal are also important. For these reasons, it is important to write your manuscript well and publish the research article in a recognized, peer-reviewed journal. In spite of the hard work put up by the researcher, the Editor and reviewer of the journal may not consider it suitable for publication. The risk of rejection can be minimized if one takes appropriate steps before and after submission.

BRIEF

- Common reasons for rejection of a manuscript
- Strategies for preparing a good manuscript
- Manuscript submission
- Understanding review process
- Tips for resubmission

CONTEXTUALIZE

Let us look at the case of Dr. X

Dr. X is a hard working and sincere faculty member, admired by his students. As per the requirement of medical council, he conducted a research study on improving formative assessment in undergraduate medical education. He conducted a qualitative study involving huge collection of data through in-depth interviews. In his enthusiasm to give exhaustive data, he included every bit of data and submitted the manuscript to a well-recognized journal with high impact factor. Unfortunately, the manuscript was returned with the following comments: "You have not mentioned about ethical aspect of conducting interview; your analysis is too shoddy; the language of the paper is also poor and not up to the mark for our international journal; We regret to inform you that your paper is rejected".

Dr. X was not only upset but almost went into depression. After 6 months, he was casually talking to his friend Dr. Y with many publications about the incident. Dr. Y told him that this type of occurrence is quite common in the initial part of our publication process. He guided Dr. X to address each of the issues pointed out by the earlier journal editor. As guided by his friend, Dr. X revised the manuscript by addressing the issues raised by the reviewers and submitted it to another Journal. Modified manuscript submitted by Dr. X got accepted after minor corrections. This incident boosted the morale of Dr. X who went on publishing several papers after this incident.

DESCRIBE

Reflecting on the episode, you will appreciate that successful submission of manuscript requires thorough understanding of the factors which lead to selection or rejection of a paper in medical education.

Common Reasons for Rejection

Choosing the over studied topic or subjects not appropriate for the journal will not attract its readership.

- In several journals, retro-prospective studies, Case reports, and studies involving small sample size etc will not be accepted.
- Use of invalid statistics analysis and absence of control group could be other reasons.

- If the data presented in the manuscript is not new or the data is not supporting the conclusion, manuscript will not be considered for publication.
- If the discussion section is written poorly in terms of grammar, language and content, the article is likely to be rejected.
- All the cited references in the manuscript should be relevant and relatively recent. They should be listed as per the journal style

If an article is rejected by a particular journal, you cannot infer that the manuscript is poor or ineffective. It only means that your article is not matching with the requirements of the journal. Rejection happens for various reasons (Ali.2010, Hesterman et al. 2018). We have listed some of the most common causes of rejection, along with some tips for overcoming these short comings in Table 1.

Table 1: Tips to overcome the manuscript rejection

SN	Reason for rejection of manuscript	How to overcome?
1.	Manuscript is not appropriate or relevant subject area for the journal/their readership.	Several journal finder tools are available to select an appropriate journal for subject matter of the manuscript.
2.	Author has not followed research & publication ethics.	Authors should follow research ethics as well as publication ethics All authors have to ensure that they approve their contribution for the final version of the manuscript.
3.	Study design and methodology are not appropriate, small sample size with invalid statistical analysis.	Author/s need to explain the methodology in detail in the manuscript and also check the statistical validity and methodology while initiating the study.
4.	Conclusion is vague and not supported by the data.	Data presentation should be represented in appropriate Tables and/ or figures. Conclusion should be written with supporting information or conclusion should be based on the results of the study.
5.	Manuscript is poorly drafted with many language errors.	One should take utmost care in editing the language or take the help of English language editor.
6.	Author has not followed the 'instruction to authors' in the journal website.	Author has to avoid Desk rejection by following the journal instructions strictly.

Selecting right journal holds the key

After completing your research work, you need to select an appropriate journal for submission of your manuscript. A separate discussion on the list of journals which are devoted to MER in India and abroad can be found elsewhere in this book.

Higher the impact factor, higher the rejection rates. Rejection may lead to frustration for the authors. You need to strike a balance between the impact factor of the journal and the quality of your manuscript. By doing so the chances of acceptance of manuscript will increase.

After choosing an appropriate journal for the manuscript, you should carefully follow the instructions to authors in the journal for preparing the manuscript in terms of word limit, number of tables and figures and style of presentation. Manuscripts are of various types like; original research papers, review articles, case reports, systematic reviews, meta-analysis, editorials, letters to editors etc. Some Journals may be interested in publishing more of particular type of articles. It may be good idea to start with submission of manuscript for a short communication or letter to the editor where the chances of rejection are less. Once you develop some confidence you may go for original articles, and then aim for review papers including systematic review and meta-analysis which is difficult in a new field of work.

If you go through the contents of journal's earlier issues, you will come to know the type of articles published in that journal. You should try to match your article with the scope of the journal. Most of the journals will allow supplementary materials to be included and it should be submitted as part of your manuscript. Editor and reviewers will look for some originality and new issue in the submitted manuscript. Journal editors will always try to improve their impact factor and citation. Unless the study involves some new issue, it is less likely to be read and cited by others. Lack of originality could be one of the reasons for non-acceptance.

Strategy for preparing a manuscript

Many suggestions have been proposed for writing scientific manuscript (Kotz & Cals. 2014, Chernick. 2012, Kramer & Libhaber. 2016, Jacob & Sahni. 2020). You can choose any one of the suitable strategies in preparing your manuscript. But you need to follow the format prescribed by the journal. Most of the well-recognized journals follow the IMRAD (Introduction, Material and methods, Results and discussion) format (Table.2).

Table 2: Checklist for enhancing the manuscript quality.

SN	Section of the manuscript	Check List
1	Title	Is the title informative and attractive like including study design?
2	Abstract	Whether the abstract include the background information, methods, results and conclusion of the study? Have you added 3-5 'Key words'?
3	Introduction	Does the introduction provide adequate background information? Is the lacuna explained properly? Did you clearly state the study objective?
4	Methods	Whether the methods are explained in detail? Is the ethical clearance provided? Did you provide the details of equipment used? Is the procedure adequately described and validated? Did you use standard methods to calculate sample size? Have you described the statistical tests used for analysis?
5	Results	Whether the results are valid, credible and described in detail? Did you present the data clearly using tables and figures? Whether the obtained results are well supported by statistical analysis?
6	Discussion	Are the results justified and compared with earlier studies? Did the discussion included the limitations of the study Does conclusion match with objective of the study?

SN	Section of the manuscript	Check List
7	Tables and figures	Whether table and figures used appropriately? Are the titles and legends are numbered and described properly?
8	References	Did you include only relevant references? Did you cite all the references in the text? Whether the references are cited and listed as per journal style?
Please note: The journals vary in their criteria for acceptance. You should be guided by the instructions to the authors. Most popularly Vancouver referencing style is used.		

1. Title should be informative, precise, and indicate the study design. It must capture the interest of the audience. Avoid abbreviations in the title of the article. One should try to indicate the objective, outcome and type of the study in the title.

   Example:

   Avoid: The effect of parental smoking on the development of lung disease in children: study of a multicentre mixed group.

   Better: Association of parental smoking and the development of childhood lung disease in Indian population: an observational study.
2. **Abstract:** It should be brief but informative. It should give a brief summary of the study. Most of the Journals expect a structured abstract. It should contain background information, objectives, methods, results and conclusion. Abstract should be followed by 3-5 'Key words' which will be used for indexing. Generally, an abstract may contain about 250 -300 words.
3. **Introduction** section is considered to be important in raising the quality of the article to next higher level. Include few paragraphs about the background information summarizing existing knowledge, evidence and lacunae. It is then followed by the purpose of study, hypothesis (if needed), the scope of the study and the research questions. The introduction should be concise and convince the readers regarding the significance and importance of the study. It should create interest among the readers to read the full article.
4. **Methods:** Methods section deals with a comprehensive description of the whole process beginning with the ethical clearance, information about the study site and the time period during which it was conducted. All relevant methodology including data collection and analysis should be clearly described. If an established method is used for investigation, suitable reference to be given. This section will also indicate the sample size calculation, ethics committee clearance and clinical trial registration details as applicable. All research studies should be approved by the respective ethics committees. In a manuscript, methods section should be written in past tense. Addition of a study flow chart will be ideal. In a randomized controlled trial, consort flow chart should be given. Flow chart will give a clear picture of the study to the reader.
5. **Results section:** It should contain observation and outcome of analysis of data using suitable statistical methods. Appropriate Tables and Figures can be used without repeating the same information in the text. Titles of Tables should be on the top and that of Figures below them. They should be suitably numbered with appropriate legends. Authors should not only list the observations but also describe the objective interpretation of the results obtained.

6. **Discussion:** You should initially highlight the significance and originality of the findings. Secondly this section should contain important findings of the study and their interpretation in comparison to the findings reported by other studies along with their references cited. Next you need to emphasize and discuss the strengths and limitations of your study which will open up new avenues for research question of future studies. Finally, briefly summarize the conclusion. You should carefully avoid exaggerating and claiming unsubstantiated study results. The last section should be devoted to offer some recommendations for future studies.
7. This should follow declarations like, acknowledgement, conflict of interest, financial support received etc.
8. **Reference listing:** All important references should be cited and listed as per journal style. It is advisable to use citation software such as Zotero, endnote, reference managers etc. References cited to be as recent as possible.
9. **Language editing and Plagiarism checking:** One should check for grammatical and spelling mistakes. It is better to take the help of a language editor if required (Desai. 2019, Adkoli & Parija. 2020). Plagiarism checking is important before submitting the manuscript since similarity to published material creates poor impression about the author. All information in a manuscript should be drafted in authors own words. Even putting sentences from one's own earlier publication will also amount to plagiarism (Debnath. 2016).

1. **Manuscript submission:** After you have chosen the appropriate journal, final version of the manuscript should be checked again before submission. The current trend is increasing number of e-journals and e-submission process, which you should get familiar with. Prepare a concise cover letter including the summary highlighting the important findings in two or three sentence justifying publication of the article (Nicholas. 2019). This will provide the important information to the editor regarding the manuscript. This cover letter has to be prepared and signed by the corresponding author of the article. All authors of the article need to sign the copyright form and also disclose the author's conflicts of interest in the manuscript. Who are all eligible to claim authorship and who should be acknowledged for their support is another important issue. The sequence of authors listing and the corresponding author need to be decided quite early, in order to avoid any misunderstanding later (Jagadeesan etal. 2021).
2. **Understanding the review process.** Once the manuscript is received by the journal editor, usually there will be two levels of review of manuscript. Initially, it will be internal peer review by the editorial team to decide whether the manuscript is the type of article that they really want to publish in their journal and if so whether it meets the standard for sending to external reviewers. Sometimes the editors may reject after initial screening and this is known as 'desk rejection'. Each journal has its rejection rate, which will be approximately 30- 70% of the manuscripts received by the editorial office. Now after completing the internal reviews, the editorial office will send the manuscript to external reviewers for assessing the quality of the article to decide publication, modification or rejection **(Fig. 1)**.

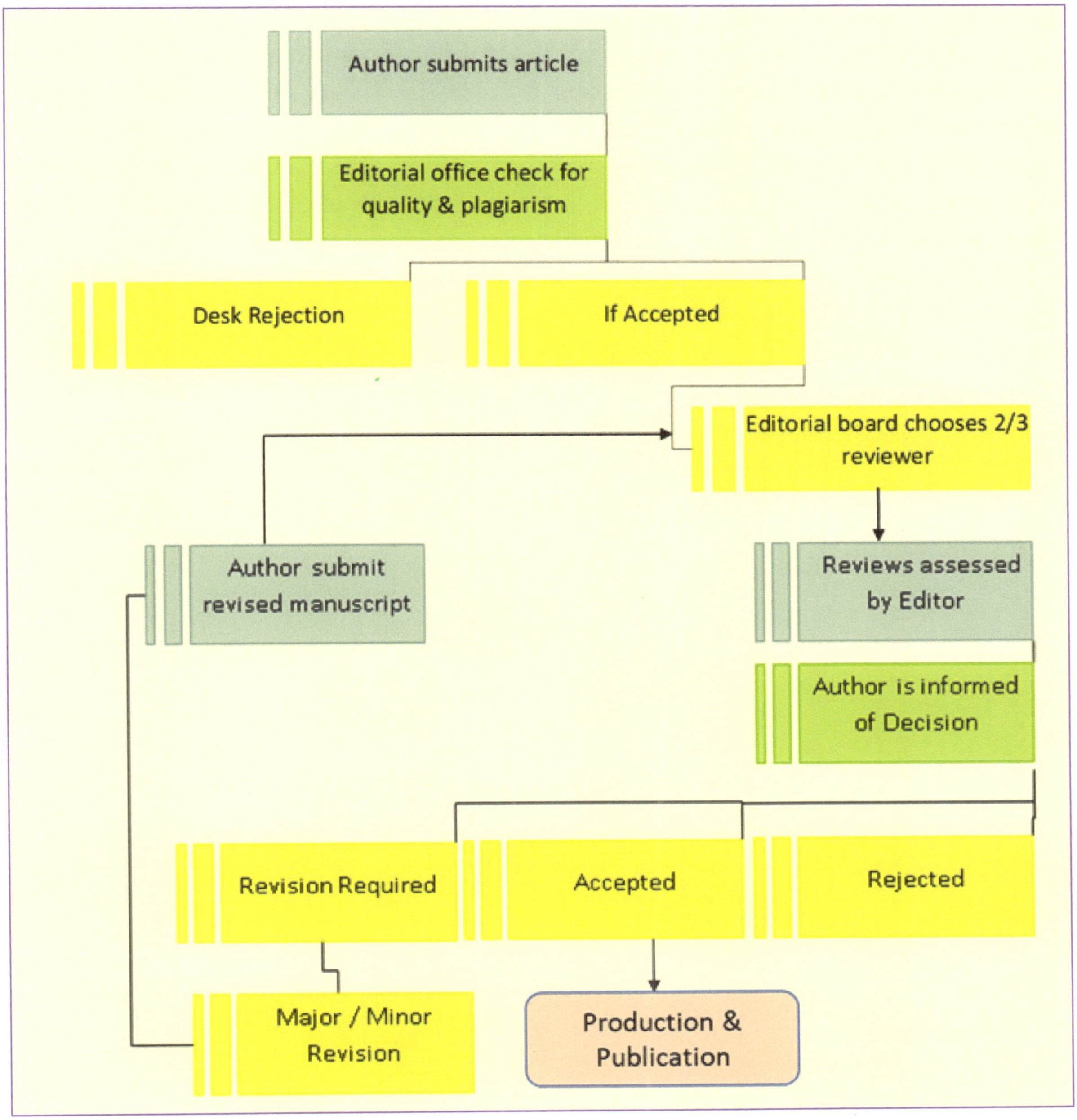

Figure 1: A flowchart showing peer review process from submission to publication

The reviewer will comment on the manuscript with regard to the following issues: -

(i) The scientific content of the manuscript

(ii) Adequacy of data for answering the research question

(iii) Whether the result obtained is original and the method used is scientifically sound

(iv) Completeness of the literature review and discussion

(v) Whether the article will be of interest to the journal readership

As author, we need to be careful to address these issues before submitting the article to the journal editorial office.

3. **Manuscript resubmission**. Once the manuscript is sent for review, reviewer will suggest either rejection or modification of the manuscript based on his observations. These comments should be carefully addressed before resubmission. In case the manuscript is not recommended for resubmission, the comments will help the author to modify the manuscript and submit it to another Journal. When the reviewer and editor suggest resubmission with modification, author should carry out suggested changes and send a covering letter giving details of changes done point vice. Unless there is adequate evidence for not making the changes, it is better to carry out the suggested changes (Sullivan. 2015). If author disagrees with reviewer, it should be clarified with suitable data and references.
4. **Enhance the readability through effective use of visual media**. Besides scientific content, the layout, design and effective use of tables, boxes, charts, diagrams, graphs, figures, flow charts and illustrations help in increasing readability of the paper (Fig. 2). Prepare manuscript which looks good, informative and also fulfils all the journal requirements. Visually attractive article is more tempting to the readers as well as reviewers. A well-organized manuscript helps to sustain reader's interest (Kotz & Cals. 2014).

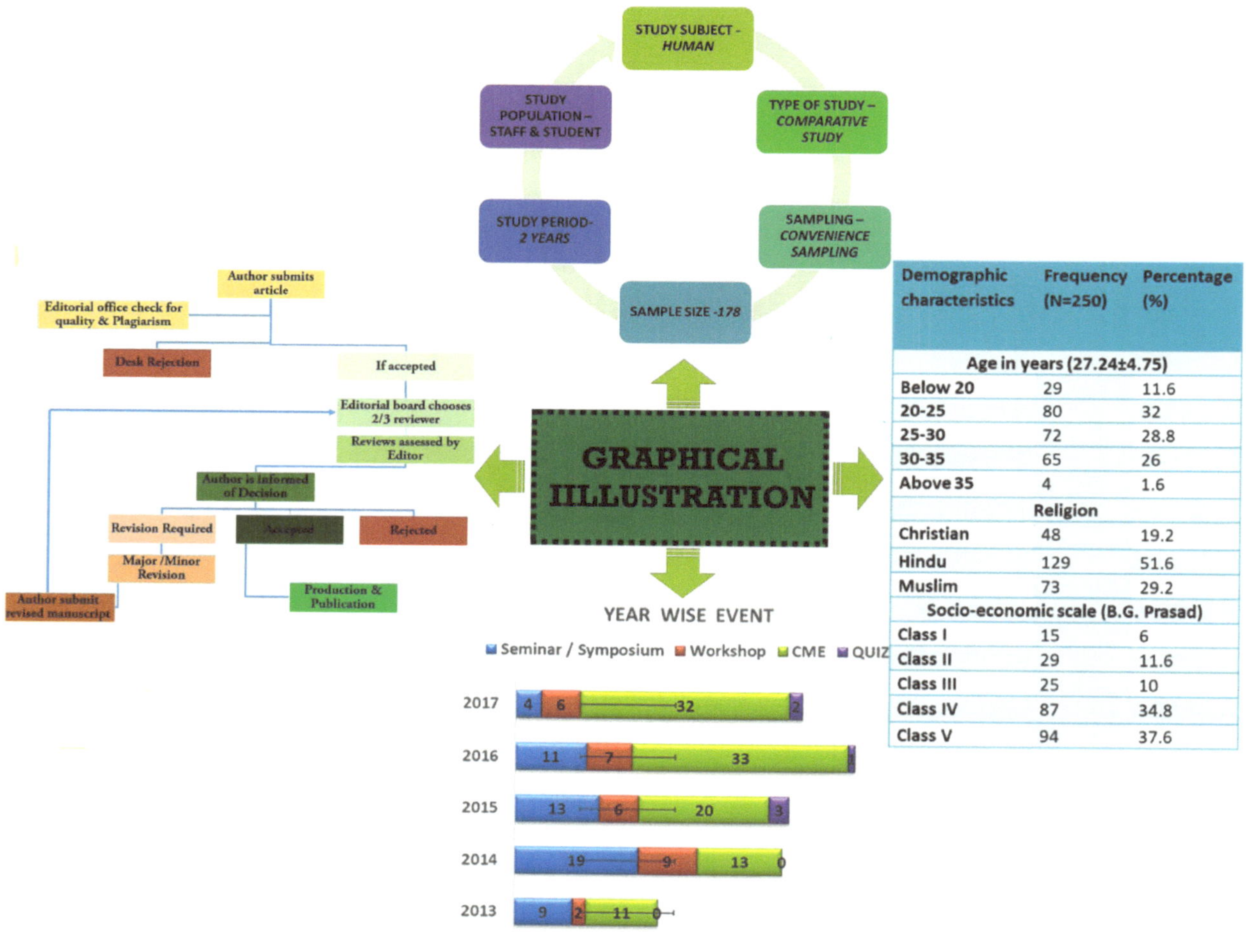

Figure 2: Illustration showing methods to Enhance the readability through effective use of visual media

SUMMARIZE

We have discussed some important issues related to publication of original articles in reputed journals. Choosing an appropriate journal, drafting the manuscript as per the journal style will increase the chances of acceptance of the manuscript. A well-researched topic and appropriately drafted manuscript taking care of the suggestions discussed will reduce the risk of rejection. In addition, reasonable and respectful responses to reviewers will also enhance the acceptance of the article. Therefore, scientific quality is the most important in consideration. Manuscript should be clear and concise so that chances of rejection will be reduced.

EVALUATE

(i) If you are a junior faculty member without any experience of research project, which type of article you would like to start?

(ii) Dr. B. who studied in Hindi medium does high quality research on effectiveness of online instruction. He sends his paper to LANCET and gets regret letter within a week. Guess two probable reasons cited by the editor.

ROAD AHEAD

1. The chapter you have read, has not dealt with enhancement of language skills in writing a research paper. If you wish to learn about this aspect, read the following article:
   Adkoli B.V., Parija S.C. (2020) Language Skills in Research Paper Writing. In: Parija S., Adkoli B. (eds) Effective Medical Communication. Springer, Singapore. *https://doi.org/10.1007/978-981-15-3409-6_14*

2. Would you like to explore more in writing each part of IMRAD structure? Read the following article:
   Jacob T.G., Sahni P. (2020) Publishing Effectively and Ethically. In: Parija S., Adkoli B. (eds) Effective Medical Communication. Springer, Singapore. *https://doi.org/10.1007/978-981-15-3409-6_11*

REFERENCES

Adkoli, B. V., & Parija, S. C. (2020). Language Skills in Research Paper Writing Effective Medical Communication (pp. 149-157): Springer.

Ali, J. (2010). Manuscript rejection: causes and remedies. Journal of young pharmacists: JYP, 2(1), 3.

Chernick, V. (2012). How to get your paper accepted for publication. Paediatric respiratory reviews, 13(2), 130-132.

Debnath, J. (2016). Plagiarism: A silent epidemic in scientific writing–Reasons, recognition and remedies. Medical Journal Armed Forces India, 72(2), 164-167.

Desai, G. (2019). How to leverage the language: A guide for medical writers in India. Perspectives in clinical research, 10(1), 37.

Hesterman, C. M., Szperka, C. L., & Turner, D. P. (2018). Reasons for manuscript rejection after peer review from the journal headache. Headache: The Journal of Head and Face Pain, 58(10), 1511-1518.

Jacob, T. G., & Sahni, P. (2020). Publishing Effectively and Ethically Effective Medical Communication (pp. 123-130): Springer.

Jagadeesan, S., Valia, A., & Panda, S. (2021). What the IJDVL expects from authors: Better writing. Indian Journal of Dermatology, Venereology and Leprology, 1-3.

Kotz, D., & Cals, J. W. (2014). Effective writing and publishing scientific papers, part XII: responding to reviewers. Journal of clinical epidemiology, 67(3), 243.

Kramer, B., & Libhaber, E. (2016). Writing for publication: institutional support provides an enabling environment. BMC medical education, 16(1), 1-5.

Nicholas, D. (2019). How to choose a journal and write a cover letter. Saudi journal of anaesthesia, 13(Suppl 1), S35.

Sullivan, G. M. (2015). What to do when your paper is rejected. Journal of Graduate Medical Education, 7(1), 1.

Section IV

Scholarship

Chapter 25

What is Scholarship?

Henal R Shah, Rashmi A Kusurkar, Avinash Supe

ABSTRACT

Educational research is a growing field, both in its scope, quality and quantity. Scholarship is driven by research and the formulation of a hypothesis that creates new knowledge. This was believed to be the gold standard of educational research. This view was a limited view of understanding educational scholarship. Boyer (1990) expanded this view to include many other activities: scholarship of discovery, application, integration, and teaching. This chapter clarifies various terms related to scholarship, and outlines the steps to conduct research, the obstacles that may be faced and suggestions to overcome them. Technology is increasingly playing a pivotal part in the conduction and publication of research. The authors suggest possibilities for the use of technology and methods to harness it. Finally, the chapter concludes with simple tips to enhance teacher's scholarship portfolio.

Key Words: educational scholarship, tips for scholarship, technology, growth of scholar

ASSESS NEED

Are you a scholar? Do you engage in scholarship in medical education? Most teachers would reply negatively to these questions. At the same time, most would affirm that they engage in scholarly work, research, and other outputs in their respective disciplines. This ambivalence implies that the transition from a clinical researcher to medical education scholarship is slow and often incomplete. Many factors such as paucity of time and competing interests may be responsible for this (Jordan et al., 2018). Lack of clarity of terms and understanding of what scholarship implies in medical education, and its benefits, are other factors.

Most medical educators engaged in a teaching institute think of scholarship as a means for research publications. (Nuthalapatyet al., 2012) In medical education, one needs to take a more comprehensive view of what constitutes scholarship and a scholar. Teachers spend a tremendous amount of time and resources on valuable activities such as the development of curriculum, assessment, and teaching. These are the bedrock for ensuring good quality graduates. Unfortunately, this work of teachers was neither appreciated nor awarded any consideration for promotion.

Ernst Boyer's work was a turning point in redefining the concept and scope of scholarship (Boyer, 1990). He identified four types of scholarship: scholarship of discovery, application, integration, and teaching. In a recent AMEE guide on educational scholarship (Cleland et al., 2021), the authors have described scholarly teaching, the scholarship of teaching and learning (SoTL) and scholarship. A scholarly teacher is reflective and uses evidence from the literature to improve her/his teaching, curriculum design, or assessment. SoTL is the process of contributing to the community of medical teachers by an organised enquiry into the learning of students and sharing the findings in the public domain. However, at times, it is difficult to demarcate the two. The scholarship is "publicly disseminated activities that advance practice and knowledge for health professions educators and/or the health professions education community" (Cleland et al., 2021). In the truest sense, scholarship implies a systematic methodology to find an answer to a problem or an issue by referring to the literature, and collecting and analysing data. Thus, scholarship includes not only publication of educational research, such as randomised controlled trials (RCTs) or bench investigations, but also public dissemination of one's work through activities such as conducting teaching workshops, giving invited lectures, and creating assessment plans.

A person may begin as a scholarly teacher and progress to SoTL or move in to other domains of scholarship. The process may be cyclical, with scholarly teaching leading to SoTL, which may lead to the scholarship of discovery. In this chapter, we shall discuss scholarship which will be expanded in the next chapter on SoTL.

BRIEF

- Educational scholarship is an important criterion for the professional growth of teachers.
- It includes not only original research, but also public dissemination of one's work through variety of activities such as conducting teaching workshops, designing instructional resources, and creating assessment plans. To qualify as scholarship, a product or innovation needs to be built on prior knowledge, be publicly disseminated, peer-reviewed and open for others to build on.
- The skills involved in scholarship development can be acquired and practiced.

CONTEXTUALIZE

Scenario: Many teachers were baffled with the outcome declared by a promotion committee in a famous institute. An associate professor in the Department of Anatomy missed an opportunity for promotion. Citing inability to fulfil the prescribed number of research publications as a problem, the committee rejected his application for advancement. He is a passionate teacher and caring mentor. Students flock to attend his class. How did such an exceptional teacher not meet the criteria for promotion? There were two important issues flagged by this decision. One was the inability of teacher to convert his strengths into research publications and other forms of scholarship. Are there avenues to achieve them? Secondly, how does one give value to the significant work done by teachers such as the passion for teaching and disseminating the art and science of teaching through invited lectures and workshops? There must be mechanisms to appreciate and award these contributions. This example underscores the need for teachers to be familiar with and practice scholarship in medical education.

DESCRIBE

Traditionally the gold standard of scholarship has always been publications of research with creation of new knowledge. This presented a limited view of scholarship. Boyer (1990) expanded this view to include many other activities of a teacher in the ambit of scholarship and worthy of being considered as a criteria for promotion (Diamond, 2002). A teacher conducts activities and takes on roles that may be beyond the current definition of scholarship.

Boyer (1990) looked beyond research and described four types of scholarship in medical education:

1. *Scholarship of discovery* includes traditional research activities and publications that broaden the knowledge of a discipline. E.g., review papers, empirical research, development of new theories or concepts in a discipline.
2. *Scholarship of integration* makes links across disciplines that foster appropriate use of concepts across disciplines. E.g. A systematic review of faculty development which is not limited to medical education, cross-disciplinary research, using practices from one discipline to inform and adapt practices in another discipline such as using gaming for robotic surgery skills development.
3. *Scholarship of application* calls for using theory in practice, including using theories or ideas from other disciplines. E.g. reviewing for journals, utilising the learnings from the publications of others to improve teaching-learning practices, creating a curriculum or teaching & learning method using constructs of theory and evidence-backed knowledge.
4. *Scholarship of Teaching* (teaching and learning) involves developing new and evidence-based ways to facilitate and assess learning. E.g. A presentation of a systematic review of the effectiveness of methods used for assessment or for a talk to sharpen leadership to improve education, innovation, and improvisations in education. SoTL will be discussed further in the next chapter.

Criteria for Educational Scholarship

Scholarship in Medical education has been defined as a tangible product such as a journal article, a book, a presentation, a durable educational product, new knowledge, or its presentation that was peer-reviewed or publicly disseminated. This definition is expanded to include products besides research articles, like webinars, presentations on curriculum evaluation, presentations of assessment programs, etc.

For an activity to be an indicator of scholarship, it needs to fulfil the following criteria (Diamond, 2002):

1. The work involves expertise in the discipline
2. The activity should have clarity of goals, preparation of good groundwork and use of appropriate methods
3. The final product has an element of reflection and is publicly disseminated
4. It must be built on prior constructs, principles, or best practices and is beyond individual utility and significance; others can build on it

5. Peer-reviewed

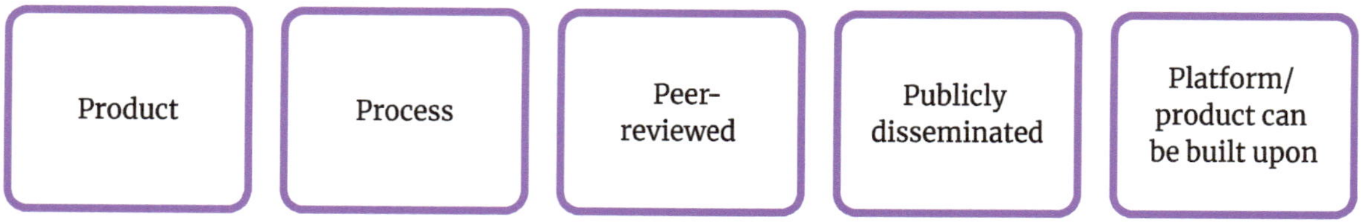

Figure 1: The five P's of scholarship

Importance of Scholarship

Educational Scholarship helps a broad spectrum of stakeholders in the education system by providing them with many answers (Fraenkel & Wallen, 2006): All stakeholders benefit differently.

1. Administrators and regulators: Learn ways to improve governance and create policies that foster learning; regulators have guidelines for comparison of standards and benchmarking
2. Teachers: Are empowered by being informed of best practices, evidence-based methods that are effective strategies
3. Students: Scholarship sheds light on pathways to achieve competency
4. Clinicians: Best practices help in clinical management
5. Community and country: Improvement of health care through the use of evidence-based strategies

How to begin a journey into scholarship

1. **Decide on an area of interest**
   To begin, reflect on the long-term professional goals and align scholarship goals to them. Break the goals down to short term, intermediate and long-term goals. Create a timeline depending on your expertise and context. The most crucial part of academic research is asking and answering important questions related to medical education. Identify a question that you are genuinely and passionately interested in. While some questions maybe suggested by others, such as a department head, others may emerge from your interactions or personal reading (Chacko & Supe, 2015)
2. **Collaborate**
   Any research project is the work of a team. Multiple skills such as proficiency in concepts and theory, educational research design, scientific writing, statistical analysis, networking are required. Involving stakeholders within and across institutions can be the key to success. Following the agreed timelines, motivating each other, and keeping the goal in sight irons out the process. Write up the research proposal.
3. **Improve standards for a scholarship**
   Glassicket al. (1997) have proposed standards for evaluating research & project proposals. These are presented here as a checklist and can be used whilst preparing your research papers.
   a. ***Clear Goals***: Is the statement of purpose clear? Are the aims enunciated? Are the research questions appropriate?
   b. ***Adequate Preparation***: Has a thorough literature review been conducted to identify the gaps in knowledge on the paper's topic?

c. ***Appropriate Methods***: Are the methods, instruments, and design appropriate for answering the research questions?
d. ***Significant Results***: Do results answer the questions and achieve the goal? Does the research add to the literature in that area? Does the research open more avenues for exploration?
e. ***Effective Communication***: Is the writing scientific, clear, and appropriate for the audience? Is the message coherent and reflect integrity?
f. ***Reflective Critique***: Do the researchers adequately reflect on their work?

Does the scholar use evidence from the literature to support or argue their case? Are limitations acknowledged and pathways for future research highlighted?

4. **Overcoming Barriers**

The barriers to scholarship are intrinsic to the study and include a lack of time and formal research training. The paucity of funds, resources, collaborators, mentors, and support by administrative leaders are other extrinsic factors that are a deterrent to scholarship. Sometimes the learners who are subject of the study may be disinclined and not consider the study valuable. Think of ways to navigate beyond this.

Table 1: Obstacles and suggestions for overcoming them

Obstacle	Solutions
Paucity of ideas	Read review articles, brainstorm.
Not sure how to conduct research, project	Get training, join others as an assistant, get a mentor.
Difficulty in data gathering	Anticipate, network, use of reminders, involve students to brainstorm on effective ways of gathering data.
Difficulty in data analysis	Consult methodological papers, books, a statistician, or expert colleagues.
Procrastination in writing	Set deadlines, break them into smaller pieces, ask colleagues/team to support.
Rejected article	Do not lose hope. Use feedback to improve and resubmit quickly.
Lack of funds	Learn how to apply for grants, know where grants are available, advocacy for increased funding in this area.

5. **Forums for publication**

Completed research can be presented and published in either paper-based or digital formats. Each has its advantages.

a. **Journals:** The choice of journal is an informed decision. It is based on the intended audience and type of study. Should it be published in a specialty or education journal? Should it be a national, regional, or international journal? Factors to consider are:
   (i) Indexed journals -The advantage of an indexed journal is that it offers a broader reach and better chances for citations and translation to other contexts. PubMed, Sciences Citation Index (SCI), Indmed, are a few indexing agents.
   (ii) National, regional, or International -The type and content of research determines the article's usefulness. If findings can be generalized across continents, one could try for

an international journal. Opting for a national journal seems more appropriate if the study is more locally relevant.

(iii) Open Access journals: The philosophy behind Open Access journals is to have a broad reach and make research available to all. However, authors may find the cost of publishing in Open Access exorbitant.

(iv) "Impact Factor" of the journal -The impact factor of a journal is calculated from the number of citations received by the articles. Whether this reflects superior research is a debatable issue. However, currently, this parameter is significant to propagate one's research and oneself as a researcher. This is a well-known but controversial parameter of a journal's reputation.

(v) Influential journals - Some journals are distinguished because of the quality of their work irrespective of their impact factor.

(vi) Specialty Journals - Medical education articles may be published in either specialty or educational journals. The deciding factor for the choice of journal is the topic of research and the target audience.

(vii) Manuscript types -Journals publish manuscript types such as original articles, reviews, editorials, brief communications, letters, viewpoints, to name a few. Check instructions for the specific manuscript type that you are attempting to write. The table below mentions a few journals, their impact factors (from the journal website or resurchify.com, 2021), accessibility and the link to instructions for authors.

Table 2: List of some Journals in Medical Education

SN	Name	Impact factor	Open Access	Instruction for authors (link)
1	Medical Education	4.570	Hybrid open access (with fee)	*https://onlinelibrary.wiley.com/page/journal/13652923/homepage/forauthors.html*
2	Academic Medicine	5.354	Yes (with fee)	*https://journals.lww.com/academicmedicine/Pages/InformationforAuthors.aspx*
3	The Clinical Teacher	0.76	Hybrid open access (with fee)	*https://onlinelibrary.wiley.com/page/journal/1743498x/homepage/forauthors.html*
4	Medical Teacher	1.93	Yes (with fee)	*https://www.tandfonline.com/action/authorSubmission?show=instructions&journalCode=imte20*
5	Education for Health	0.73	Yes	*https://www.educationforhealth.net/contributors.asp*
6	SEAJME		Yes	*https://seajme.sljol.info/author/login/?submit=True*
7	Teaching & Learning in Medicine	1.848	No	*https://www.tandfonline.com/action/authorSubmission?show=instructions&journalCode=htlm20*
8	BMC Medical Education	1.831	Yes	*https://bmcmededuc.biomedcentral.com/submission-guidelines*
10	JAMA Network Open	5.71	Yes	*https://jamanetwork.com/pages/for-authors*

SN	Name	Impact factor	Open Access	Instruction for authors (link)
11	Perspectives on Medical Education	2.27	Yes	*https://www.springer.com/journal/40037/submission-guidelines*
12	Medical Science Educator	0.54	Yes	*https://www.springer.com/journal/40670/submission-guidelines*
13	Health Education Journal	0.938	Yes (with fees)	*https://journals.sagepub.com/author-instructions/HEJ*
14	Nurse Education in Practice	1.614	Gold (with fee)	*https://www.elsevier.com/journals/nurse-education-in-practice/1471-5953/guide-for-authors*
15	International Journal of Medical Education	1.76	Yes	*https://www.ijme.net/authors/*

Speciality Journals where articles related to medical education are also published:

1. Academic Emergency Medicine
2. Academic Psychiatry
3. Advances in Physiology Education
4. Cell Biology Education
5. Family Medicine Journal
6. J. General Internal Medicine
7. Indian Journal of Pediatrics
8. Indian Journal of Gastroenterology
9. JAPI, FOGSI Association journals
11. Journal of Pharmacology and Pharmacotherapeutics
12. Anatomical Sciences Education
13. American Journal of Pharmaceutical Education
14. The New England Journal of Medicine
15. National Medical J India
16. Journal of Rural & Remote Health
17. Journal of Post Graduate Medicine

b. Digital platforms

Clearing houses or Web Portals. Many professional and educational associations have started their web portals. All educational and other material is peer-reviewed and posted on these websites. Educational tools for measurement and such resources can be submitted to clearinghouses. Please find some of the links below:

(i) AAMC: Repository for Peer-Reviewed Educational Materials: www.aamc.org/members/gea/cube.htm

(ii) Alliance for Academic Internal Medicine Educational Tools: www.im.org/AAIM/tools/default.htm

(iii) Society of Teachers of Family Medicine: www.edserv.musc.edu/prn/resource

(iv) American Physiologic Society: www.the-aps.org/education
(v) Association of Surgical Educators: www.surgicaleducation.com/educlear/index.htm
(vi) Association of Professors of obstetrics & gynaecology: www.apgo.org/resourcenetwork
(vii) Council on Medical Student Education in Pediatrics: www.unmc.edu/community/comsep
(viii) MedEdPortal: www.mededportal.org
(ix) MedEd*Publish:https://www.mededpublish.org/home*

Others: Blogs, social media can also serve as channels for disseminating information.

6. **Handling setbacks such as rejection**
Whilst it is disappointing to receive a rejection, one must view the feedback as a source for improving one's current and future work. Poor writing, poor problem definition, inadequate data or statistical analysis are common causes of rejection. (Bordage, 2001) [Please refer to the chapter on "How to enhance the acceptance of your manuscript?" for further pointers.]

Role of departments and institutions in fostering educational research

Research does not occur in a vacuum. Nurturance by the institution, department and professional bodies facilitates the growth of research. Help may be available in many ways. (Fincheret al., 2000)

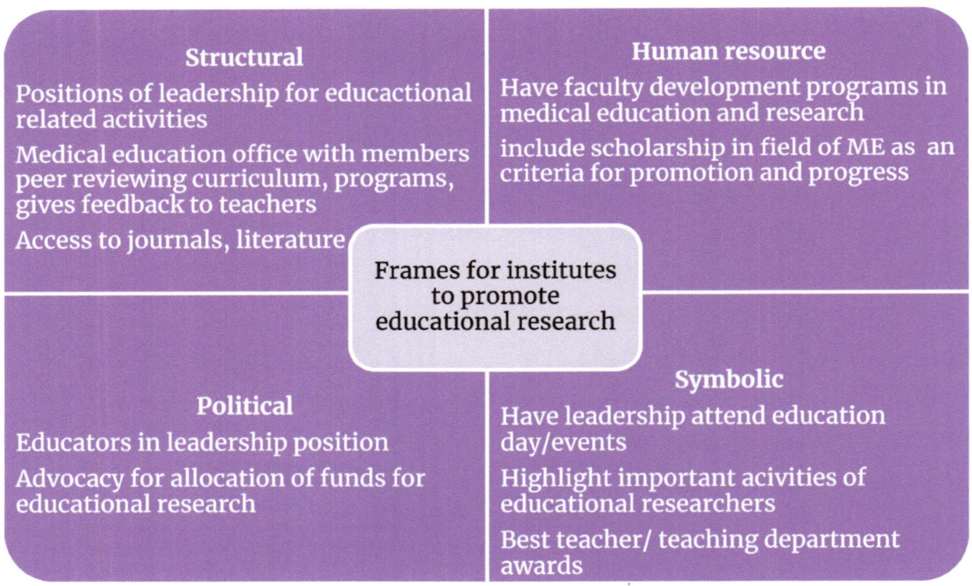

Figure 2: The ways institutes can offer help

Role of technology in research

The digital scholarship aids educational scholarship activities by facilitating the flourishing of the creative and reflective aspects. It has opened the following avenues (Goh & Sanders, 2019).

1. Open Access and non-peer-reviewed outputs: These allow for broader dissemination, especially in low resource settings. Open access journals may have an established pre-publication or post-

publication peer-review process. Non–peer-reviewed scholarly outputs, including research and teaching, are often presented as conference proceedings. Some of these may be peer reviewed.

2. Social media such as Facebook, WhatsApp, Instagram, and Twitter, may be used to present educational research. FOAM (Free Open Access Meducation) which includes blogs, podcasts, videos, Virtual Reality (VR) and Augmented Reality (AR) is helpful as teaching aids especially where traditional training is deficient.
3. Digital analytics is used to measure numerous online activities. Google Analytics and Altmetric are free online platforms that compute the number of open access publications and social media comments. This data gauges the utility and popularity of the scholarly output.

Understanding Bibliometrics and digital analytics

Measurement of impact is one of the critical yet controversial issues in educational scholarship. Traditionally this is referred to as bibliometrics. In the digital world, the terms for the impact are altmetrics, cyber metrics or webometrics. They play a role in obtaining grants and awards, criteria for promotion, and university ranking. Please find some examples of impact measurement below. (Roemer & Borchardt, 2012)

General resources:

1. Google Scholar citations is a free service which facilitates authors to create their profile and provides h- index and i-10 index. H index is based on a scientist's most cited papers and reflects productivity and impact. The number of citations helps in calculating i-10 (at least 10 citations). The utility of the h index is to compare researchers of similar career length in a similar field or subject. It gives a snapshot of the scholar'sprofile *Access: http://scholar.google.com/intl/en/scholar/citations.html*
2. SCImago Journal and Country Rank: Scopus runs a free website to provide two metrics; SCImago Journal Rank (SR based on citations and influence) and Source Normalized Impact per Paper (SNIP) *Access: http://www.SCImagojr.com*
3. Scopus is a paid subscription database. Metrics include standard options such as several times cited and h-index, SJR. and SNIP. They also have an "Altmetric for Scopus, "which is a third party application displaying mention of paper across social media. *Access: http://www.scopus.com*
4. Web of Knowledge, which includes the web of Science, was the pioneer in this field. It provides h-index, impact factor, Eigen factor, and field-based journal rankings. Though mired in controversy, they are considered the gold standard in traditional bibliometrics. *Access: http://www.webofknowledge.com.*

Altmetric resources

1. **Altmetrics.org.** is a free and central website for information about the growing altmetrics approach. Altmetrics is the study of new metrics based on the Social Web for analysing and informing scholarship. (Roemer & Borchardt, 2012). It may look at factors such as the number of views, discussions, citations, saves and recommendations. Altmetrics.org uses new online tools for calculating impact. *Access: http://altmetrics.org.*
2. **Impact Story.** It is a free, open-source tool designed to support URL-based publishing through the aggregation of online altmetrics. Users create collections of materials and the material is assigned impact categories, such as generally/highly "saved,""cited,""recommended," or "discussed." This resource is precious for scholars publishing in non-traditional venues or with scholarship too new to have accumulated traditional citations. *Access: http://impactstory.it/.*

3. **PLoS Article-Level Metrics.** Public Library of Science (PLoS) is an open-access journal repository. PLoS offers Article-Level Metrics, which measure the influence of individual PLoS articles, the times it is downloaded, mentioned in social media and blogs. PLoS also tracks internal article metrics, such as comments, notes, and ratings. The drawback is that it is only available for PLoSarticles. *Access: http://article-level-metrics.PLoS.org/.*
4. **Publish or Perish.** PoP is a free, downloadable program that gathers data from Google scholar based on the author's name. PoP can calculate numerous metrics besides the h-index. *Access: http://www.harzing.com/pop.htm.*
5. ReaderMeter is a free tool that focuses on readership and not citations. It gathers data by processing readership from Mendeley. Each report provides information such as an author's"HR-Index,""GR-Index,""Total Bookmarks," and "Top Publications by Readership." *Access: http://readermeter.org/.*

Scholarship in COVID times

The COVID-19 pandemic has produced a tsunami of changes in the field of teaching and implementing the curriculum. Notwithstanding the current difficulties, the need for engaging in medical research persists. In the current context, action research, having quick iterative cycles of design and research, would help substantiate the transformational change that is happening and is required. (Goh & Sandars, 2020) The use of open access and digital media would facilitate rapid dissemination that is essential in current times. Institutional support and involvement would be necessary to achieve this goal.

Growth as a Scholar

Just as skill acquisition has a process from novice to expert, the growth of a scholar may be charted similarly. One begins as a novice and gradually becomes proficient. This awareness will guide the choice of journal or platform for presentation. In the process of growth, be aware of the goal, celebrate milestones and achievements along the way. These activities bolster motivation and sensitise the researcher to one's strengths and weaknesses.

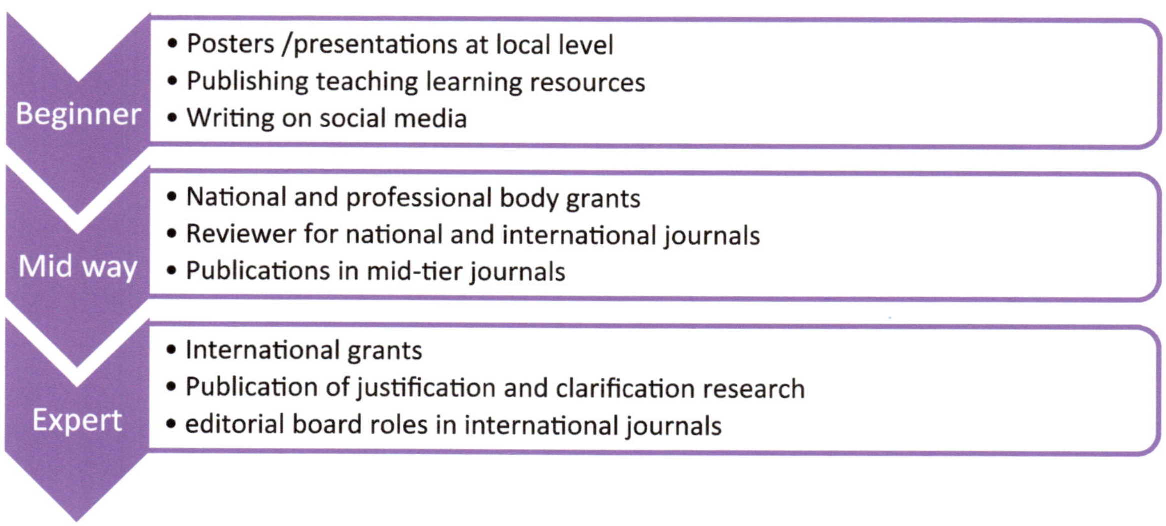

Figure 3: Growth of a Scholar

Status of Scholarship Today

Educational scholarship has become viable with the development of processes to facilitate growth. Faculty training, grants and scholar programs are budding. There is a change in the promotion criteria where teaching innovations and other SoTL are accepted. New awards and recognitions are evolving, as is the broader availability for dissemination. Most pertinently, new faculty tracks are being considered.

SUMMARISE

We suggest you make a list of critical points you have gathered from this chapter and jot them down below for reference.

EVALUATE

Reflect on where you place yourself on the ladder of research?

How can one take steps to convert one's activities into scholarship?

Do a SWOT analysis to understand your strengths and context

- What are one's strengths? What is the scholar passionate about and does well? What resources are available? Who can collaborate or mentor?
- Weaknesses: What needs improvement in individual scholarship skills? What resources are lacking?
- Opportunities: What opportunities are present? What strengths can one leverage? What trends can be capitalized?
- Threats: What are the threats preventing the teacher from doing scholarship?

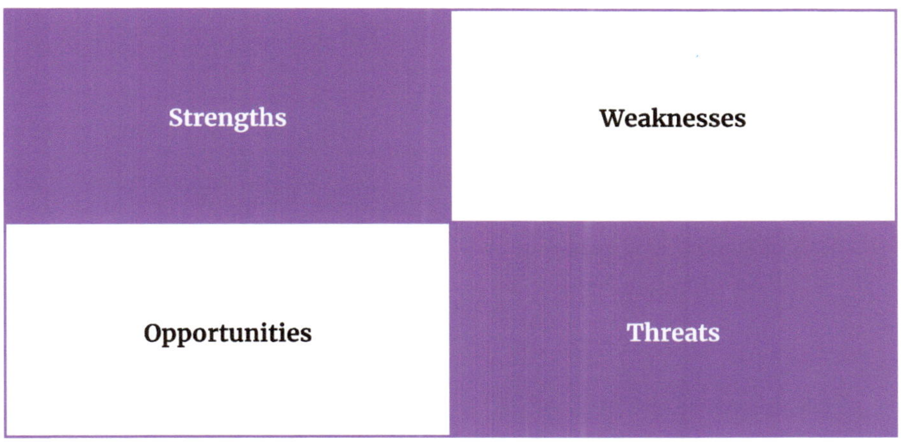

Figure 4: SWOT analysis

ROAD AHEAD

Educational scholarship has come to age in most parts of the world. However, a recent study revealed that most published literature shows that Asians, Africans and South Americans are underrepresented as authors. (Buffone, 2020). The institute must promote faculty development to facilitate growth in educational scholarship. The institution's role, attitude, help, and how it makes resources available would make this path easier to tread.

Improving the quality of studies is the next agenda. Whilst opportunistic studies are simpler to conduct, planned systematic research with robust designs to ensure outcomes may yield more valuable results.

Besides discovery, we need to consider working with other disciplines to promote the scholarship of integration. Leadership, including that of the Academy of Health Professional Education, must promote interdisciplinary work. The upliftment is possible by designing innovative research and funding processes dedicated to interdisciplinary work. In order to flourish, Interprofessional education and integrative research need support from health universities. Training specialists in translational research is another critical step. The scientific community must push for efficient ways for showcasing the importance of its work to the community.

On an individual level, how can one move ahead? One needs to make a concrete plan. The following template can be used to plan further. (Santen, Peterson & Wolff, 2019; Sullivan, 2018)

Table 3: Ten tips to help the progress of a scholarship

SN	Define Goals - Short, intermediate, and long term	
1	Scholarship progress.	Tips.
2	Identify topic for research.	Read, collaborate.
3	Decide a topic.	Based on context, interest.
4	Form a team.	Decide who will be partners.
5	Write a precise scientific research proposal.	Use Glassick's criteria to refine.
6	IRB approval.	As per the committee.
7	Implement research.	Celebrate small wins.
8	Analysis and writing.	Take help if required for analysis Keep writing scientific and simple.
9	Decide journal.	Based on the type of research and context.
10	Hurdles.	Troubleshoot Keep motivation going.
11	Publication.	Celebrate and prepare for the next project.

REFERENCES

Bordage, G. (2001). Reasons reviewers reject and accept manuscripts: the strengths and weaknesses in medical education reports. *Academic medicine*, 76(9), 889-896.

Boyer, E. L. (1991). Scholarship Reconsidered: Priorities of the Professoriate. Princeton, NJ: The Carnegie Foundation for the Advancement. *Metropolitan Universities.*

Buffone, B., Djuana, I., Yang, K., Wilby, K. J., El Hajj, M. S., & Wilbur, K. (2020). Diversity in health professional education scholarship: a document analysis of international author representation in leading journals. *BMJ open*, 10(11), e043970.

Cleland, J. A., Jamieson, S., Kusurkar, R. A., Ramani, S., Wilkinson, T. J., & van Schalkwyk, S. (2021). Redefining scholarship for health professions education: AMEE Guide No. 142. *Medical Teacher*, 1-15.

Chacko T and Supe A. (2015). "Scholarship in Medical Education" in The Art of Teaching Medical Students. Eds Bhuiyan PS, Rege NN & Supe AN. (3rd Edition). Elsivier, Mumbai. Pp. 448-460.

Cook, D. A. (2010). Getting started in medical education scholarship. *The Keio journal of medicine*, *59*(3), 96-103.

Cook, D. A., Bordage, G., & Schmidt, H. G. (2008). Description, justification and clarification: a framework for classifying the purposes of research in medical education. *Medical education*, *42*(2), 128-133.

Diamond, R. M. (2002). Defining scholarship for the twenty-first century. *New Directions for Teaching and Learning*, *2002*(90), 73-80.

Fincher, R. M. E., Simpson, D. E., Mennin, S. P., Rosenfeld, G. C., Rothman, A., McGrew, M. C.,... & Turnbull, J. M. (2000). Scholarship in teaching: an imperative for the 21st century. *Academic medicine*, *75*(9), 887-894.

Find Impact Factor. Resurchify. (2021). https://www.resurchify.com/impact-factor.php.

Fraenkel, J. R., Wallen, N. E., & Hyun, H. H. (1993). *How to design and evaluate research in education* (Vol. 7). New York: McGraw-hill.

Glassick, C. E., Huber, M. T., & Maeroff, G. I. (1997). *Scholarship Assessed: Evaluation of the Professoriate. Special Report*. Jossey Bass Inc., Publishers, 989 Market Street, San Francisco, CA 94103.

Goh, P. S., & Sandars, J. (2019). Digital Scholarship–rethinking educational scholarship in the digital world. *MedEdPublish*, *8*.

Goh, P. S., & Sandars, J. (2020). Rethinking scholarship in medical education during the era of the COVID-19 pandemic. *MedEdPublish*, 9.

Jordan, J., Coates, W. C., Clarke, S., Runde, D., Fowlkes, E., Kurth, J., & Yarris, L. (2018). The uphill battle of performing education scholarship: barriers educators and education researchers face. *Western Journal of Emergency Medicine*, *19*(3), 619.

Nuthalapaty, F. S., Casey, P. M., Cullimore, A. J., Dugoff, L., Abbott, J. F., Chuang, A. W.,... & Wolf, A. (2012). To the point: a primer on medical education research. *American journal of obstetrics and gynecology*, *207*(1), 9-13.

Roemer, R. C., & Borchardt, R. (2012). From bibliometrics to altmetrics: A changing scholarly landscape. *College & Research Libraries News*, *73*(10), 596-600.

Santen, S. A., Peterson, W., & Wolff, M. (2019). Turning Your Educational Work into Scholarship. *AEM education and training*, *3*(1), 79-80.

Sullivan, G. M. (2018). A toolkit for medical education scholarship. *Journal of graduate medical education*, *10*(1), 1.

Chapter 26

Scholarship of Teaching and Learning (SoTL)

Rashmi A Kusurkar, Henal Shah, Avinash Supe

ABSTRACT

Scholarship of Teaching and Learning (SoTL) refers to teachers understanding pedagogical principles of teaching and learning, reading literature on this topic, collecting evaluation data from students, presenting findings to colleagues, being open to critique and using the insights generated to improve one's teaching. Making one's findings public and open to critique is what distinguishes SoTL from scholarly teaching. SoTL does not have standard definition in the literature in spite of several authors suggesting a standardization in order to get the maximum benefit from SoTL in terms of student learning. Integration of SoTL in leadership and vision, policy and planning and organizational structures in medical education can go a long way in having impact with SoTL. One can engage in SoTL either individually or through a community of practice. The latter has several advantages like sharing of expertise and scholars inspiring each other through their work. SoTL in medical education misses meaningful contribution from the Global South countries. The reasons for this need investigation and as a community we need to be more inclusive in our scholarly practices.

Key Words: scholarship; teaching; learning; scholarly activity; medical education, health professions education

ASSESS NEED

Generally, doctors are expected to start teaching without any formal training in teaching. During this process doctors can have many questions about the teaching-learning process, student motivation and engagement, assessments, competency training and so on. At such times, they do not know who to turn to. They are trained for conducting and understanding research in their own disciplines, but have no idea how to view the education that they provide and the evidence from educational research through a critical lens, which is a completely different cup of tea. (Cleland et al. 2021) Teaching in a scholarly manner and engaging in scholarship of teaching and learning (SoTL) are important components of teaching competency.

BRIEF

- Teaching, scholarly teaching, scholarship of teaching and learning (SoTL) and educational scholarship are distinct entities.
- Scholarly teaching includes viewing one's own teaching practices through a critical lens and using pedagogical principles and evidence-based insights to improve them.
- SoTL includes making one's investigation into problems public and open to critic and taking feedback to improve.
- Teachers can engage in SoTL individually or through participating in a community of scholars/ teachers.

CONTEXTUALIZE

A colleague and a fellow educator of the first author, Dr. Inge van Wijk, developed a 4-year graduate entry medical program at the Faculty of Medicine Vrije Universiteit, Amsterdam, the Netherlands. It was an MD-program focused on research with elements which were different from the regular 6-year medical education program. At the heart of this program was the creation of a close-knit learning community. As the Educational Director of this program, Dr. van Wijk did not limit herself to developing the program, but also collected and analysed evidence to evaluate the program and pinpoint its strengths and weaknesses. Most of the times her hypotheses about how and why the program worked were supported through the evidence she generated. Dr. van Wijk presents her work on this program annually at the Netherlands Medical Education Association (NVMO) and the Association for Medical Education in Europe (AMEE) conferences. She is open to critique on her work and obtains feedback from national and international colleagues. She uses this feedback to improve the program. This is a great example of scholarship of teaching and learning (SoTL). Had Dr. van Wijk restricted herself to collecting and evaluating evidence for herself, it would be classified as scholarly teaching. The element of sharing work with colleagues and making it public and open to critique, made it SoTL. (*https://www.researchgate.net/profile/Inge_Wijk*)

Could you think of examples among your colleagues who have followed a similar trajectory? What would you advise a colleague who wants to engage in SoTL?

DESCRIBE

What is SoTL? How to move from teaching to scholarly teaching to scholarship of teaching and learning

What is teaching? As medical educators all of us are involved in teaching. When a teacher teaches without evaluation of and reflection on her pedagogical practices, she is said to limit herself to 'teaching'. What is scholarly teaching? If an educator questions his teaching techniques, reads up the literature on teaching and learning to clear his doubts and answer his questions, collects evidence in the form of evaluation and feedback from students and uses the literature and feedback to improve his teaching, he is said to engage in 'scholarly teaching'. What is then scholarship of teaching and learning (SoTL)? In addition to the things mentioned under scholarly teaching, if an educator presents her data analysis to peers and colleagues at local, national and international forums, i.e. she makes her knowledge public, she is said to engage in SoTL. Scholarly teaching derives from the literature and knowledge on teaching practice, while SoTL contributes to it. The differences between these three concepts are depicted in Figure 1. (Cleland et al. 2021)

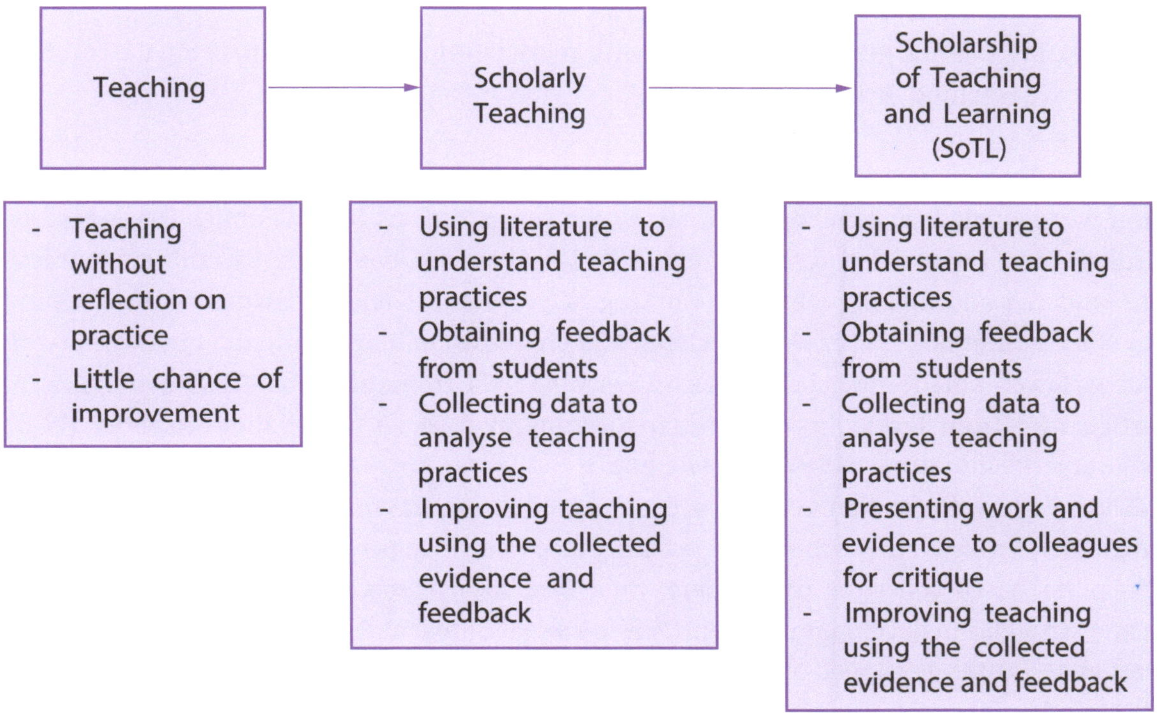

Figure 1: Differences between teaching, scholarly teaching and SoTL

A synthesis of the literature on SoTL

In 1990, Boyer introduced the concept of scholarship of teaching. His intention was to provide teaching its rightful status at Universities, as teaching was considered only second to research and deemed unimportant. (Boyer, 1990) He introduced the idea that teachers should, apart from their discipline-specific knowledge, be aware of the literature and knowledge on teaching-learning practices and use this to improve their own practice.

There has been much confusion about what scholarly teaching versus SoTL entails and getting a consensus has been rather difficult. The biggest difference between scholarly teaching and SoTL is that in SoTL, the teacher makes her work public and open to critique. (Hutchings & Shulman, 1999; Shulman, 1998; Smith, 2001; Kreber, 2002) Authors of SoTL papers highlight that having a standard definition of SoTL is pre-requisite to extracting the full potential of SoTL.

Six challenges have been identified in SoTL work. (McKinney, 2006) SoTL currently focuses on:

a) how teachers should teach instead of how student can learn,
b) undergraduate students, while it is equally important in graduate students,
c) classroom level work, while it is relevant at program/departmental levels as well,
d) students only as research subjects, while students can actually enhance and help in growing SoTL,
e) Global Northern notions of education, while more participation and perspective from the developing countries/Global South is much desirable,
f) within institution and within discipline work, which needs to be done across institutions and disciplines, and,
g) doing analysis and getting the results, while more effort needs to go into using the results to improve teaching-learning.

In 2021, if we view medical education journals or platforms such as MedEdPublish (*www.medepublish.org*), MedEdPortal (*www.mededportal.org*), etc., it is clear that SoTL has moved towards student learning, graduate students and lifelong learning, working at programme and departmental levels, providing students voice within SoTL, cross-institutional and cross-disciplinary work and application-oriented SoTL. But we haven't made much progress in integrating SoTL from the Global South contexts as we still miss participation from developing countries in meaningful ways, i.e. in how they can add to the body of knowledge and the literature on SoTL. (Naidu, 2021)

SoTL is fraught with problems of non-acceptance and de-valuation by discipline-based researchers. Adendorff (2011) reported that scholars of teaching faced negative perceptions about their work among their discipline-based colleague researchers, their own insecurities about building expertise in this domain and struggles in developing an identity as a scholar of teaching. (Adendorff, 2011)

Myatt et al. (2018) developed a framework for Facilitating Institutional Conversations about SoTL (FIC- SoTL). They describe integrating support for SoTL at the Leadership, Policy and Planning and Organizational Structure levels is necessary to harness the full potential of SoTL at the institutional level. (Myatt et al, 2018)

The new developments in SoTL center around:

a) Growing SoTL through communities of practice or learning communities - This seems to be more effective, time-efficient, and impactful than trying to do it at an individual level. (Bailey et al., 2021; Fanghanel et al., 2015; Ramani et al., 2021a), and
b) Using learning analytics for boosting SoTL – Learning analytics refers to the measuring/collecting, analyzing and reporting of learner data to understand how learners learn in their contexts and how this process can be optimized. (Long & Siemens, 2011) Generally learning analytics is used at a university level, i.e. across faculties, which translates into a big sample size and data (Big Data) over different types of learners, learning environments and philosophies. This allows for the possibility of drawing strong scientific conclusions and can even lead to uncovering new trends in teaching and learning. Using data collected through learning analytics can give a strong boost to SoTL, as the ultimate goal of SoTL is improving student learning. (Bronnimann et al., 2018)

How to engage in SoTL at an individual level?

SoTL starts with being curious about your teaching-learning practices. Pay attention to the questions that come to your mind. What is going well? What can go better? What can I do to make things better? Go back and read the literature related to your questions. Learn from the published knowledge and apply it in your practice. Collect data to test your hypothesis and evaluate the changes that you have made. Take feedback from your students about your teaching. Share your findings with your peers and colleagues and get their critical input. Use this input to make improvements or innovations.

How to engage in SoTL through participating in a community of scholars/ teachers?

It can be lonely and confusing to embark on the SoTL journey. You don't have to do it by yourself. Being a part of a community of scholarly teachers can be highly inspiring and supportive in your objective. Try to look for such a community in your immediate surroundings or in your local/national professional association or in an international context. If such a community is not easy to come by, you can also initiate it yourself among like-minded educators. Participation in a community of scholars/ teachers has been proposed to function as a formative evaluation of one's SoTL through receiving peer feedback on one's work. (Smith, 2001b) Ramani et al. have described tips for initiating, growing and sustaining a community of educators/scholars. (Ramani et al. 2021a) For initiating a community it is important to formulate and elaborate a shared vision. For growing the community, it is important to plan concrete activities that are centered around SoTL and distinguish leader and follower roles in rotation. For sustaining the community, it is important to develop an identity as a group/community and establish strong mutually beneficial relationships which keeps the community members engaged. (Ramani et al. 2021a)

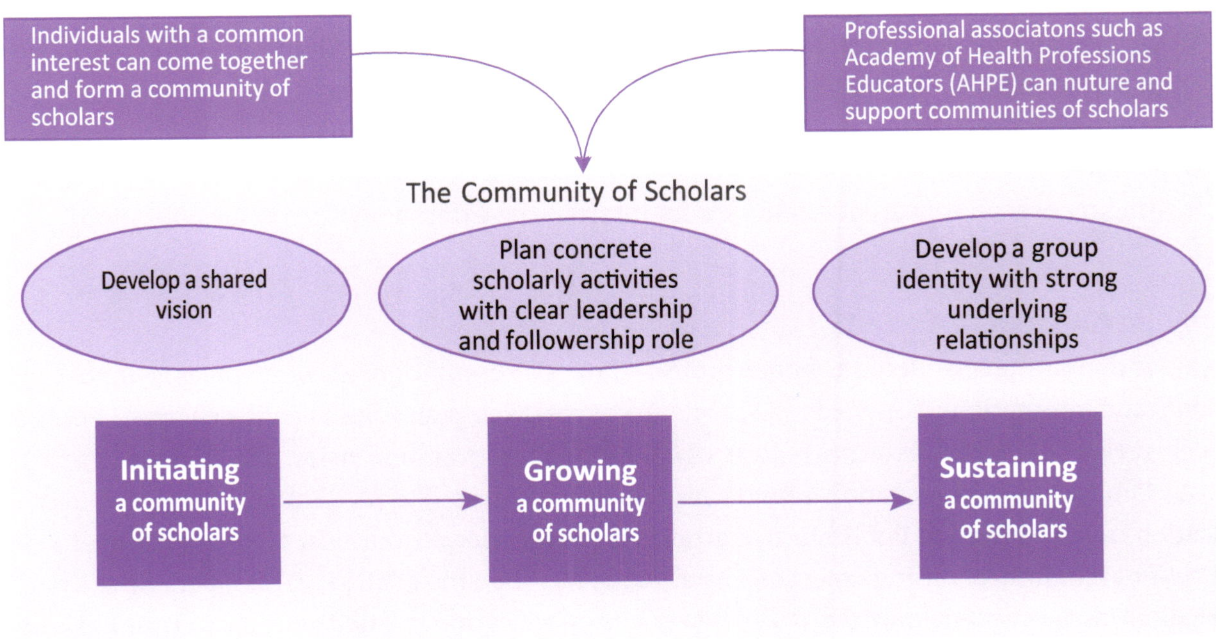

Figure 2: The principles for initiating, growing and sustaining a community of scholars (based on Ramani et al. 2021a)

Being part of an international community of scholars, known as 'Mentors Across Borders', the first author (RAK), can highly recommend participating in such an endeavor. (*https://bei.brighamandwomens.org/mentors-across-borders*) This community was initiated by Dr. Subha Ramani after collaboratively conducting a speed mentoring workshop at the AMEE conference 2019. The faculty who conducted this workshop found it inspiring to work together and exchange expertise with global educators. Owing to their shared vision of building scholarship, this group formed what is called 'Mentors Across Borders'. This community has so far published 7 journal articles through collaborative writing, conducted several workshops and mentoring sessions for faculty and students across the world and conducted Twitter chats on interesting Health Professions Education topics (#HPEMentorChat, Twitter handle - @Mentors_Borders). RAK experiences this community of educators/scholars as a critical friend, a supportive partner and an inspiring peer.

Sharing expertise around a particular domain lies at the heart of a community of practice. (Wenger et al. 2002) Communities of scholars may engage in what is called collaborative writing. Ramani et al. have provided tips on successful collaborative writing divided across three areas: the individual writer, the writing team and the scholarly product. (Ramani et al. 2021b) Professional organizations/associations such as Academy of Health Professions Educators (AHPE) can stimulate, guide and sponsor communities of practice for SoTL through, e.g. setting up Special Interest Groups (SIGs). The Association for Medical Education in Europe (AMEE) has many SIGs and also a community of Associate Fellows and Fellows, which can be considered communities of practice (*www.amee.org*).

Examples of activities in SoTL

- Writing up and conducting an evaluation project related to teaching-learning.
- Disseminating its findings at different scientific forums like conferences, symposia, etc.
- Writing articles on educational innovations and curricular reforms individually or with a community of practice.
- Writing reports on educational activities for internal and external reviews or accreditation.

How can one evaluate SoTL?

Outcomes that can be considered as evidence of SoTL are: 1) Presentations at conferences, symposia (local, national and international), invited talks, 2) Chairman or discussant roles at conferences, 3) Publication of peer-reviewed internal/external reports of educational innovations, vision and mission, curriculum, etc., 4) Publication of innovation reports on public platforms like MedEdPublish, 5) Publication of education-related blogs, 6) Publication of articles in peer-reviewed journals, 7) Membership of a cross-institutional committee on any aspect of education, 8) Membership of a SIG, 9) Membership of a national curriculum/assessment committee, 10) Reviewer role on education-related journals, 11) Journal Editorial Board roles, 12) Invitation as Faculty at other than parent institutes, 13) Fellowship of professional bodies like AMEE, etc.

What is its relevance in growth and promotions of a teacher?

This aspect of SoTL is not yet fully developed. In spite of Boyer's efforts, as long ago as in 1990, to promote and value teaching as a profession, many institutions do not value and recognize SoTL activities as evidence of scholarship. Discipline-based scholarship is valued at the cost of SoTL, as promotions are given only on the basis of disciplinary and research-related achievements. Some institutions have special teacher-tracks or education tracks for their teachers to grow in SoTL. (Cleland et al., 2021) These tracks generally move along Assistant Professor to Associate Professor to Professor trajectory. The level of achievement required varies from local to international, and within a small course to a pan-curricular or across institutions perspective. As described by Myatt et al., SoTL needs to be integrated into the policy and planning, and leadership and vision of an institution, to get its due credit. (Myatt et al., 2018) In case institutions are not ready to change their promotions criteria, national associations like the AHPE should take up the work of educating and convincing institutional heads and the National Medical Commission of India.

Since 2009, in India, publications in indexed journals have been made obligatory for promotion to Associate Professor and Professor in medical colleges. In 2017, the General Body of Medical Council of India ruled that only 1 publication in medical education in an indexed/national journal will be recognized as on par with a discipline-specific publication, and hence be considered as a criterion for promotion. (MCI Meeting, 2016-2017) There is an urgent need to expand this recognition of medical education publications in the future guidelines for placements and promotions.

SUMMARIZE

SoTL involves reading the literature for known pedagogical practices, using it to improve own teaching, viewing one's teaching work critically, collecting data and feedback from students and peers and opening up one's work to critique. SoTL can be done at an individual level or through joining a community of practice. The community of practice can be local, national or international. SoTL contributes knowledge to the field of education. SoTL activities must be valued as promotion criteria.

EVALUATE

This section is meant to encourage the readers to reflect and self-evaluate their learning at the end of the chapter. The following assignments may help in this process:

Make a list of all the questions that have kept you thinking through your teaching experience. Read the literature to find out if your questions have already been answered in the literature. Try to convert your questions into simple research questions. Think about what data from which participants you will need to answer these questions. Collect data and analyse it. Check your interpretation of the results with a biostatistician or a methodology expert. Write up your work in the form of a scientific article. Present your work to colleagues at your institution or partner institutions. Present your work at a local, national or international conference.

ROAD AHEAD

SoTL needs to grow in Universities over the world but growing it in developing and the Global South countries deserves special attention. (Kusurkar, 2022) Currently the medical education literature and practice is dominated by Global North scholars. (Kusurkar, 2022) This is clearly seen in a paper published on the history of medical education. (Ten Cate, 2021) Global South educators frequently create educational innovations in a very non-supportive and financially constrained context, but for reasons not really well-known, their work does not reach the Global North world. The Global North could hugely benefit from the Global South perspective on teaching and learning. For this it needs to be more inclusive in its practices.

SoTL also needs to be integrated into policy and planning and leadership development and vision of an institution. But this can be challenging and needs support from the top management.

For more information on SoTL and to engage in SoTL, you can check out the following links and resources:

- *https://bei.brighamandwomens.org/mentors-across-borders*(For applying to become Mentors at large)
- *https://bei.brighamandwomens.org/mab-scholarship*(Resource on scholarship)
- *http://www.amee.org/fellowship*(For applying to become AMEE Associate Fellow/Fellow)
- Follow #HPEMentorChat on Twitter
- Follow #MedEdChat discussions on Twitter, for archived chats check out *http://www.allianceforclinicaleducation.org*

REFERENCES

Adendorff, H. (2011). Strangers in a strange land–on becoming scholars of teaching. London Rev Educ., 9(3):305–315.

Bailey E, Le Vin A, Miller L, Price K, Sneddon S, Stapleton G, Wolfe L. (2021). Bridging the transition to a new expertise in the scholarship of teaching and learning through a faculty learning community. Int J Acad Dev. Ahead of Print. *https://doi.org/10.1080/1360144X.2021.1917415*

Boyer, E.L. (1990). Scholarship reconsidered: priorities of the professoriate. Lawrenceville (NJ): Princeton University Press.

Bronnimann, J., West, D., Huijser, H., Heath, D. (2018). Applying learning analytics to the scholarship of teaching and learning. Innov High Educ., 43:353–367.

Cleland, J.A., Jamieson, S., Kusurkar, R.A., Ramani, S., Wilkinson, T.J., van Schalkwyk, S. (2021). Redefining Scholarship for Health Professions Education. AMEE Guide number 142. Med Teach., 43 (7): 824-838.*https://doi.org/10.1080/0142159X.2021.1900555*

Cox, M.D. (2013). The impact of communities of practice in support of early-career academics, International J for Acad Develop., 18(1):18-30. DOI: 10.1080/1360144X.2011.599600

Fanghanel, J., Pritchard, J., Potter, J., & Wisker, G. (2015). Defining and supporting the scholarship of teaching and learning (SoTL): A sector-wide study. Executive summary. York: Higher Education Academy.

Hutchings, P. & Shulman, L. (1999). The scholarship of teaching: new elaborations, new developments. Change, 31:10-15.

Kreber, C. (2002). Teaching excellence, teaching expertise, and the scholarship of teaching. Innov High Educ., 27(1):5-23.

Kusurkar RA. (2022). The leaky pipeline: The leaky pipeline of publications and knowledge generation in medical education. Persp Med Educ. (In Press).

Long, P., & Siemens, G. (2011). Penetrating the fog: Analytics in learning and education. EDUCAUSE Rev., 46(4), 31–40.

McKinney, K. (2006). Attitudinal and structural factors contributing to challenges in the work of the scholarship of teaching and learning. New Dir Inst Res., 129:37–50.

MCI Meeting, No. MCI-6(2)/2016-Med./MCI General Body 7th Session (Continuing 143rd Session) Minutes Of The General Body Meeting Held On 29th March, (2017). Retrieved on 7th June 2021 from: *https://www.nmc.org.in/MCIRest/open/getDocument?path=%2FDocuments%2FPublic%2FPortal%2F-Meetings%2FGeneral%20Body%2F2017%2F03%2F29%2FMNGB-29.03.2017.pdf*

Myatt, P., Gannaway, D., Chia, I., Fraser, K., McDonald, J.2018. Reflecting on institutional support for SoTL engagement: developing a conceptual framework, Int J Acad Dev., 23(2):147-160.

Naidu T. (2021). Modern Medicine is a colonial artifact: Introducing decoloniality to medical education research. Acad Med., 96:S9–S12.

Ramani S, McKimm J, Findyartini A, Nadarajah VD, Hays R, Chisolm MS, Filipe HP, Fornari A, Kachur EK, Kusurkar RA, Thampy H, Wilson KW. 2021a. Twelve Tips for Developing a Global Community of Scholars in Health Professions Education. Med Teach., 43(8):966-971.*10.1080/0142159X.2020.1839034*

Ramani S, McKimm J, Forrest K, Hays R, Bishop J, Thampy H, Findyartini A, Nadarajah VD, Kusurkar RA, Wilson K, Filipe H, Kachur E. 2021b. Co-creating scholarship through collaborative writing in Health Professions Education. AMEE Guide 143. Med Teach. https://doi.org/10.1080/0142159X.2021.1993162

Shulman L. S. (1998). Chapter 1, In: P. Hutchings (Ed.) The course portfolio: how faculty can examine their teaching to advance practice and improve student learning (Washington DC, American Association for Higher Education).

Smith, R. 2001a. Expertise and the scholarship of teaching. New DirTeach Learn., 86:69–78.

Smith, R. 2001b. Formative evaluation and the Scholarship of Teaching and Learning. New Dir Teach Learn., 88:51–62.

Ten Cate, T.J. (2021). Health professions education scholarship: The emergence, current status, and future of a discipline in its own right. FASEB Bioadvances, 3:510–522. DOI: 10.1096/fba.2021-00011

Wenger E, McDermott RA, Snyder W. (2002). Cultivating communities of practice: a guide to managing knowledge. Boston (Ma): Harvard Business School Press.

Chapter 27

Unlocking Intellectual Property Right (IPR) in Health Care Higher Education

M. Senthil

ABSTRACT

Intellectual Property Right (IPR) in Health Care Higher Education Many people says it's an emerging filed in medical education. I would rather say Health professional educators have been kept under dark about this field for decade or so. Now to match the global economy and growth lot of light has been through to this IPR to create important among the young India. This chapter will briefly tell about the need of IPR and our presence in the world in terms of innovation and invention. The chapter discuss the need for Innovation Eco System in health care higher education and how to start innovation ecosystem at institute level and department level. A brief description of different types of IPR available in India like Copyright, Patent, Trademark, Industrial Design, Layout Design and Geographical indication has been focused in the section road map to IPR. This IPR chapter unlocks the Patent, Copyright, Industrial Design, and trademark filing process with appropriate examples and illustrations. The important outcome of any IPR work is to do a technology transfer, this chapter will slightly touch up How to start the process of technology transfer, present eco system in India and the need to promote the concept of start-ups among faculty and students.

Key Words: copyright, patent, trademark, industrial design, intellectual, property, technology, innovation, invention, ecosystem

ASSESS NEED

Why Intellectual Property Right?

Global competitiveness has redefined business strategies worldwide and the focus has certainly shifted to examining how our knowledge resources can reposition our stand in the world market. It means that process of wealth creation is changing from resource based to knowledge based i.e. it now depends on brainpower and our ability to create, to sell, to explain and to solve problems. As a result, in future wealth would out of our brains rather than the ground. And the goods and services being created by our brainpower would be marketed in the global village[1]. Now a basic question that needs to be answered is how to protect this property of knowledge Prior to this we need to think that how knowledge could be converted into property? Knowledge being abstract there are only two ways of turning knowledge into property. One way is secrecy, which is used to protect three types of information, namely trade secrets, know – how and rituals. Another way is Intellectual Property Laws, including Copyright, Patent, Registered Industrial Design and Trademark, legislation and conventions.

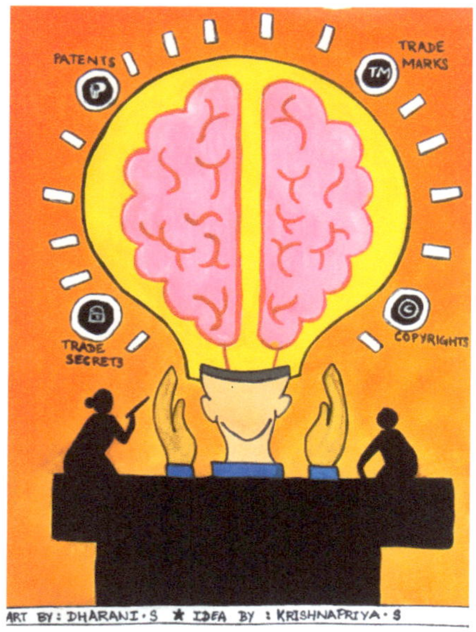

Why Intellectual Property Right Matter?

Reward for intellectual creation	• Monetary • Professional • Recognition
Encouragement and growth	• Creativity is encouraged • Industrial growth
Recognition of protection	• The ensure protection and recognition for unwritten and unrecorded cultural expressions

Why Intellectual Property Right in Health Professional Education?

Intellectual Property in Health care will help us in developing indigenous product which is the need of the hour in terms of raising medical bills and health care expenditures in the country. In today's scenario 90% of our health care solutions like equipment, instruments and even the guidelines are imported. Only in Pharm industry we are the biggest manufactures for the world, but the formulations are imported. So Intellectual Property is the heart of our Indian health system as it has to sustain the financing model of growth and development.

BRIEF

What is Intellectual Property Right?
Who can file Intellectual Property Right?
How to Kick Start Innovations
Government support
Different types of IPR

- Patent
- Copy right
- Trademark
- Industrial Design
- Geographical Indicator

IPR in Medicine and Higher Education
Technology transfer and commercialization of IPR

CONTEXTUALIZE

Mr. Innovation has added a feather in his cap; namely he has successfully patented a device which has travelled and become popular in a distant location.

Let us see what he has to say about his patent.

"Universal Back Resting Device (UBRD)" it was an accidental invention, which started in 2012 with a rectangular board used as a head rest for our Public health dentistry outreach activities. In 2015 a FB comment "Low Cost Dental Chair "for our Nilgiris outreach program made us file the UBRD patent in 2015. Today UBRD is a granted & commercialized patent for public use. Recently department of community dentistry school of dentistry, university of IOWA, USA has ordered UBRD for their outreach program. In a nutshell the UBRD invention started in 2012 at a school outreach in Karaikal today it has reached United States of America."

DESCRIBE

What is Intellectual Property Right?

Intellectual property Right (IPR) is a term used for various legal entitlements which attach to certain types of information, ideas, or other intangibles in their expressed form. The holder of this legal entitlement is generally entitled to exercise various exclusive rights in relation to the subject matter of the Intellectual Property. The term intellectual property reflects the idea that this subject matter is the product of the mind or the intellect, and that Intellectual Property rights may be protected at law in the same way as any other form of property. Intellectual property laws vary from jurisdiction to jurisdiction, such that the acquisition, registration or enforcement of IP rights must be pursued or obtained separately in each territory of interest.

Intellectual property rights (IPR) can be defined as the rights given to people over the creation of their minds. They usually give the creator an exclusive right over the use of his/her creations for a certain period oftime[2].

Who can file Intellectual Property Right?

Intellectual property is an intangible creation of the human mind, usually expressed or translated into a tangible form that is assigned certain rights of property. Examples of intellectual property include an author's copyright on a book or article, a distinctive logo design representing a soft drink company and its products, unique design elements of a web site, or a patent on the process to manufacture chewing gum[2].

How to Kick Start Innovations

Innovations in Health Care are the need of the hour for the growth and development of the country. Innovations at health care can be made possible only by a very good health professional educator. To begin innovations can start at your own work place weather in a class room, clinics, preclinical labs or department we should create a good eco system where students can be given an environment for an innovative thinking.

Innovation needs to be started in health professional education to make India a Developed Country and to create a Profile for the country. We are very young independent country but all this 75 years we had been recognized by most of countries has a service related country whereas we depend on other countries for work, which need to be changed if at all we want our nation to be a developed country in a decade or so.

Keeping this mind the government has started various schemes and polices like.

- Start-up India Stand-up India
- Atma-nirbhar Bharat Abhiyan (Self-reliant India Mission)
- Be Vocal on Local Products
- Make for the World
- Skill India
- New Educational Policy - 2020

The process

To Start innovations the health professional educator should focus on the following accepts like Platform, Inclusion, Eco-system, Drivers, Discourse.

Platform	• Change in Mind-set • Egotistic approach to WIN WIN WIN approach • Friendly and a team leader attitude
Inclusion	• Ready to accept changes • Encourage STUPID question in class room/clinics • Be available to the students
Ecosystem	• Provide autonomy and flexibility in the classroom/clinics • Simple encouraging words like "good "nice" "well done" "try better" "good idea" "good question • Develop polices for a good innovation eco systems
Drivers	• Encourage Multidisciplinary & Collaborative approach • Accept the generational change
Discourse	• Encourage debate, discussion among students • Identify best practices among students

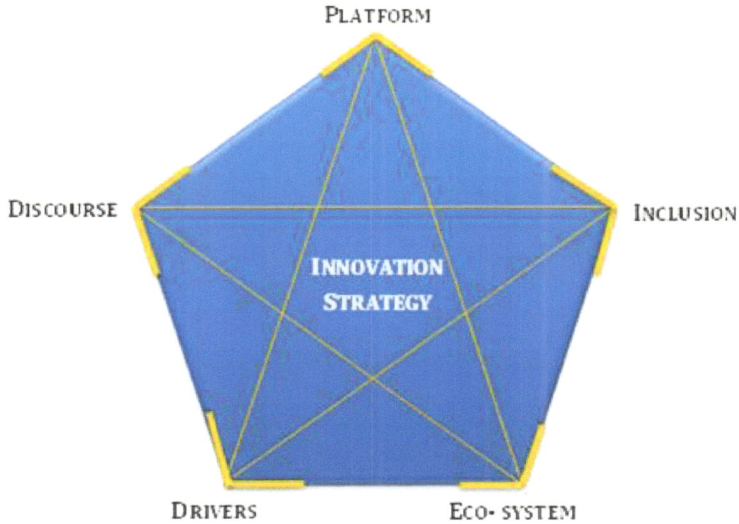

The five-pronged focus will foster innovations by:

- Democratizing Information
- Identifying and empowering domain experts
- Ensuring institutional autonomy, freedom, flexibility, accountability and transparency
- Increasing faculty and students participation at all levels
- Improving Governance & Planning

Different Types of IPR[2]

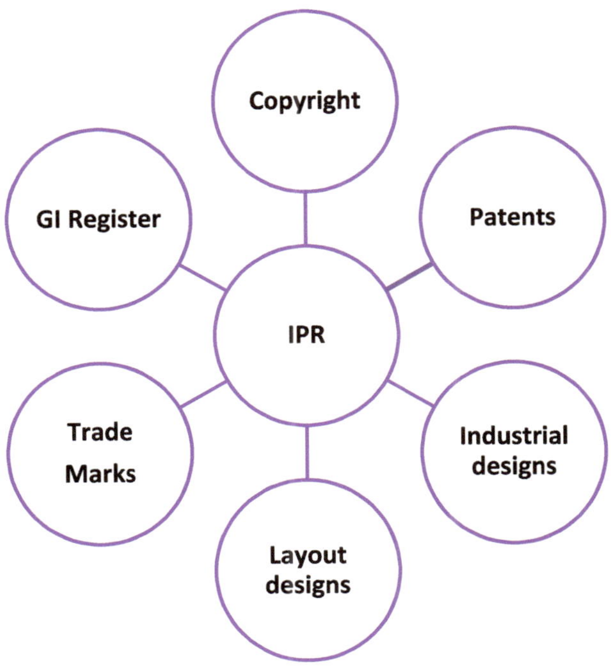

1) Patent

What Is A Patent?

Patent is an exclusive right granted by the Authority (Govt. of India) to the applicant for a limited period in lieu of full disclosure of his/her invention.

What Is Required for Patent?

Three Statutory Pillars of PATENTABILITY

1. Novelty (new)
2. Inventive Step (non-obvious)
3. Industrial Applicability (utility)

Invention must be

- Relate to a Process or Product or both
- Be new (Novel)
- Involve an inventive step
- Be capable of industrial application
- "Invention" means a new product or process involving an inventive step and capable of industrial application.

Invention must not be

- Published in India or elsewhere.
- In prior public knowledge or prior public use within India.
- What is claimed must be different from what is already known.

"NEW" MEANS A feature of an invention that

- Involves technical advance as compared to the existing knowledge
- Has economic significance
- Makes the invention not obvious to a person skilled in the art
- "Would a person with ordinary skills have thought of the alleged invention?". If the answer is "no", then the invention is non-obvious.

Industrial application

- Invention is capable of being made or used in any kind of industry

I Have an Invention What to Do Next?

Publishing

- Publish in newspapers, media, journals, magazines, websites, etc.
- You will get publicity if the published invention is interesting.
- If you file the patent application after publishing, you will not get patent right, because the novelty of the invention is lost through publication.

Patenting

- You can first file the patent application in Patent Office.
- You can publish your invention after filing the patent application.
- The patent office will also publish your invention in their journal.
- Hence, you will get both publicity and monetary reward through patents.

Patent Application Processing

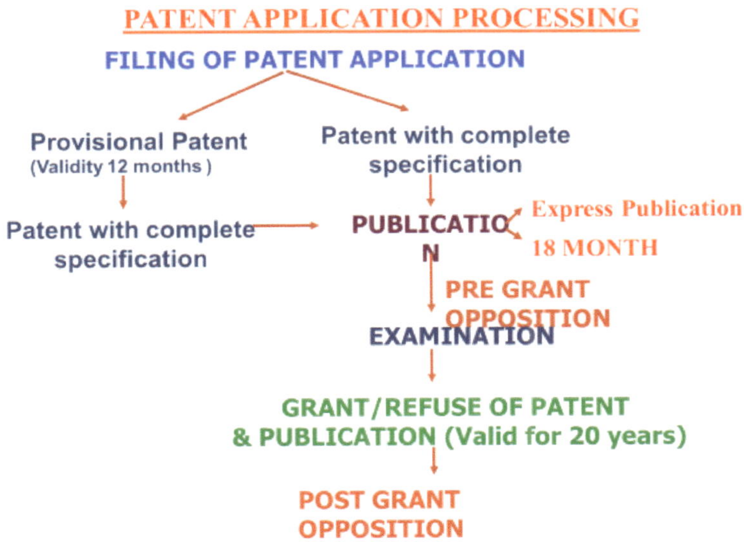

Provisional Patent (Validity 12 months)

- A provisional patent specification is basically a preliminary application which is filed before filing a usual patent.
- It explains the invention in a broad manner.
- It is the document which may be filed before a Complete Specification
- It is called "provisional" since it is incomplete and a predecessor of a complete specification which comes later.
- Although it is not mandatory, it is highly recommended as it has a lot of benefits for the inventor.

Patent with complete specification has to be have the following details in the application

- Title of the invention
- Field of invention
- Use of invention
- Prior art
- Aim of the invention
- Summary of the present invention
- Brief description of drawings
- Statement of invention
- Detailed description of invention
- Drawings & worked examples
- Claims
- Abstract

What are not Inventions?

- Invention Against Natural Laws.
- Discovery of scientific principle, abstract theory and new property – (Micro-organism).
- New use of a known substance - Second medical use not permissible.

- Substance obtained by mere admixture (Physical admixture)
- Method of agriculture or horticulture.
- Mere arrangement or rearrangement of known devices.
- Any process for: medical human beings or animals Surgical Treatment to render them free/Cure from disease or to increase prophylactic Diagnostic, Therapeutic outcomes

2) Copyright

What is copyright?

The legal right granted to an author, composer, playwright, publisher, or distributor to exclusive publication, production, sale, or distribution of a literary, musical, dramatic, or artistic work.

What does it do?

Gives authors or artists the legal right to exclude others from using their works.

What is protected?

- Literary Works (All Text Including Computer Software)
- Musical Works
- Dramatic Works
- Choreographic Works
- Pictorial, Graphic, & Sculptural Works
- Motion Pictures & Other Audiovisual Works
- Sound Recordings
- Architectural Works

What is not protected?

- Ideas, Concepts, Or Discoveries
- Titles, Names, Short Phrases, And Slogans
- Works That Are Not Fixed In A Tangible Form Of Expression Such As Improvised Speech Or Dance
- Works Consisting Entirely Of Information That Is Commonly Available And Contains No Originality
- Anything Written Or Created By The Government

What rights does the owner control?

Rights to:

- Make copies of the work
- Distribute copies of the work
- Perform the work publicly (such as for plays, film, or music)
- Display the work publicly (such as for artwork, or any material used on the internet or television)
- Make "derivative works" (including making modifications, adaptations or other new uses of a work, or translating the work to another media)

How long does copyright protection last?

- For the life of the author, plus 60 years if the applicant is individual
- 95 years for corporations

Copyright Application Processing

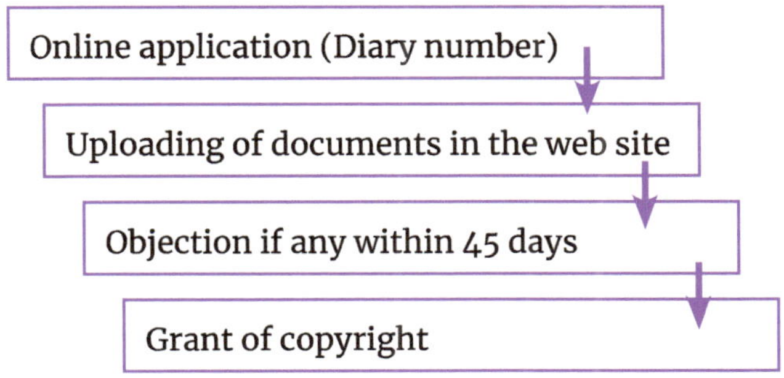

3) *Industrial Design*[12]

An industrial design relates to the appearance of an article, which results from features such as the lines or colors of the article or its ornamentation.

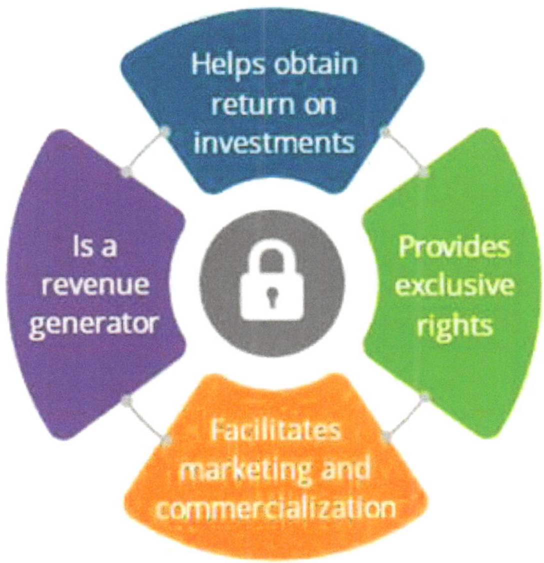

Benefits of protection of Industrial Design

What kind of protection does an industrial design right offer

The owner of a registered industrial design has the right to prevent third parties from making, selling or importing articles bearing or embodying a design which is a copy, or substantially a copy, of the protected design, when such acts are undertaken for commercial purposes.

What kind of products can benefit from industrial design protection?

Industrial designs are applied to a wide variety of products of industry and handicraft items: from packages and containers to furnishing and household goods, from lighting equipment to jewelry, and from electronic devices to textiles. Industrial designs may also be relevant to graphic symbols, graphical user interfaces (GUI), and logos.

4) Trademark

A trademark is a distinctive sign that identifies certain goods or services produced or provided by an individual or a company.

What is a trademark?

A trademark can be any word, phrase, symbol, design, or a combination of these things that identifies your goods or services. It's how customers recognize you in the marketplace and distinguish you from your competitors.

The word "trademark" can refer to both trademarks and service marks. A trademark is used for goods, while a service mark is used for services.

A trademark:

- Identifies the source of your goods or services.
- Provides legal protection for your brand.
- Helps you guard against counterfeiting and fraud.

A common misconception is that having a trademark means you legally own a particular word or phrase and can prevent others from using it. However, you don't have rights to the word or phrase in general, only to how that word or phrase is used with your specific goods or services.

For example, let's say you use a logo as a trademark for your small woodworking business to identify and distinguish your goods or services from others in the woodworking field. This doesn't mean you can stop others from using a similar logo for non-woodworking related goods or services.

Another common misconception believes that choosing a trademark that merely describes your goods or services is effective. Creative and unique trademarks are more effective and easier to protect.

5) Geographical Indicator (GI) Register[12]

A **geographical indication** (GI) is a name or sign used on products which corresponds to a specific geographical location or origin (e.g., a town, region, or country). The use of a geographical indication, as an indication of the product's source, acts as a certification that the product possesses certain qualities, is made according to traditional methods, or enjoys a good reputation due to its geographical origin.

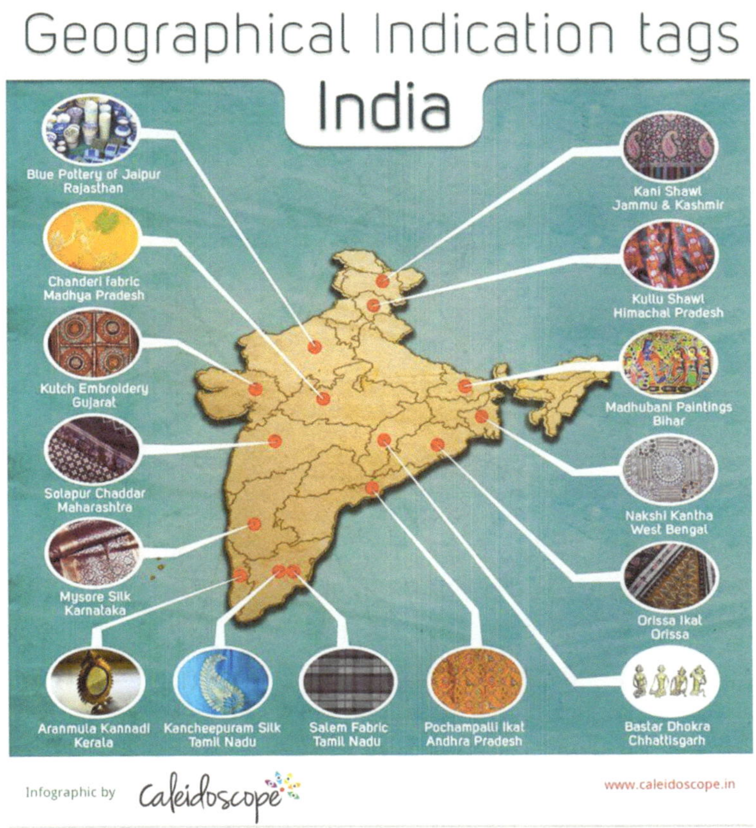

6) Technology Transfer and Commercialization of IPR

Technology transfer, also called transfer of technology (TOT), is the process of transferring (disseminating) technology from the person or organization that owns or holds it to another person or organization. These transfers may occur between universities, businesses (of any size, ranging from small, medium, to large), governments, across geopolitical borders, both formally and informally, and both openly and secretly.

Need for TT and Commercialization[15]

The main objectives of technology commercializing include leveraging R&D outcome and intellectual assets, raise the accessibility of scientific outcome to broad range of consumers, development of new services and products ready for commercialization, and last but not the least, to intensify industrial competition. The transfer can originate either due to technology push (through research) or market pull (through industry). The international scope of technology commercialization may encompass developed nations, developing nations and other countries with economy transition.

Process of TT

- Step 1: Invention Disclosure
- Step 2: Evaluation
- Step 3: Patent Application
- Step 4: Assessment and Marketing
- Step 5: Licensing of Patents
- Step 6: Commercialization.

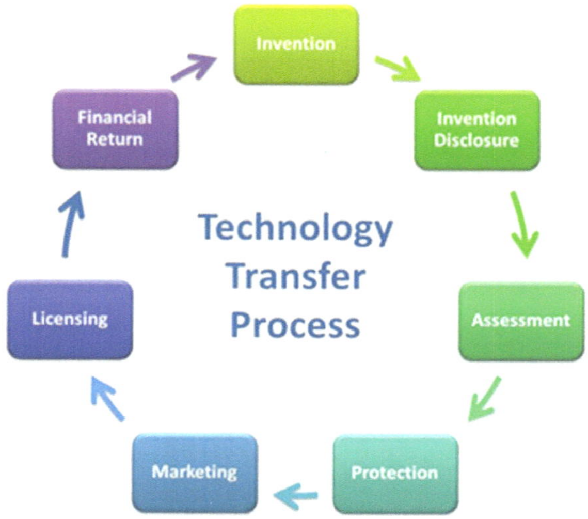

Role and scope of health care Start-ups in IP

A widening gap between the needs of care seekers and traditional healthcare services has emerged as a major challenge. It adds to the unaffordability and inaccessibility of healthcare. All the factors have collectively contributed towards the growing healthcare startup ecosystem with the innovative solutions.

SUMMARIZE

This chapter has explained the need of Intellectual Property in Higher Education for growth and development of the country with following key points:

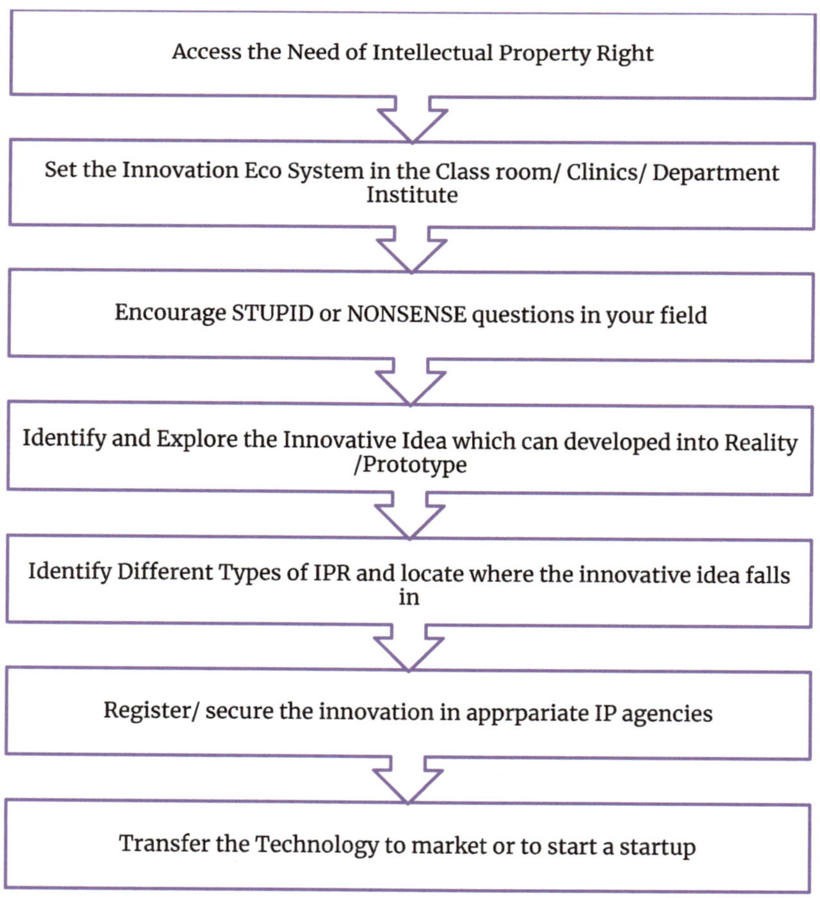

EVALUATE

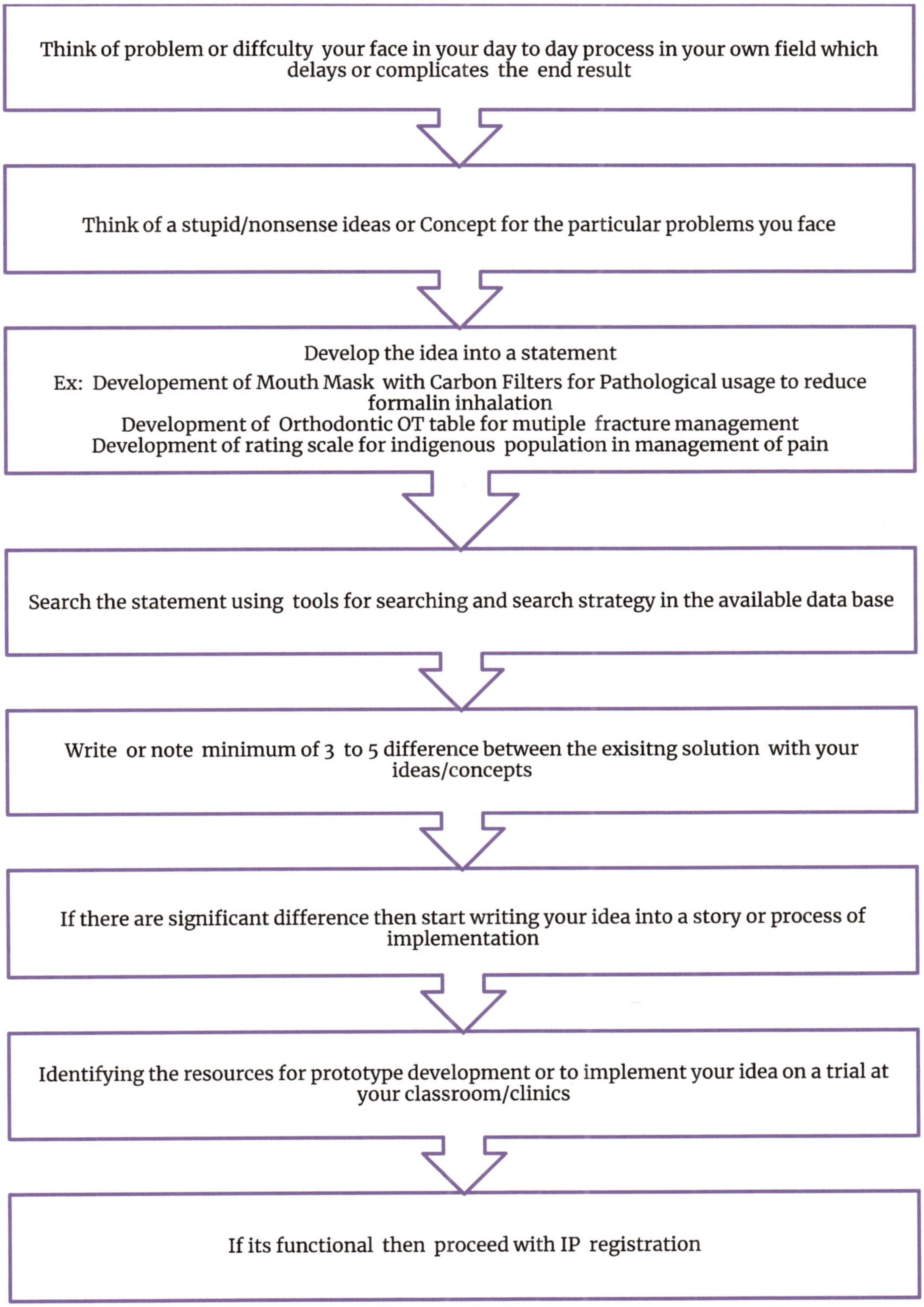
Think of problem or diffculty your face in your day to day process in your own field which delays or complicates the end result
Think of a stupid/nonsense ideas or Concept for the particular problems you face
Develop the idea into a statement
Ex: Developement of Mouth Mask with Carbon Filters for Pathological usage to reduce formalin inhalation
Development of Orthodontic OT table for mutiple fracture management
Development of rating scale for indigenous population in management of pain
Search the statement using tools for searching and search strategy in the available data base
Write or note minimum of 3 to 5 difference between the exisitng solution with your ideas/concepts
If there are significant difference then start writing your idea into a story or process of implementation
Identifying the resources for prototype development or to implement your idea on a trial at your classroom/clinics
If its functional then proceed with IP registration

ROAD AHEAD

In the world of innovation, India has an old reputation: it remains a minnow when it comes to patents. If over 600,000 applications were filed in the US and more than twice that number in China in 2017, in India, there were only 46,600 and patent grants came to just over 12,000 in a country of 1.37 billion people. To make matters still more difficult is the fact that India has spent just 0.7% of its gross domestic product (GDP) in 2016-17 on research & development. In contrast, Japan, the US and China have spent 3.2%, 2.8% and 2.1%, respectively in the same time period . In a nondescript building on a narrow, congested lane in central Mumbai, the Office of the Controller General of Patents, Designs and Trademarks is bent on changing this. It wants to make filing patents cheaper and granting patents faster, which, it hopes will result in more applications.

The road ahead for patents is paved with research and funding. While Indian companies, including startups, universities and research institutes need to direct their attention towards generating more patents; if India has to emerge as a hub of inventiveness, it also calls for increased spending on research and development.

REFERENCES

Carla Tardi (2021), Trademark, Retrieved from *https://www.investopedia.com/terms/t/trademark.asp*

Copyright law of India (2021), Retrieved from *https://en.wikipedia.org/wiki/Copyright_law_of_India*

Designs (2020), Retrieved from*https://ipindia.gov.in/designs.htm*

Geographical Indication (2021), Retrieved from*https://en.wikipedia.org/wiki/Geographical_indication*

History of Indian Patent System (2021), Retrieved from *https://ipindia.gov.in/history-of-indian-patent-system.htm*

Indian trademark law (2021), Retrieved from *https://en.wikipedia.org/wiki/Indian_trademark_law*

Industrial Designs (2021), Retrieved from https://www.wipo.int/designs

JyothiDatta PT (2019), TB survivors file challenge to prevent J&J from extending patent life on Bedaquiline, Retrieved from *https://www.thehindubusinessline.com/companies/tb-survivors-file-challenge-to-prevent-jj-from-extending-patent-life-on-bedaquiline/article26212539.ece*

LexOrbis(2019), IP Case Compilation 2019, Retrieved from *https://www.lexorbis.com/pdf/IP_Cases_2019.pdf*

Mangal S (2005), Intellectual Property Rights: Indian Scenario, Journal of Business Administration online, Vol. 4 (1), Spring

Patent Expert Issues(2021), Layout Designs (Topographies) of Integrated Circuits, Retrieved from *https://www.wipo.int/patents/en/topics/integrated_circuits.html*

Rajkumar S. Adukia (2015), Handbook on intellectual property rights in india, Retrieved from http://caaa.in/Image/34_Hb_on_IPR.pdf

Ravi, R, Janodia, M.D (2021), Factors Affecting Technology Transfer and Commercialization of University Research in India: a Cross-sectional Study. J Knowl Econ (2021), Retrieved from *https://doi.org/10.1007/s13132-021-00747-4*

Seetharaman G (2019), Patents crucial for India to bridge tech gap with US and China, Retrieved from https://economictimes.indiatimes.com/tech/internet/pending-patents-key-to-bridge-vast-tech-gap-with-us china/articleshow

The Copyright Act (1957), Retrieved from *https://copyright.gov.in/Documents/CopyrightRules1957.pdf*

The Patents Rules (2003), Retrieved from E-Version of Indian Patents Act, 1970, *https://ipindia.gov.in*

Trademark basics (2021), Retrieved from *https://www.uspto.gov/trademarks/basics/what-trademark*

ADDITIONAL INFORMATION

Global Scenario of IP filing in India[6]

In the world of innovation, India has an old reputation: it remains a minnow when it comes to patents. If over 600,000 applications were filed in the US and more than twice that number in China in 2017, in India, there were only 46,600 — and patent grants came to just over 12,000 in a country of 1.37 billion people. In a nondescript building on a narrow, congested lane in central Mumbai, the Office of the Controller General of Patents, Designs and Trade Marks is bent on changing this. It wants to make filing patents cheaper and granting patents faster, which, it hopes will result in more applications.

The path to patents is paved with research and funding. While Indian companies, including startups, universities and research institutes need to direct their attention towards generating more patents if India has to emerge as a hub of inventiveness, it also calls for increased spend on research and development (R&D).

India spent just 0.7% of its gross domestic product (GDP) in 2016-17 on R&D. Meanwhile, Japan, the US and China spent 3.2%, 2.8% and 2.1%, respectively, in 2017, according to the Organisation for Economic Co-operation and Development (OECD). India wants to more than double its R&D expenditure to at least 2% of GDP by 2022.

India has still not woken up fully to the significance of intellectual property rights (IPR), particularly patents, and their commercial implications. Patent filings and grants in India are dominated by foreign applicants: they filed two-thirds of patent applications in 2018-19, and got four-fifths of grants, according to the Office of Controller General of Patents, Designs and Trade Marks. In India, Qualcomm, the US chipmaker, topped both patent filings and grants in 2018-19. It made 1,559 applications, more than six times the filings of Tata Consultancy Services (TCS), the top Indian company on the list. Qualcomm was granted 405 Indian patents in 2018-19, four times the patents assigned to state-owned Bharat Heavy Electricals Ltd (BHEL), the Indian company with the most patent grants last fiscal.

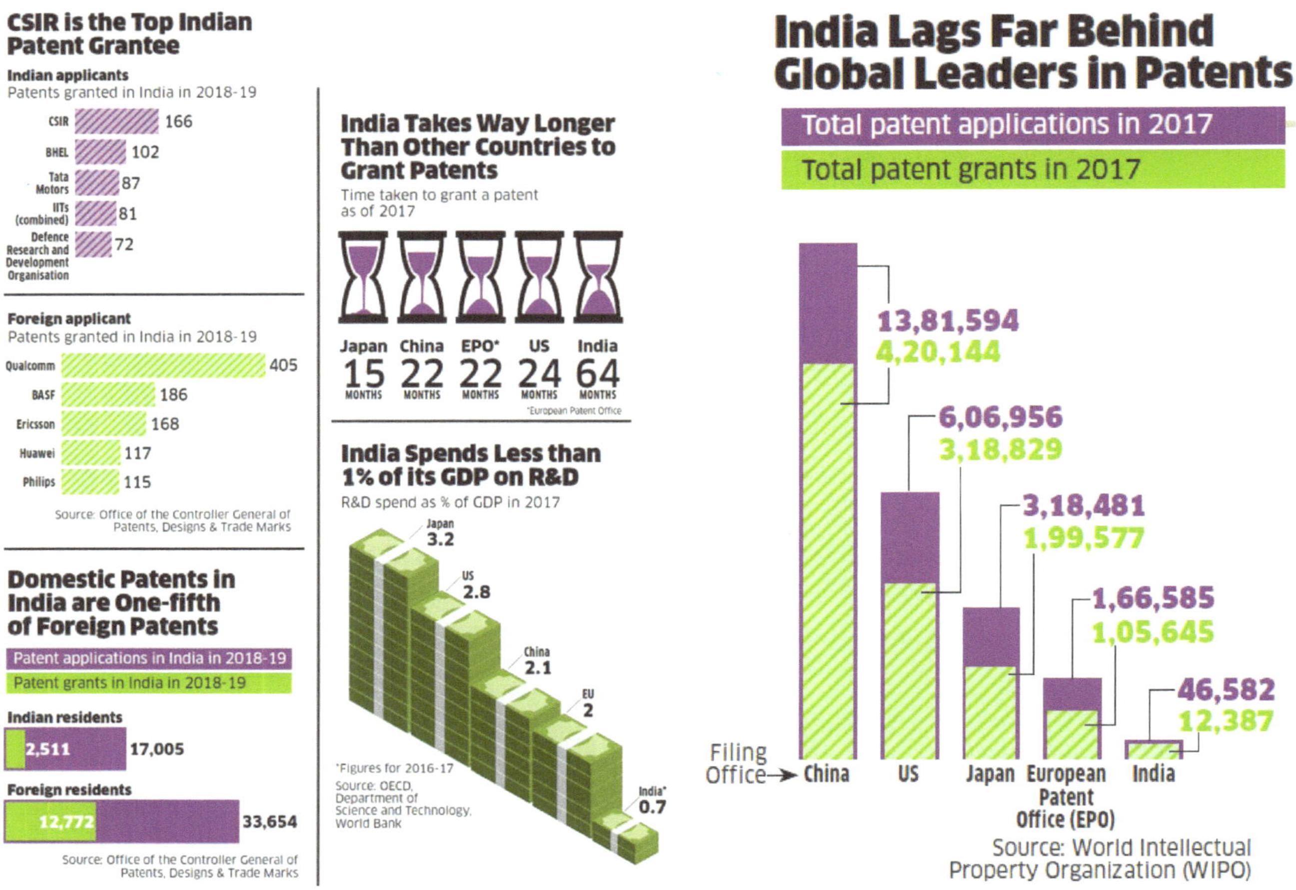

IP infringement case scenarios in India Health Care

Trademark

Glenmark Pharmaceuticals Ltd. v. Curetech Skincare and Galpha Laboratories Ltd[17].

Court: High Court of Bombay

Case No: Notice of Motion (L) No. 1890 of 2018 in COMIP (L) NO. 1063 of 2018

Order dated: 28thAugust, 2018

Issue: Whether a defendant being a habitual offender can be asked to pay exemplary damages?

Judgement: The dispute concerned the Plaintiff's product Candid-B, an anti-fungal cream, and a similar drug being sold by Defendant No. 2 named Clodid-B ("impugned mark"). In addition to the adoption of similar word mark, the Defendant No. 2 had also copied the trade dress, color scheme, art work, font style and even manner of writing of the Plaintiff's product. The Defendant No. 2 stated that the impugned mark was adopted by mistake and chose not to contest the suit. The Defendant No. 1, being just the contract manufacturer for Defendant No. 2, also chose to submit to the decree. While decreeing the suit in favour of the Plaintiff, the Court considered the fact that the Defendant No. 2 is a habitual offender. The counsel for the Plaintiff produced a prior judgment of the Delhi High Court [Win-Medicare Pvt. Ltd. Vs. Galpha Laboratories Ltd. & Ors.], wherein it was categorically observed by the Delhi High Court that Defendant No. 2 is a habitual offender. It was also noted by the Court that various pharmaceutical companies have instituted infringement cases against Defendant No. 2 and most of them have obtained injunction orders. Over and above the infringing activities, the Defendant No. 2 was also found to be a violator of FDA regulations. In many instances, the medicinal products of Defendant No. 2 were found to be of "Not of standard quality/Spurious" by Central Drugs Standard Control Organization. In view of the repeated violations, the Court, as a matter of deterrence, slapped an exemplary cost of Rupees One Crore Fifty Lakhs on Defendant No. 2. Along with this cost, the Court also ordered the furnishing of personal undertakings to the Court from all the Directors of Defendant No.2 to the effect that they would withdraw and destroy all products bearing the impugned mark and its variants from the market; apply for cancellation of manufacturing permission for products bearing the impugned mark; shall conduct business in accordance with FDA rules and regulations and would not indulge in infringing activities qua products of not only the Plaintiff but other pharmaceutical companies also.

Patent Infringement

Merck Sharp & Dohme Corporation & Anr.v. Aprica Pharmaceuticals Private Limited[17]

Court: High Court of Delhi

Case No.: CS (OS) 1236/2013

Order Dated: November 14th, 2017

Issue: Whether the Defendant's launch of ECOGLIPT in the Indian market would lead to infringement of the Patent right of the Plaintiff in SITAGLIPTIN?

Judgement: The Court was of the view that Defendant's product blatantly infringed and completely contravened Plaintiff's patent right. Although the Defendant had not launched the product commercially, still the court felt that there was reasonable apprehension that launching the product could cause irreparable damage to the Plaintiffs which could not be compensated in terms of money. The suit was, thus, decreed in favour of the Plaintiffs and against the Defendants along with the actual costs. The Plaintiff was also given the liberty to file the exact amount of money incurred in the adjudication of this suit.

Novartis vs Cipla[17]

The two judges bench (division bench) of the Delhi High Court has upheld the decision of a single judge restraining Cipla from selling generic version of Novartis patent on respiratory drug containing 'INDACATEROL' or 'INDACATEROL Maleate' marketed under the name ONBREZ. Cipla challenged the decision on three main issues a) Novartis is not manufacturing the drug in India thus not making use of Patent b) public interest is not being served on account of import of a small quantity and price difference between Novartis and Cipla's drug c) right to restrain a third party from infringement (*Section 48*) is subject to working of Patent (*Section 83*).

Brief facts:

1. Cipla launched generic version of Novartis patented drug sold under the mark ONBREZ containing 'INDACATEROL' in October 2014.
2. Cipla had priced its generic versions of the drug, at Rs. 130 per pack of ten tablets, compared with Rs. 677 for Onbrez.
3. Novartis filed a suit for patent infringement seeking an injunction against Cipla's generic version of ONBREZ, alleging infringement of its patent over INDACETROL.

4. The single judge of Delhi High Court granted temporary injunction restraining Cipla from selling its generic version. At the same time giving Cipla liberty to have the injunction order modified if they file a petition for Compulsory license and it was decided in their favour.

Patent Monopoly

Patent challenge mounted against J&J's attempt to extend monopoly on high-priced anti-TB drug[16]

Two tuberculosis survivors have filed a patent challenge on Johnson and Johnson's TB drug Bedaquiline. Nandita Venkatesan from Mumbai and Phumeza Tisile from South Africa have filed a challenge at the Mumbai Patent Office to prevent the company from extending its monopoly on the patented drug, a note from humanitarian organisation Médecins Sans Frontières (MSF – Doctors without Borders) said, adding that they were supporting the case.

Both individuals had survived drug-resistant TB (DR-TB), but lost their hearing because of the toxicity of the treatment. "They are now fighting to ensure that newer drugs like Bedaquiline – which are safer and more effective – are made affordable and accessible to everybody with DR-TB, to replace painful and toxic drugs that need to be injected," the note said.

The J&J patent application being challenged is for the salt form of Bedaquiline, which does not merit patenting under India's patent law, the MSF note said. If granted, J&J's monopoly on Bedaquiline would be extended from 2023 to 2027, delaying entry of generics by four additional years. This strategy of 'patent ever-greening' by filing additional, often unmerited patents, is commonly used by corporations to extend monopolies on their drugs beyond the standard 20 years.

"Preventing this patent barrier is expected to encourage TB drug manufacturers from India to enter the market with generics and supply Bedaquiline at lower prices to national TB programmes and TB care providers globally," it added.

About 558,000 people developed DR-TB in 2017, but only 25 per cent of them were treated. The standard DR-TB treatment in most countries has included drugs that need to be injected daily and are associated with several serious side-effects. The cure rate is only 55 per cent, the note explained.

"I lost my hearing when I was 24 because of the brutal side-effect of an injected DR-TB drug," said Nandita Venkatesan, who completed her treatment in 2015. "I was devastated by this loss, which took a heavy financial, emotional and mental toll on me. How many more people will have to die or go deaf, waiting to access safer and more effective drugs that can save their lives, without such devastating side-effects? With this patent challenge, we want to prevent an extension of the patent monopoly that will continue to block people from accessing more affordable generic versions of Bedaquiline."

Chapter 28

Institutional Strategies to Promote Scholarship in Health Professions Education

P V Vijayaraghavan, Latha Ravichandran, Narasimman Swaminathan

ABSTRACT

Scholarship of Teaching-Learning (SoTL) is gaining attention in Health Professions Education (HPE). Recognising and rewarding SoTL requires good governance at the institutional level. Developing and implementing appropriate strategies forcreating a culture among faculty members holds the key. This chapter discusses various factor that contribute to developing an appropriate eco-system or educational environment; these include institutional vision and mission, transparent policy, procedures, effective supportive system, appropriate recognition and reward structure that can improve the SoTL at the institute level. The chapter draws from the authors' personal experience of scholarship development and aims to provide a base for reflection on the institutional governance to promote SoTL

Key Words: educational scholarship; governance; leadership; policy; procedures; teaching; learning

ASSESS NEED

Scholarship of Teaching Learning (SoTL), in Health Professional Education (HPE) has gained attention in the recent past. In a editorial Singh T and Gupta P (2021) proposed that SoTL should be considered as a criteria for promotion of medical teachers in India. However, promoting SoTL among the Health Professions educators is challenging. There are several factors that affect such a move. Lack of educational research skills, preoccupation with teaching or clinical duties, lack of dedicated time, lack of recognition or weightage to educational research and absence of supportive structure including staffing and financial resources are often cited as the main barriers to SoTL. Good governance at the institutional level can play a vital role in achieving the desired goal. Developing strategies to facilitate and steer scholarly teaching towards SoTL across health profession educational institutes is therefore the need of the hour. Understanding the role of institutional support will help educators to convert their scholarly teaching into educational scholarship.

Health professions education in India, is quite a complex system in terms of structure and regualtions involved. Both Central and State Governments exercise control over the educational system run by the public and private sector. While the medical colleges are regulated by the National Medical Commission, dental, nursing, pharmacy and allied health sciences institutes are being regulated by their respective councils. Many of the health professions institutes come under the jurisdiction of universities which are again of different types. They are accountable to the UGC, and subject to assessment and accreditation by the National Assessment and Accreditation Council (NAAC). The medical colleges under the health sciences universities, therefore, face additional challenge of understanding and applying SoTL. However, irrespective of the type of institute, for ensuring the purpose of the quality of training, enhancing the scholarship of faculty remains a universal agenda. In this chapter, we discuss various aspects of institutional support in promoting SoTL.

BRIEF

- Good institutional governance plays a vital role in promoting SoTL
- Academic freedom, shared governance, transparent rights and responsibilities, meritocratic appointment are the principles of good governance in academic institutions
- Creating community of practices, mentoring, providing opportunities to develop skills required for scholarly work and implementing transparent policies, to promote SoTL at institutional level are key to success
- Recognising SoTL through transparent and appropriate appraisal system will promote SoTL

CONTEXTUALISE

The co-author of this chapter (LR), was identified by the leadership to facilitate the curriculum development initiative of the undergraduate (MBBS) medical curriculum in the institution in association with the Harvard Medical International (through MOU) and also to participate in faculty development programs. The result was an innovative integrated curriculum for the undergraduates. The outcome of this experience led to the institution being recognised as the Nodal Centre for faculty development by the then Medical Council of India (MCI, now National Medical Commission, NMC) with her appointment as Co-convener of the Nodal Centre.

The experience gained by her was supported by the institution by nominating her as the member of the Medical Council of India Faculty and curriculum development committees for the competency based undergraduate curriculum. The outcome was her contribution to the national curriculum and also to lead the faculty training of nearing 3000 medical faculty over a decade.

This expertise was utilised for internal development by her appointment as the Chair of the Curriculum Committee and Secretary of the medical education unit that has now evolved into Department of Medical Education. The outcome was scholarly projects and publications in medical education. For example, our recent publications in peer reviewed journals.

The institution supported her by nominating her to educational scholarships, the FAIMER fellowship, and Advance Course in Medical Education. The outcome was establishment of the Centre for Health

Professionals Education and the position of Associate Dean Education to oversee the educational activities of the university including other health sciences. This triggered more faculty pursuing fellowships and PhD in medical education, resulting in capacity building and scholarship in health professions education.

The institution now aiming at international visibility, accreditation and collaboration, her scholarship has been extended to International Fellowship in Medical Education (IFME) that offers scholarship for master's in medical education at Keele University.

Throughout her career in Health Professional Education, she is mentored by accomplished, seniors then Dean Education and Director Academic Administration of the Institute, later as Vice-Chancellor of the University.

DESCRIBE

Governance: Meaning and Importance

Governance includes policies and procedures intended to establish norms and develop strategies towards agreed institutional goals. The good governance ensures accountability, transparency and stakeholders' participation and successful implementation. Governance also signifies the standards, values and directions set by the institution through which stakeholders are involved in a transparent, inclusive and responsive manner towards institutional vison and mission (UNESCO, 2015). Within the context of higher education institutions governance can be defined as "the means by which universities and other higher education institutions are organized and managed".

In broader term the characteristics of good governance includes participation, consensus oriented, accountable, transparent, responsiveness, effective and efficient. The principles of good governance in higher education institutes includes academic freedom, shared governance, transparent rights and responsibilities, meritocratic appointment, financial stability and accountability (Mulinge et al., 2017).

Academic freedom allows faculty members to practice scholarly teaching which in turn will result in SoTL. Shared governance provides equal opportunities to the faculty members to participate in decisions which affect them both direct and indirect. Well defined merit system should be in place selection and promotion of faculty members. This principle of good governance shall be the key to promote SoTL in health professional institutes. Recognising and rewarding scholarly teaching and scholarship of teaching are critical as it contribute towards institutional mission and vision.

Health Professions Institutes should have well defined governance to promote scholarly activities of its stakeholders. Through the governance structures, routine teaching and learning preparation, delivery and assessment can be converted as educational scholarship if they are shared to a larger audience after peer review process. Higher education institutes should recognise educational scholarship to enhance quality and stakeholder's satisfaction (Chacko, 2021). The performance appraisal system recommended by University Grants Commission (UGC) provides importance to teaching learning. Institutes shall consider these guidelines in order to promote SoTL.

Creating a community of practice

Members of community support and motivate each other's by developing and sharing resources. In the long run members of the community develops stronger bond and commits to achieve the common goals as a team. Established communities of practice can positively influence faculty members to understand scholarly teaching learning (Kensington-Miller et al., 2012). Planned activities of such peer groups need to be facilitated by appropriate governance. Health professional education units of the institutes can be such communities, to promote SoTL. Establishing and nurturing health professional education units might influence scholarly teaching and SoTL positively.

Integrating various education units as health professional education unit will provide opportunities to develop communities of practice. Medical Education Units will be able to handhold and mentor the educational units of other health professionals to scholarly of teaching and SoTL.

The authors of this chapter, involved in training of faculty members were approached by a neighbouring institute to train their teachers in online methods during COVID pandemic. A short online course was created to train the educators in using Google classroom and the impact of training was assessed using a retro-pre questionnaire. There was a significant improvement in participants' perceived competencies using various features of Google classroom. The findings of this was published in a peer reviewed indexed journal. Creating and delivering a course in a short time was feasible because of the involvement in the FDPs at institutional level. This is an example how scholarly teaching could be effectively transferred as SoTL. (*https://doi.org/10.1016/j.jtumed.2020.11.003*,) The co-authors' Institution has a defined policy on FDP, which provided adequate exposure to faculty members to scholarly teaching. Creating a community within the institute might positively influence SoTL.

Promoting the scholarship opportunities in education among the faculty members is vital as it improves the quality of core teaching learning. In their recent editorial Singh T and Gupta P, discussed the need for promoting SoTL (Singh & Gupta, 2021). It is important that Higher Education Institutes provides adequate opportunities and create conducive atmosphere to its faculty members to engage in scholarly activities.

Role of Faculty Development Programs (FDP)

As we reflect, scholarly teaching is the foundation for SoTL, institutes should focus on training faculty members through structured faculty development programs. The faculty members of HPE have limited training in pedagogy, erstwhile Medical Council of India and recently National Medical Commission introduced mandatory faculty development programs (FDP) at the basic, advanced level and curricular implementation support programs. The objective of these FDPs is to improve the quality of medical education by training the faculty members. The details of the FDPs conducted by Sri Ramachandra Medical College & Research Institute, (Nodal centre) Chennai, are provided in the table below.

	Number of FDPs	Number of Faculty members trained
Pre-revised Basic Course Workshop (BCW) at nodal.	29	743
Revised BCWs conducted at medical colleges with onsite observers from nodal centre.	70	1603
AETCOM module (from January 2015 to December 2018).	10	251

Faculty members trained implemented innovative teaching methods and converted them as SoTL. For example "One minute preceptor" as a method of PG teaching was implemented by a faculty member and the impact was published in peer reviewed journal (Ravichandran et al., 2019). Facilitating scholarly teaching practices among faculty members through training, mentoring and appropriate recognition will be the key to SoTL (Patel, 2014). Creating a centre or unit of HPE to promote scholarly teaching might serve as a base to promote SoTL at institutional level. The FDPs should cultivate critical inquiry skills on teaching learning method.

Faculty empowerment strategies are considered as one of the key indicators under the criterion governance leadership and management, for accreditation by the National Assessment and Accreditation Council (NAAC). It insists on regular faculty development programme and transparent performance appraisal. Institutes shall consider educational research publications as one of the key performance indicators in faculty appraisal, which will promote SoTL at institutional level.

Mentoring

Kensington M and colleagues suggested mentoring as a method to inculcate SoTL among early career academicians. Shadowing an expert might improve critical inquiry skills and lead to SoTL. Institute should provide such opportunities by creating community of practice. One-on-one dialogues and consultations with educational experts and accomplished academic leaders might facilitate scholarly activities. Structured coaching sessions in the form of peer mentoring seems to be effective in promoting scholarly activities. Establishing a HPE unit at the institute level might serve this purpose. However, this requires further research prior to generalisation (Kensington-Miller et al., 2012).

> In our institute, Medical Education Unit is well established with experienced faculty members. The success of the MEU is transmitted to other health professionals by creating educational units. MEU is mentoring other Health Professional education units. Currently Sri Ramachandra Centre for Health Professionals Education functions as a team in imparting quality education. Senior members of MEU hand hold the other units in conducting FDPs and educational research. (*https://stel.bmj.com/content/6/6/351*)

Creating transparent policies and procedures to promote SoTL

Institute should have a clear policy to promote SoTL. An analysis of Canadian Medical Institutes policies on promoting educational scholarships, revealed wide variations and lack of clarity (Van Melle et al., 2014). It is important to create awareness among educational leaders regarding the importance of SoTL. SoTL shall include any forms of peer reviewed research and innovation in HPE. The dissemination of such findings shall be through publications or through conference presentations. The objective of any SoTL is that it can be replicated in a scalable way through institutional policies, presenting the finding of educational research in discipline specific as well as HPE conference can be considered for recognitions. Attending and sharing the findings of HPE research with the larger audience can also be considered as SoTL. (Haslett, 2009) such as analysing journal publications. However, this snapshot survey uses attendance at higher education conferences as a measure. Attendances were analysed at three conferences in the UK between July-December 2008. The country in which each conference delegate was based and (for Wales only. Participation in conference will lead to self-reflection about individuals teaching skills and promote critical inquiry. Recognising through institutional award will encourage faculty members to improve SoTL.

The institutional policies to promote SoTL shall

- be able to differentiate SoTL from other scholarships
- define career path for the educators
- focus on all possible appropriate outcomes of SoTL rather only on publications
- reasonable awards and recognition for SoTL activities at institutional level

Creating support structures

Several challenges in promoting educational scholarships are identified. Lack of time, inadequate knowledge and skills in educational research and lack of administrative support were some of the challenges documented in the literature (Lehmann, 2014). Goldszmidt MA et al through a mixed method study identified the support requirements in promoting SoTL. Lack of educational research skills among the faculty members were identified as an important barrier. This study also identified that merely having an advanced educational degree may not be sufficient to promote educational research (Goldszmidt et al., 2008) there is a paucity of literature addressing how to support those who wish to do so.\nAIMS: The purpose of this study was to explore faculty involvement in and support needs for pursuing education scholarship.\nMETHODS: A purposive sample of 108 medical faculty with an interest in medical education were invited to participate in a two-phase, mixed-methods study (survey and focus groups. Providing appropriate training and resources to facilitate SoTL is important. Training faculty members in educational research methods apart from routine FDPs might improve the scholarly activities.

We run monthly journal club (JC) through HPE, which focus on educational publications. Members of various health professions participate in this club to discuss the published innovative practice. Educational research methods are deliberated in detail during JCs. The impact of this journal clubs is noticed by increased number of publications in peer reviewed journals and conference presentations.

Higher Education Institutes should encourage disseminating scholarly activity to a wider audience through publications and presentations. This could be possible by creating a community of educators interested in SoTL within the institute (Williams et al., 2013) the authors provide a conceptual model along with examples of practical strategies for overcoming resistance to change within institutions. The paper provides examples from a variety of different international contexts to show how incentives and other non-coercive measures can motivate faculty and administrators to weave SoTL into institutional fabrics.\nDrawing on social network theory and the concept of communities of practice, the paper presents a model with attendant strategies for disseminating SoTL values and practices across all three levels of post secondary institutions: the micro, the meso, and the macro. The authors argue that for SoTL to take root in organizational cultures, there must be 1. Creating a centre for Health Professions Education can be considered as a priority measure to promote SoTL. In his editorial Chacko VT, suggested the measures to be considered at institutional level to promote SoTL (Chacko, 2021).

Since 2019 at our institute, we established teaching excellence award with the following objectives:

- Recognise the teaching excellence both as individuals and teams
- Showcase the institutes commitment towards quality teaching – learning
- Encourage scholarly activities in teaching and learning
- Inspire and nurture the faculty members in Health Professions Education

We created a transparent process and criteria to assess the nominees. We were able to identify the faculty members with potential towards scholarly publication. We observed that the faculty members' involvement in educational research is improved as evidenced by increased number of publications and conference presentations. For instance, in last year's simulation conference four members of SRIHER presented their findings and the abstracts are published indexed journal. We will be able to analyse the impact of this initiative in due course.

SUMMARIZE

- Creating the culture of SoTL in Health Professions Education institutes is mandatory though it is challenging. It is possible to promote SoTL through good governance which includes institutional commitment and leadership skills.
- Establishing a community of practice to promote SoTL seems to be effective based on our experience. However, this requires further research.
- Promoting health professions education requires high commitment equally from the organisation and the faculty members. It is the responsibility of the institute to create conducive environment to carry out educational research.

EVALUATE

Reflect: Does your institute have a policy to promote educational scholarship? If yes, how does it benefit you as Health Professions Educator? If no, will you attempt to propose one such policy to the leadership?

Based on the strategy discussed in this chapter prepare an outline of steps which you would like your administration to take for enhancing the overall scholarship development? What problems do you anticipate and how do you resolve them?

ROAD AHEAD

Based on our experience and available literatures institution support in the form of good governance is vital in promoting SoTL

Strategies to be considered to promote SoTL at Institutional Level:

- Developing and implementing well defined policies to promote SoTL
- Facilitating a community of practice by establishing Health Professions Education Unit with dedicated faculty members
- Providing administrative support
- Training faculty members in educational research methods
- Allocating dedicated time to carryout educational research
- Creating necessary infrastructure including technology e.g
- Recognising SoTL through incentives
- Promoting innovative teaching methods like Blended Learning
- Identifying and nurturing talents
- Providing leadership roles to the deserving faculty members to promote SoTL

For further understanding of Governance you may refer the following links:

1. *https://hea.ie/assets/uploads/2018/01/governance_framework-15.5.17.pdf*
2. *https://codesria.org/IMG/pdf/3-_the_governance_of_higher_education.pdf*
3. *https://www.boardeffect.com/en-gb/blog/the-importance-of-good-governance-in-higher-education/*

REFERENCES

Chacko, T. V. (2021). The Scholarship of Teaching: Why India should promote it for promotion & tenure. Journal of Education Technology in Health Sciences, 4(1), 1–4.

Goldszmidt, M. A., Zibrowski, E. M., & Weston, W. W. (2008). Education scholarship: It's not just a question of "degree." Medical Teacher, 30(1), 34–39. https://doi.org/10.1080/01421590701754136

Haslett, S. (2009). Higher education conference attendendance and engagement with the scholarship of teaching and learning: A Welsh perspective. Journal of Applied Research in Higher Education, 1, 66–73. https://doi.org/10.1108/17581184200900015

Kensington-Miller, B., Brailsford, I., & Gossman, P. (2012). Developing new academic developers: Doing before being? International Journal for Academic Development, 17(2), 121–133. https://doi.org/10.1080/1360144X.2011.616049

Lehmann, S. W. (2014). The ADMSEP Education Scholars Program: A novel approach to cultivating scholarship among psychiatry educators. Academic Psychiatry: The Journal of the American Association of Directors of Psychiatric Residency Training and the Association for Academic Psychiatry, 38(3), 364–367. https://doi.org/10.1007/s40596-014-0090-2

Mulinge, M. M., Arasa, J. N., & Wawire, V. (2017). The Status of Student Involvement in University Governance in Kenya: The Case of Public and Private Universities. CODESRIA. https://doi.org/10.2307/j.ctvh8r378

Patel, F. (2014). Promoting a culture of scholarship among educational developers: Exploring institutional opportunities. International Journal for Academic Development, 19(3), 242–254. https://doi.org/10.1080/1360144X.2013.805693

Ravichandran, L., Sivaprakasam, E., Balaji, S., & Swaminathan, N. (2019). Effectiveness of the 1-Minute Preceptor on Feedback to Pediatric Residents in a Busy Ambulatory Setting. Journal of Graduate Medical Education, 11(4 Suppl), 204–206. https://doi.org/10.4300/JGME-D-19-00440

Singh, T., & Gupta, P. (2021). Can We Consider Scholarship of Teaching Learning Rather than Focusing Only on Publications for Recognition of Medical Teachers by National Medical Commission? Annals of the National Academy of Medical Sciences (India), 57(01), 01–02. https://doi.org/10.1055/s-0041-1728179

Swaminathan, N., Govindharaj, P., Jagadeesh, N. S., & Ravichandran, L. (2021). Evaluating the effectiveness of an online faculty development programme for nurse educators about remote teaching during COVID-19. Journal of Taibah University Medical Sciences, 16(2), 268–273. https://doi.org/10.1016/j.jtumed.2020.11.003

UNESCO. (2015, May 26). Concept of Governance [Text]. International Bureau of Education. http://www.ibe.unesco.org/en/geqaf/technical-notes/concept-governance

Williams, A. L., Verwoord, R., Beery, T. A., Dalton, H., McKinnon, J., Strickland, K., Pace, J., & Poole, G. (2013). The power of social networks: A model for weaving the Scholarship of Teaching and Learning into institutional culture. Teaching & Learning Inquiry, 1(2), 49–62. https://doi.org/10.20343/teachlearninqu.1.2.49

Chapter 29

Scholarship of Integration and the future of Medical Education and Research (MER)

Suptendra Nath Sarbadhikari, Bhagyajyoti Priyadarshini, L V Simhachalam Kutikuppala, Shanthan Jodavula, Saranya Mukherjee, Vamsi Krishna, Sadhna Sharma, Amy Price and Rakesh Biswas

ABSTRACT

Scholarship of integration is meant to make connections within and between disciplines to result in a new knowledge or practise. Applied to medical education, it aims to distribute the fruits of academic activities to benefit patient care, which in turn, facilitates the construction of new knowledge translated into practice. The students are the immediate users, whose outcomes are both driven and measured by assessment. Patients are the ultimate beneficiaries; whose needs are of foremost consideration. The advent of new digital technologies in e-learning and assessment makes it possible for bridging the gap between the patient care expectations and student learning outcomes.

In this chapter we describe a comprehensive model of integration, which is compatible with the new vision of India (to bring synergy between Modern/Western Medicine with traditional Systems of medicine practised in India (AYUSH – Ayurveda, Yoga and Naturopathy, Unani, Siddha and Homeopathy) for optimizing health care delivery.

We have demonstrated a working prototype for scholarly integration in medical education and research framework, showcasing student user driven, patient centered assessments of learning outcomes driving health care outcomes. It includes predominantly, user driven case based blended learning ecosystem (CBBLE), and patient centered assessment, with other elements: problem mapping, evidence-based audit, peer review, peer assessment with online portfolio system. It highlights a participatory action research framework and learning ecosystem that thrives in transparency, accountability and real time evidence-based audit of education and practice.

In addition, we have reported a SWOT analysis and offered suggestions for further exploring our prototype model especially in Indian and other similar settings.

Key Words: scholarship; integration; patient centred learning; medical education, medical practice, research, connections

ASSESS NEED

This is a postulated effective tool to tackle the problem statement highlighted in the chapter primarily around two broad categories and its subcategories:

a) Current disintegration of Medical education and practice

   Medical student and faculty engagement in rote memorization through an arcane curriculum that promotes plagiarism and diminishes scholarship, which is disconnected from:

   Patients who continue to suffer due to lack of student and faculty engagement with them in a broader empathic meaningful manner.

b) Long overdue National Medical integration of health care delivery through methodologically diverse streams of interventions:

   India's traditional and tribal systems of Medicine have been historically neglected due to undue hype created by an ancient but dominant Western mode of Medical education that does not allow for critical thinking and current evidence but instead embroils our students and teachers in inflexible and systems dependent thinking.

The current West has moved on globally, and we aim to move beyond the colonial past that hinders students and teachers from learning and developing clinical practice that meets the needs of India.

WHO are the intended audience for this chapter?

All beneficiaries of Medical education including the primary beneficiary also known as patients or care seekers as well as caregivers ranging from medical students, their teachers and practicing physicians as well as medical education and practice researchers and administrators.

WHAT issues does this chapter address?

Medical education research is a tool to eventually improve patient outcomes as patients are the ultimate beneficiaries of Medical education.

For most medical students and teachers medical education begins with their entry to medical school and begins with an introduction to the dead body and this cadaveric teacher bares it's innards for all budding health professionals to learn the various components of the individual human system even while they attend parallel classes on physiology and biochemistry to further learn how this anatomic structure functions in a living human in all it's fascinating internal molecular and cellular complexity.

Again, in the next year they learn pathology which describes how a body is structurally ravaged by illness at a cellular and molecular level often historically unravelled after death. Finally they are introduced to the whole alive human being in their later clinical years where they learn to apply the knowledge of yester years to a living complex human being with his her complex network of problems rooted either in his her environment or genes.

However this was not always how medicine was historically learned and this current curricular methodology of putting dry factual content before the student gets to experience learning in the context of the entire human, undermines the very ethos of medical education which is essentially to help health professionals improve patient care outcomes.

Consequently, one main problem statement theme for this chapter is the current "disintegration of Medical education with practice" and the tool that it aims to resolve the problem with is scholarly integration of Medical education and research.

The other problem that this chapter addresses with the same tool is the current issue of national medical integration, which has reached a tipping point due to a reigning Covid chaos that has fast tracked all diverse interventions with varying methodological backgrounds into battling one single disease. Essentially, we need to move past pandemic crisis to meet other medical needs even within a pandemic or endemic crisis.

Scholarship of integration in Medical education and research: what it is and what it isn't

Scholarship of integration in medical education and research makes connections within and between disciplines, locating knowledge in a broader context giving meaning to specific discoveries. It aims to distribute the fruits of academic discovery to benefit specific individual members of society also known as patients who in turn help academics to multiply the construction of new knowledge translated into practice. It is vital that academic institutions and medical schools remain relevant in an era when the production of knowledge is increasingly recognized as a social collaborative activity. (Hofmeyer *et al* 2007).

a) Current disintegration of Medical education and practice
   Medical student and faculty engagement in rote memorization through an arcane curriculum. (Lal 2016) found rote learning tends to promote plagiarism and diminish scholarship, which is disconnected from:
   Patients who continue to suffer due to lack of student and faculty engagement with them in a broader empathic meaningful manner.
b) Long overdue National Medical integration of health care delivery through methodologically diverse streams of interventions (Shankar 2015, WHO 2018, NITI Aayog 2019, Srinivasan 2020):
   India's traditional and tribal system of Medicine have been historically neglected due to undue hype created by an outdated but dominant Western mode of Medical education that is inconsistent with Indian culture, patient needs and preference and which ill prepares our future physicians to engage with empathy, critical thinking and collaboration as this model leans heavily on hierarchal structures that do not allow for the development of flexible minds and resilient hearts needed for the practice of medicine in the century.

Quoting Shankar (2015): "long-term strategy involving radical changes in medical education, research, clinical practice, public health and the legal and regulatory framework is needed, to innovate India's public health system and make it both integrative and participatory. India can be a world leader in the new emerging field of "integrative healthcare" because we have over the last century or so assimilated and achieved a reasonable degree of competence in bio-medical and life sciences and we possess an incredibly rich and varied medical heritage of our own."

Although current West has moved on globally, it is time now for Indian medicine to rise to meet the challenges of today's world and put aside the dogmas and the colonial subservience that continues to haunt our education and practice.

Our proposed tool of scholarly integration enables shared knowledge through a participatory framework and includes practical methods to guide institutional change along with reporting and evaluating them.

At the outset one must clarify that scholarship of integration is not the same as scholarship of teaching and learning also known as SOTL and borrowing from an excellent recent editorial (Singh and Gupta 2021), SOTL as identified by Felten (2013), thrives on five principles:

1. inquiry focused on student learning,
2. grounded in context,
3. methodologically sound,
4. conducted in partnership with students, and (
5. appropriately public.

Singh and Gupta's editorial (2021) contributes very interesting questions.

"How such a scholarship can be evaluated? Should it focus on output or outcome?"

The answer to the first would be open access self-publication in one's own online learning portfolio such as even an online question paper designed can be shared for evaluation among peers as here: *http://medicinedepartment.blogspot.com/2021/05/online-blended-bimonthly-assignment.html?m=1*

The above link to our online test for the month of May 2021 is essentially a student user driven, real patient centered, experiential sharing of individual patient data in the form of patient centered questions for solving and helping those individuals.

The competencies tested are: "The questions below cover the entire spectrum from anatomy, physiology to diagnostic, therapeutic uncertainty to resolve one disease theme and predictably move from symptoms to diagnosis and treatment challenges. For traditional classification purposes we have classified the questions into anatomical areas.

Most questions test the reading comprehension skills of the examinee and some prior familiarity with medical terms and strategies and also more importantly assesses their ability to use online search tools toward better expression of their learning points in the form of answers that are again made available open access for post publication peer review.

In summary the answers to the following questions in this online question paper will assess the examinee's competencies in empathically dealing with:

- Clinical problem solving
- Medical terminologies familiarity including areas of anatomy, physiology, pathology
- Current EBM strategies for managing diagnostic and therapeutic uncertainty."

Although unlike last month it doesn't test the competencies for familiarity with Empathy, Humanities and ML AI.

Q10 looks at another topical area and that is "medical education" itself where students are also encouraged to think about their learning process.

The answer to the second would surely be outcomes but not just on student learning but also in the context of Medical education directed toward its ultimate beneficiaries, that is the patients themselves, through a framework that enables driving of patient outcomes through student learning outcomes and a real time clinical audit trail that allows us to join the dots between the two.

The above would bring us closer to scholarship of integration in Medical education and research which is not just about integrating scholarship of teaching learning with the scholarship of discovery but is all about integration of patient centered societal goals with teaching and learning.

BRIEF

Scholarship of integration in Medical education and research: what it is and what it isn't:

- Scholarship of integration in medical education and research makes connections within and between disciplines, locating knowledge in a broader context giving meaning to specific discoveries.
- It aims to benefit individual patients, who in turn help academics to facilitate the construction of new knowledge translated into practice.
- Working prototype for scholarly integration includes student user driven, patient centered assessments of learning outcomes driving health care outcomes.
- Other elements are case based blended learning ecosystem (CBBLE), and patient centered assessment, with other elements: problem mapping, evidence based audit, peer review, peer assessment with online portfolio system.
- Scholarship of integration enables shared knowledge through a participatory framework and includes practical methods to guide institutional change along with reporting and evaluating them.
- Scholarship of integration focuses on outcomes not just on student learning but also in the context of Medical education directed toward its ultimate beneficiaries, that is the patients themselves, through a framework that enables driving of patient outcomes through student learning outcomes and a real time clinical audit trail that allows us to join the dots between the two.

CONTEXTUALIZE

The corresponding author of this chapter [RB] began with a few ideas, in 2002, at Manipal College of Medical Sciences, Pokhara, Nepal. There he encouraged his medical students to record their individual patients' narratives. In 2008, the first conceptual model for CBBLE (case based blended learning ecosystem) was developed, called as UDHC (User Driven Health Care). This reaffirms the fact that CBBLE had a strong component of offline connection and locality that was blended to requirements of the online users. The motto behind developing CBBLE as a subset of UDHC was to build a case-based reasoning database that would serve as a platform for health care providers as well as patients to make best decisions for individual cases by comparing and learning from the cases with the data-base of other individual patients with similar trajectories. The concept of CBBLE (Podder *et al* 2018) was presented by one of our Elective students at Medical Education Conference at AIIMS, Bhubaneswar in January 2020 and by another student at a medical college in California in early 2021. The pandemic, seemingly a big loss for education, proved to be a blessing in disguise to strengthen our system, as it drove newer opportunities to explore online learning with non-BMJ elective students, who added a considerable amount of data to our work around scholarship of integration. The pandemic was well utilized by taking classes globally where we regularly connect with our students live during morning rounds and also encourage them to make individual case presentations and also record it in their portfolios. Many of these case reports, from the Student Electives, are available in BMJ Case Reports Archives at PubMed Central.

So, it can be said that the snow-ball effect was achieved in a steady, dedicated manner. The destination looks unpredictable, especially due to the pandemic and all the visible and non-visible constraints, yet it is being traversed with proper planning and a zeal to bring about a positive change. The mushrooming of problem statements and solutions at different places at different times, is being tackled with both a vertical and horizontal approach. All these efforts had made it possible for our proposed model of Scholarship of Integration to stand where it is today. In this chapter some snippets from this evolving and ongoing real story are presented.

Individual integration of different roads to healing

One of our expert patients has published another paper (Young *et al* 2011) with our team members where she elaborated on her cure and the integration of multidisciplinary interventions that was brought about to effect it. She subsequently utilized the power of online integration to provide a voice to similar stories from many patients around the world.

Quoting her version from the paper: "the large doses of prednisone I took to try to resolve my ***ITP*** (Idiopathic Thrombocytopenic Purpura), plus the usual factors of age, hormones, and genetics resulted in a diagnosis of ***osteoporosis***. For both of these conditions, I am sorting through the medical hype, trying to determine the validity and meaning of the sometimes-conflicting diagnostic tests, and weighing the different approaches for improving my health. What I'm finding is no different from what I found 20 years ago. The treatments suggested by the endocrinologists and alternative doctors are often very different. The patient experiences do not match the published literature. There are significant pharmaceutical profit motives that may skew the diagnosis, research, and treatment suggestions (Shomon, 2000). Once again, I'm balanced in the middle with one foot in the conventional world and one in the alternative world, trying to find a secure and reliable place to heal. And there are millions of us who feel this way."

Pandemic driven acceleration of scholarship of integration between different ways of knowing and doing in healthcare

The current chaos in modern medical healthcare reflects a failure of evidence based medical education and research directed at the end beneficiary of Medical education, that is the patient and the time is ripe for scholarship of integration to develop the optimal adaptive systems framework for it.

Quoting verbatim from a recent essay in Lancet global health particularly focused in India although very relevant globally,

"Academic institutions and professional medical societies should reflect on their roles. A range of recommendations and treatment algorithms from norm-defining medical institutions and societies are circulating on social media. These institutions are notable by their failure to share the evidence that informs these recommendations, discuss nuances of implementation, or present conflicts of interests of those involved in developing these recommendations." (Bhaumik et al 2021)

National Medical Integration and the role of scholarship of integration in Medical education and research:

> Hundred years ago, independent research in Ayurveda on scientific lines was planned with the establishment of the "Jatiya Ayurbigyan Vidyalaya" in 1921, (also known as Calcutta National

Medical College) founded as a product of the Non-cooperation movement and was inaugurated by Subhas Chandra Bose. Calcutta National Medical College was nationalized in 1967 and was perhaps the first private medical college in India to be nationalized.

More here:*https://medicinedepartment.blogspot.com/2021/06/national-medical-integration-and-role.html?m=1*

More about it in the description but before that a quick look at the history of "integration of medical education and research" from 200 years in India with the British integrating their system of Western Medicine with that of the pre-existing Indian system with near total demise of the Indian system.

Hundred years later there is a pandemic driven resurgence (Anand and Patwardhan 2021) toward another attempt at integration and scholarship of integration in medical education and research can go a long way to connect these different ways of knowing and doing healthcare through a patient centered framework that is described below.

DESCRIBE

WHY (the need to connect different ways of knowing and doing in healthcare)?

To put the current disintegration of Medical education and practice into context, we need to first understand individual patient requirements and societal requirements to gain further insights into medical practice and how it can be integrated with medical education.

We share below an illustrative example from one of our online expert patients that we have published before (Biswas et al 2008)

The details are available here: *https://medicinedepartment.blogspot.com/2021/06/part-1-contextualizing-need-for.html?m=1*

HOW (is scholarship of integration, a framework for transparent and accountable healthcare and education)?

The problem statement for this chapter as also mentioned above in the introduction is the current "disintegration of Medical education with practice" and the tool that it aims to resolve this problem is with scholarship of integration in Medical education and research.

The chapter will now proceed to describe how this can be done through a current working prototype of student user driven, patient centered assessments of learning outcomes driving health care outcomes and also provide a historical overview of how this developed in different Indian Medical colleges through a faculty coordinator and his students and patients.

Evolution of a model for patient centered, scholarship of integration in Medical education and research

The participatory case based blended learning ecosystem CBBLE framework that is a model for a patient centered, scholarship of integration in Medical education, has been actively evolving since a few decades in different medical colleges in India and has been described in detailed timeline in the link below:

http://medicinedepartment.blogspot.com/2021/06/evolution-of-model-forpatient-centered.html?m=1

Working prototype of a scholarly integration of medical education and research framework

The working prototype shared here is a minimalistic, user driven learning framework that enriches pre-existing curricular and assessment infrastructures instead of dramatically attempting to change it but aims at effecting a slow transformation.

More here: https://*medicinedepartment.blogspot.com/2021/06/working-prototype-of-scholarly.html?m=1*

Student user driven, patient centred assessment prototype

In this module our readers can see how the patient data captured in the previous module was utilized in a monthly summative assessment test for the same batch of students to test their competencies in patient care related to clinical problem solving through empathic patient data capture and continuity of communication.

More here: *https://medicinedepartment.blogspot.com/2021/06/student-user-driven-patient-centred.html?m=1*

Gradual integration of traditional with competency driven curricula in a patient centered learning framework

The definition of competency for a medical student health professional is: "habitual, consistent and judicious use of communication, knowledge, technical skills, clinical reasoning, emotions, values, and reflections in daily practice for the benefit of the individual being served" (Epstein and Hundert 2002)

Scholarship of integration driven by shared online learning portfolios promoting formative, 'reading comprehension and creative writing' scholastic competencies in peer review/assessment

This form of online portfolio based formative assessment of competency can be improved upon and rapidly scaled to all medical colleges in India. This is an evidence based formative and summative assessment of the learning competencies of 2016 MBBS batch posted in the department of Medicine online **from May 2020 to March 2021 and ward postings from Feb 2021 to first week of March 2021.** The formative assessment is from each UG student's logged competency around patients (evidence) evaluated regularly from date of joining. The formative assessment has been divided into non-verbal which assesses their competency in procedural domains including empathic communication and body language (video evidence links shared where captured) and verbal which assesses their ability to communicate their patient centered work, evidenced in their day-to-day E logs.

More here:*https://medicinedepartment.blogspot.com/2021/06/scholarship-of-integration-driven-by.html?m=1*

Peer to peer review/assessment of Online assignments in E logged learning portfolios

Unfortunately in our soon to be past (and largely current) offline system of medical (and other) education, we inadvertently reward students for stealing by giving the best marks in theory answer papers to the best copy pasted answers from memorized text books thus encouraging a hitherto unrecognized form of plagiarism but the real world of 'virtual shared learning' cannot tolerate sharing of unoriginal work. More here (in a conversational learning module):

https://medicinedepartment.blogspot.com/2021/06/peer-to-peer-reviewassessment-of-online.html?m=1

Evidence based medical assessments drive student learning outcomes

This is not just evidence based medical education with evidence of correlation between awarded marks (quantitative learning outcomes) versus process of assessment (qualitative data capture inputs to drive assessment) but also an attempt to integrate Medical education with practice by putting the patient at the centre of Medical education.

Here is a description of an Indian patient's 'quest' for cure taking him away from mainstream medicine and making him embrace other streams, including Ayurveda. The patient finds a respite, although short lived, as it worsens again and makes him again having to approach mainstream medical practitioners. In this narrative, an endoscope is put inside the patient's colon, followed bymedicines that are manufactured by the big pharmaceutical industry.

More here: *https://medicinedepartment.blogspot.com/2021/06/evidence-based-medical-assessments.html?m=1*

Making connections between different ways of knowing and doing

In the above framework of what is just one stream of healthcare delivery among other delivery frameworks, we cite below a patient centered example of another closely related healthcare delivery framework that the British subjugated 200 years back. More here: *medicinedepartment.blogspot.com/2021/06/making-connections-between-different.html?m=1*

The box sums this up:

Empathic Narrative of a 35-year-old UC Patient

April 15, 2021

This current case report shows the empathic narrative of a 40 yr old male in his own words, on his 15 years journey with Ulcerative Colitis

"What can be more painful than having a disease well diagnosed, but not responding to any treatment? And when it combines with having to consume endless medicines and spending hours together in the toilet with no improvement, it's worse than a nightmare. My journey with Ulcerative Colitis was the same, past 15 years. It all started in the year 2004, when I had regular episodes of abdominal pain, followed by bowel evacuation with blood and mucous. When I consulted a local hospital, I was put on a bunch of medicines without any proper diagnosis. Symptoms went on increasing day by day. I then consulted a gastroenterologist, who performed Colonoscopy, and gave the diagnosis of Ulcerative Colitis. Chills went down my spine when I have read about the disease over internet.

I was already suffering with neck pain, lower back pain and headaches for years, and this added up now. I was started on steroids and few other medications. The doctors believed that

Contd...

the painkillers (NSAID) which I used continuously for my pains could have possibly triggered this. No dose of steroids gave me any relief, so were other drugs. I went on changing doctors for opinions, to check whether the diagnosis or the treatment was going well or not. It only made things more complicated, as every doctor asked for a series of fresh investigations before commenting anything. Any little variation in food used to trigger severe episodes of mucoid stools and abdominal pain. Headaches were a regular menace. Any oral medication for one issue used to trigger another problem.

My family life and social life got badly affected. The need to rush to toilet frequently made me stick to home, unemployed. I tried working from home for a while, but I was in a state of mental depression thinking round the clock about the disease and reading about it. I was in a feeling of becoming a financial burden for my family, after which I silently went on consuming steroids and other medicines, probiotics and immunosuppressants from 2004 to 2016. Ten years have passed away with endless endoscopies, colonoscopies, biopsies and blood tests. Everything was pointing towards the same diagnosis. I had to undergo blood transfusion too in the middle, as my Hemoglobin levels have fallen low. It alters between 6-8 gm. Moving out of home was a herculean task.

On advice of a friend and in search of cure with a hope, I retorted to Ayurveda treatment in the year 2016. I was evaluated and advised a few medications and therapies/treatments to be undergone. As I was skeptic towards AYUSH systems (for the bad experience I had with Homoeopathy), I was given contacts of other patients of UC at the hospital. It's only after speaking to them, I could get courage to proceed further. Things went well for 2-3 years, and as my abdominal pain and episodes of stool evacuation reduced greatly, I was optimistic. Its then that things started to go out of the track again. Slowly my symptoms went on increasing day by day, and accordingly necessary changes were made in my treatment schedule, but in vain.

I was back to the state of mental depression, when one day the treating doctor said I may have to restart modern drugs for a while to control acute episodes. I was greatly depressed, not only because of this, but on seeing other patients getting cured. I didn't know what was going wrong in my case. There were many sleepless nights, thinking and reading a lot about this disease, and searching for a possible cure, but in vain. The worst phase of my life started in the year 2020, wherein I started to spend 4-6 hours in the toilet. I never expected that my health condition could deteriorate to such extent. No medicine was working, and slowly suicidal thoughts took over my mental status.

At this moment again, I have approached another hospital on the advice of the Doctor treating me, and they planned to start a drug called Azathioprine, only after using steroid for a week. Cursing my fate, I have started it again.... "

By the patient's Ayurveda Physician:

> On the evening of 5th day after starting steroid, the patient fell down unconscious while walking around casually. He was immediately rushed to a hospital, and on the way had a seizure activity. CT Brain revealed Bifrontal hemorrhagic Infarction. Necessary management was initiated. He continued to be in vegetative state with no significant response. Re-evaluation with MRI Brain revealed extensive cerebral edema, and he was planned for craniectomy. As the financial burden went on increasing, he was shifted to a Government Hospital, and there the patient finally lost his fight.

Above was a description of HOW scholarship of integration in medical education and research practice has been operational in some medical colleges in India through patient and student-centred connections between their individual learning requirements toward better health care outcomes.

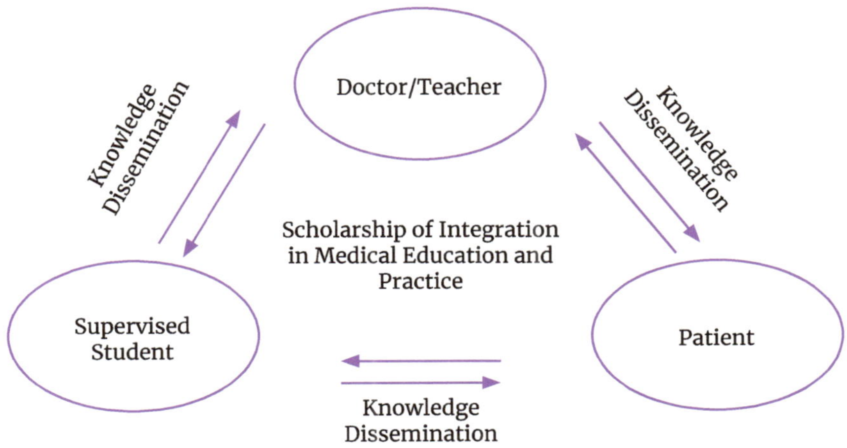

Figure 1: Scholarship Integration and the Future of Medial Education and Research

Now we shall proceed to engage our readers to EVALUATE the above described process, again through a patient centered medical education lens and describe the ROAD ahead.

SUMMARIZE

This chapter has contextualized and described a working prototype for scholarly integration in medical education and research framework showcasing student user driven, patient centered assessments of learning outcomes driving health care outcomes.

Some restatement from B Brief section.

The working prototype described in this chapter tackles the above problem statements head on and describes a participatory action research framework and learning ecosystem that thrives in transparency, accountability and real time evidence-based audit of education and practice.

So WHAT?

- **(S)trengths:** Promising solution to current felt need that can bridge gaps in healthcare learning competencies as well as address patient outcome complexities.
- **(W)eaknesses:** Quasi-experimental and complex study design and consequent potential of study sample selection bias. (Workarounds: ensure transparent and accountable online documentation of entire process that is naturally subject to external peer review in real time)
- **(O)pportunities:** Potential to scale into a sustainable model of practice-based learning toward improving patient outcomes.
- **(T)hreats:** Participant motivation leading to study attrition, patient privacy and confidentiality (Workarounds: regular motivational meets with participants of both groups with real-time transparent documentation of the interaction that transpires between all the stakeholders)

To appreciate the experiment fully, the comfort zone of printed books has to be forsaken and the hyperlinks mentioned in the chapter have to be visited repeatedly.

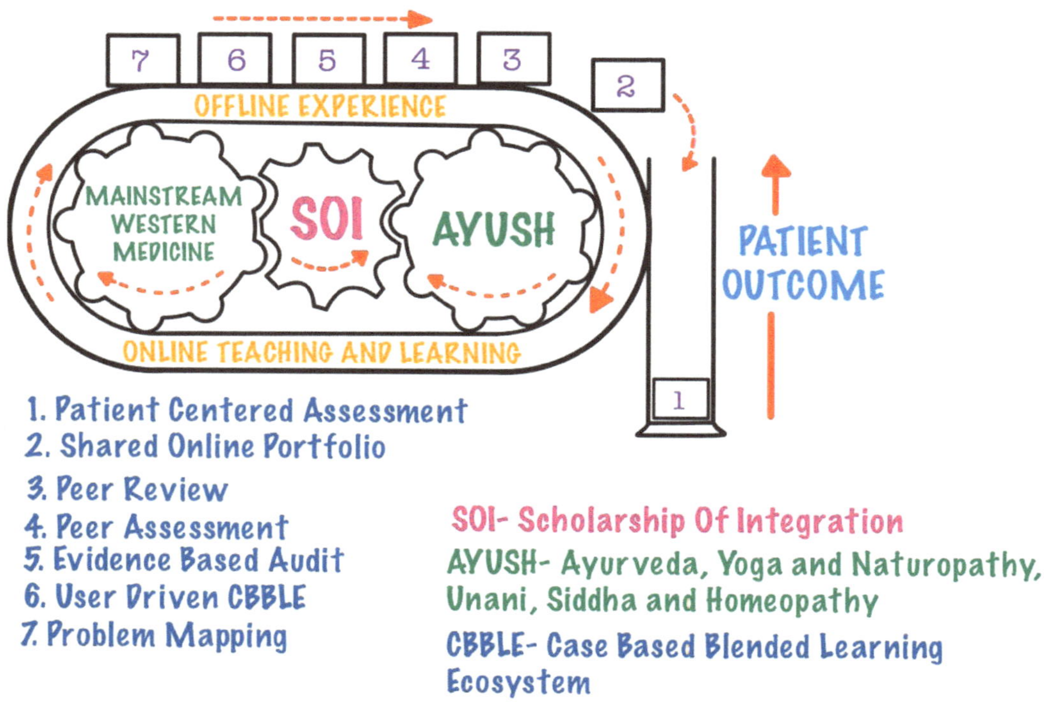

Figure 2: Working model of Scholarship of Integration with its major pillars and outcomes

EVALUATE

The essential premise behind scholarship of integration in Medical education and research as portrayed in this chapter has been around making connections between patients, medical students (who in the expanded definition of lifelong learners are also known as practicing doctors as well as faculty) More here: *http://consciousnotebooksequel.blogspot.com/2014/?m=0*

What is the first step toward developing competency in making connections? In the medical student driven real example of connecting to patients what were the necessary competencies that came from medical training than from premedical upbringing?

The next driver toward making connections in scaling scholarship of integration is an often-neglected tool also known as peer review/assessment. Traditionally assessments have always been between higher authorities also known as teachers assessing a lower powered student while in the real-world humans assess each other all the time and all humans thrive on feedback.

Here: *https://medicinedepartment.blogspot.com/2021/06/medicine-department-paper-for-june-2021.html?m=1*

Is the Medicine assessment online assignment for June 2021 that aims to evaluate the examinees aptitude for?

a) scholarship, which is reflected in their ability to read comprehend, analyze, reflect upon and discuss captured patient centered data as in their 'original' answers to the assignment for May 2021.

b) scholarship of integration, which is reflected in
   1) their ability to connect with and capture patient centered data (as already demonstrated by many of the 2019, 2017, 2016 batch students who have captured it in their E logs as a part of their formative assessment)
   2) their ability to connect with and engage in shared learning with their peers through peer review feedback.

Here is a link to an answer by one of the 2019 batch students, where she provides peer review feedback to ten students answering the May 2021 question as a part of her answer to the June 2021 question 1:

http://riddhibhalla25.blogspot.com/2021/06/general-medicine-monthly-assignmentjune.html

Can regular student driven peer review/assessment of patient centered learning in medical students create the much-needed change in not just improving scholarship in individual students and faculty but improve overall collective learning outcomes as well as health care outcomes?

ROAD AHEAD

Scholarship of integration is a movement that will grow organically and is also as old as civilization only it has been currently augmented by technology that facilitates human connections and scholarship through improved asynchronous communication. More here:*https://medicinedepartment.blogspot.com/2021/06/introduction-to-evolution-of-human.html?m=1*

One of the amazing transformations that we can look forward to in the near future is tremendous improvement in "individual patient data" based reasoning systems that will give new meaning to precision medicine, which shall make the process of healthcare cognition accessible, transparent and accountable to larger populations. Considerable headway is happening in this direction detailed in this paper where in addition to the "traditional differentiation between implicit and explicit knowledge, it outlines the concepts of general and individual knowledge and connects general knowledge with the "frame problem," a fundamental issue of artificial intelligence, as well as individual knowledge with another important paradigm of artificial intelligence (AI), case-based reasoning (CBR), a method of individual knowledge processing that aims at solving new problems based on the solutions to similar past problems." More has been described by Pantazi *et al* (2004).

This will all begin with the simple step as described in the chapter, of making the first connection between a lifelong medical student and patient, toward empathic data capture and representation in a shared database and as soon as an individual patient data is shared, the data is matched with similar past patients illness trajectories and triangulated toward an optimal diagnostic and therapeutic plan for the current patient data shared.

This plan for every individual patient may not remain restricted to a single stream of medicine but will be able to effortlessly integrate different ways of knowing and doing medicine.

Current medical education is rather narrow and restricted mostly to clinical rounds and textbook gospels, whereas the rate of doubling of medical knowledge is currently around 72 days. (Densen 2011)

The real world scenario is changing from research to innovation and tele-medicine to informatics for which the students are not prepared at all. Recent example include official government notifications for the practice of Telemedicine in India for modern medicine and AYUSH disciplines. (Sarbadhikari and Pradhan 2020) The Ministry of Health and Family Welfare has been recommending Standards for EHRs since 2013 but adoption is yet be adequate. (Sarbadhikari 2019) Therefore, integration can be started early, even in pre-med schools where integration becomes part of learning and assessment.

Goh and Sandars (2020) have noted that currently there is a focus on rapid cycles of research to inform teaching, with local and wider dissemination using newer rapid approaches to publication and social media, and acceptability of these changes by institutions. Sarbadhikari (2020) has envisaged the renewed role of communication in this digital age, which has been suddenly hastened by the COVID 19 pandemic. Park *et al* (2020) believe that there is a lot of work to be done for supporting the balancing of multiple hierarchies across clinical education. However, it can and should be a worthwhile field to explore if and when both individual and organization find a mutually productive space to thrive. The COVID-19 pandemic has shown that the public health concern is a medical as well as a social problem. There lies the importance of bringing the world's scientists together to find effective solutions for controlling the pandemic. By applying novel research frameworks, interdisciplinary and trans-disciplinary collaboration are most likely to manage a pandemic's consequences and recurrences. (Moradian *et al.*, 2020)

Monash University, and the Teaching Academy of Vermont University both are offering excellent online resources for integration of medical education and scholarship.

There is one long standing lacuna in current medical education. An average student/scholar of Mainstream Western Medicine doesn't even know ABCs of AYUSH systems, whereas AYUSH scholars have a better idea on available contemporary modern practices. Isn't it a core need that scholars of modern medicine too need to know the basics of AYUSH systems, for the betterment of patients?

Some of these diversities may be well addressed by a Clinical Terminology System like SNOMED CT. India has already developed AYUSH Extensions for SNOMED CT and the Ministry of AYUSH is also hosting online electronic health records.

How Electronic Health Records (EHRs) and Clinical Terminology Systems such as SNOMED CT are being welcomed by AYUSH Ministry:

Example of assessing need: SNOMED International has released the AYUSH Extension: *https://mlds.ihtsdotools.org/#/viewReleases/viewRelease/600189*

And *https://www.nrces.in/download/files/pdf/doc_SnomedCT-IndiaAYUSHExtension-ReleaseNotes_Current-en-US_IN1000189_20210226.pdf*

Contextualizing: AYUSH Ministry has an EHR: *http://ehr.ayush.gov.in/ayush/*

Although there have been publications for such plans: *https://www.ncbi.nlm.nih.gov/pmc/articles/PMC5607391/*

And *https://pubmed.ncbi.nlm.nih.gov/29526234/*

Does any health professional educator in India know about these?

Acknowledgements: To all our patients and students
(As this chapter is mostly about them and our efforts to boost and integrate their scholarship).

Specifically, we would like to dedicate it to our current UDHC (User driven Healthcare) core students who have performed scholarship of integration with near perfection and would be a shining example of it in the near future. Also, specifically our patients in the UDHC CBBLE (case-based blended learning ecosystem) group from rural remote and even urban locales of India and elsewhere globally without whom there wouldn't have been any scholarship of integration in healthcare.

REFERENCES

Anand A, Patwardhan B. Whose Duty Is It Anyway? Annals of Neurosciences. June 2021. doi:10.1177/09727531211009800

Bhaumik S, John O, Jha V. Low-value medical care in the pandemic-is this what the doctor ordered? Lancet Glob Health. 2021 Jun 2: S2214-109X (21)00252-7. doi: 10.1016/S2214-109X (21)00252-7.

Biswas R, Case Study Approach to Healthcare, Super Lecture, 2013, Available at: *http://www.pitt.edu/~super1/lecture/lec50421/001.htm*

Biswas R, Martin CM, Sturmberg J, Shanker R, Umalso known as nth S, Shanker S, Kasturi AS. User-driven health care - answering multidimensional information needs in individual patients utilizing post-EBM approaches: a conceptual model. J Eval Clin Pract. 2008 Oct;14(5):742-9. doi: 10.1111/j.1365-2753.2008.00998. x.

BMJ Case Reports Archives, PubMed Central: *https://www.ncbi.nlm.nih.gov/pmc/journals/1299/*

Densen P. (2011). Challenges and opportunities facing medical education. *Transactions of the American Clinical and Climatological Association*, *122*, 48–58.

Epstein RM, Hundert EM. Defining and assessing professional competence. JAMA. 2002 Jan 9;287(2):226-35. doi: 10.1001/jama.287.2.226.

Felten P. Principles of good practice in SoTL. Teaching and Learning Inquiry 2013; 1 (01) 121-125

Goh P-S, Sandars J, 2020, 'Rethinking scholarship in medical education during the era of the COVID-19 pandemic', MedEdPublish, 9, [1], 97 *https://www.mededpublish.org/manuscripts/3116*

Hofmeyer, A., Newton, M., & Scott, C. (2007). Valuing the scholarship of integration and the scholarship of application in the academy for health sciences scholars: recommended methods. *Health research policy and systems*, *5*, 5. *https://doi.org/10.1186/1478-4505-5-5*

Lal P. From rote to reasoning: The paradigm shift required in medical entrance examination and beyond! MAMC J Med Sci 2016; 2:1-5

Monash University, Scholarship of Integration, High quality interdisciplinary collaboration, Available at: *https://www.monash.edu/medicine/mcshe/about/integration*

Moradian, N., Ochs, H.D., Sedikies, C. et al. The urgent need for integrated science to fight COVID-19 pandemic and beyond. J Transl Med18, 205 (2020). *https://doi.org/10.1186/s12967-020-02364-2*

NITI Aayog. (Nov 2019). Health System for a New India: Building Blocks – Potential Pathways to Reform, Available at: *https://niti.gov.in/sites/default/files/2019-11/NitiAayogBook_compressed_1.pdf*

Pantazi, S. V., Arocha, J. F., & Moehr, J. R. (2004). Case-based medical informatics. BMC medical informatics and decision making, 4, 19. *https://doi.org/10.1186/1472-6947-4-19*

Park, S., Berlin, A. & Kelly, M. Clinical educational scholarship: polarized or integrated? Perspect Med Educ 9, 137–138 (2020). *https://doi.org/10.1007/s40037-020-00597-x*

Podder V, Dhakal B, Shaik GUS, Sundar K, Sivapuram MS, Chattu VK, Biswas R. Developing a Case-Based Blended Learning Ecosystem to Optimize Precision Medicine: Reducing Overdiagnosis and Overtreatment. Healthcare (Basel). 2018 Jul 10;6(3):78. doi: 10.3390/healthcare6030078.

Sarbadhikari S, Ch. 18, The Future of Communication in a Digital World, In, Parija SC and Adkoli BV, Eds, Effective Medical Communication: The A, B, C, D, E of it, Springer, 2020, ISBN:978-981-15-3408-9, Chapter DoI: 10.1007/978-981-15-3409-6_18

Sarbadhikari SN, The Role of Standards for Digital Health and Health Information Management, *Journal of Basic and Clinical Research*, 2019, **6**(1):1, Available at: *https://jbcr.net.in/JBCR-VOL-6-issue-1-2019-20/current-issues-volume-VI-issue-1-1.html*

Sarbadhikari SN, Pradhan KB, The Need for Developing Technology-Enabled, Safe, and Ethical Workforce for Healthcare Delivery, *Safety and Health at Work*, 2020, **11**(4): 533-536.https://doi.org/10.1016/j.shaw.2020.08.003

Shankar D. (2015). Health sector reforms for 21st century healthcare. Journal of Ayurveda and integrative medicine, 6(1), 4–9. https://doi.org/10.4103/0975-9476.154214

Shomon MJ, Living Well with Hypothyroidism: What Your Doctor Doesn't Tell You... That You Need to Know, 2000, WmMorrowPB

Singh S and Gupta P, Can We Consider Scholarship of Teaching Learning Rather than Focusing Only on Publications for Recognition of Medical Teachers by National Medical Commission? Annals of the National Academy of Medical Sciences (India) 2021; 57(01): 01-02, DOI: 10.1055/s-0041-1728179

Srinivasan R. (2020). Healthcare in India – Vision 2020: Issues and Prospects, NITI Aayog Reports, Available at: *https://niti.gov.in/planningcommission.gov.in/docs/reports/genrep/bkpap2020/26_bg2020.pdf*

Tejaswini, The integration of eLearning in medical education, 19 December 2020, Available at:*https://www.wemakescholars.com/blog/the-integration-of-e-learning-in-medical-education*

The Teaching Academy, Resources for Medical Education Research and Scholarship, Available at: *https://www.med.uvm.edu/teachingacademy/datacollection/medical-education-resource-list*

World Health Organization (WHO). (2018). Technical Series on Primary Health Care, Brief: Integrating Health Services, Available at: *https://www.who.int/docs/default-source/primary-health-care-conference/linkages.pdf*

Young JW, Thapaliya P and Sapkota S, Caught in the Middle: The Divide Between Conventional and Alternative Medicine, International Journal of User-Driven Healthcare (IJUDH), 2011, 1:9. DOI: 10.4018/ijudh.2011010105

Chapter 30

Medical Education Research in India: The Dialogues and the Way Forward

Balachandra V. Adkoli, Payal Bansal

ABSTRACT

This chapter is an attempt to capture the ongoing dialogues in medical education research in India and identify the way forward, extracting from the key messages of various chapters of this book. The major challenges lie in identifying and prioritizing the future research needs, ensuring methodological rigor, breaking the silos within and across the profession, and forming a community of scholars in a spirit of international cooperation.

We outline four major areas of dialogue: research versus scholarship (identity issue); medical education research (MER) versus health professions education research (HPER) (scope issue); quantitative versus qualitative approaches (methodological issues) and internal motivation versus external assessment (accreditation issue).

We conclude that transformation of MER into health professions education research (HPER) is a much needed step which requires concerted efforts, committed leadership and a catalytic role played by national and international networks. This will ultimately lead to a research and innovation ecosystem to support nation building, effective health care and wellbeing of the people.

Key Words: medical education research; health professions education; innovation ecosystem; mentoring; community of practice; networking; interprofessional education;

ASSESS NEED

Thinking about the future of any human pursuit is extremely fascinating and exciting. Wisdom says that past, present and future are a seamless continuum in the timeline. The future is built on the present, and the present is derived from the past. Medical Education Research (MER) in India is an area of recent interest, amid the wave of changes happening in the field of medical education, prompted by the regulators.

Traditionally, in India and many countries of Southeast Asia, medical education and health care systems have toed divergent ways. This is because of multiple regulators controlling education and multiple authorities who are responsible for delivering health care. The Lancet commission's report (Frenk et al, 2010) emphasized that the health professionals for 21st century must transform education to strengthen their health systems in an interdependent world. This is perhaps more relevant when the world is reeling under the COVID pandemic. It is therefore necessary that the medical colleges and health sciences universities in India should adopt a holistic approach to connect patient care, education, and research under one rubric (Adkoli, Parija, 2019).

The theory and practice in MER have been discussed in detail throughout this book. In this concluding chapter, we restate the key messages emerging from the various chapters to give a future direction. In this process, we envisage a much broader role for MER to embrace the whole spectrum of health professions education research. However, this agenda is vested with four major dialogues: research versus scholarship (identity issue); medical education research (MER) versus health professions education research (HPER) (scope issue); quantitative versus qualitative approaches (methodological issues) and internal motivation versus external assessment (accreditation issue).

We conclude that the future of MER depends upon a concerted and coordinated effort on part of all health professionals to break the silos, come together and reimagine our systems in line with the bigger picture of research and innovation ecosystems in India.

BRIEF

- Key messages emerging from the book applied to current scenario in India in the background of international developments
- Ongoing dialogues
- Research versus scholarship: need to support all types of scholarship: Teaching, Research, Application, and Integration - the identity dialogue
- MER versus HPER: Professional versus interprofessional; specialization versus integration- the scope dialogue
- Quantitative, Qualitative and Mixed Methods Research: Theory versus Practice – the methodology dialogue
- internal motivation versus external assessment – the accreditation dialogue
- Role of international networks and organizations

CONTEXTUALIZE

The health sector in India is presently grappling with the task of achieving universal health care. Towards this end, the strengths of all systems of medicine currently being practiced are being explored. Besides, the COVID 19 pandemic has posed additional challenges in terms of health care delivery. Medical Education Research (MER) in this context must address the projected needs of the country, its policy aspirations, and the goals to achieve universal health and wellbeing of the people.

The National Medical Commission (NMC) which replaced the MCI in 2019, has initiated reforms such as strengthening infrastructure, opening more medical colleges, especially in remote areas, increasing student intake and optimizing utilization of National Board of Examination (NBE) system to expand postgraduate training. The competency based MBBS curriculum introduced from 2019 onwards, with a large scale national Faculty Development Programs (FDPs) has met with challenges posed by the COVID pandemic forcing the medical colleges to resort to online teaching, whose quality and effectiveness is yet to be established.

The 3000-year-old Indian system of medicine with a holistic approach to health and well-being, has now changed into a "modernised" approach with a structured fixed curriculum. Moreover, the curricula of these plural systems of medicine and allied health sciences education are controlled by multiple regulators which work in silos. The National Education Policy (2020) has come out with a bigger picture of research and innovation ecosystem in a knowledge society.

Reflect for a minute. What should be the focus and direction of research related to education of health professionals? Is this situation a cause of concern or a window of opportunities for promoting health professions education research (HPER)?

DESCRIBE

Recapitulation of the key messages

1. Medical Education Research has benefitted from theories derived from educational research, which traditionally use quantitative and qualitative approaches to tackle problems and issues in medical education. This field has grown significantly, across the globe during the last 70 years, and deserves to be recognized as an independent field of health professions education scholarship, satisfying the all the four scholarship criteria identified by Boyer (1990): teaching, discovery, application, and integration (ten Cate, 2021; Weiss et al, 2022)
2. However, the geographic distribution of contributions in this field, is highly skewed, with most contributions coming from USA, UK, Canada, Netherlands and Australia, in contrast with Asia, Africa and South America (Buffone, 2020). Of late, contributions have started emerging from the non-western countries including India (Weiss et al, 2022)
3. MER in India is still at a nascent stage due to various reasons. The obstacles include time constraint due to heavy clinical workload, lack of motivation, lack of systematic training in research methodology, absence of collaborative work or community of scholars, lack of support from governance, shortage of suitable forums to showcase the work done, and lack of weightage given to MER and Scholarship of Teaching and Learning (SoTL) for promotion (Anshu & Supe, 2022; Shah et al, 2022; Kusurkar et al, 2022; Vijayaraghavan et al, 2022).
4. The authors have suggested several measures for improvement such as focusing on relevant and useful problems, using theory driven approach, robust methodologies (McConnel & Kahlke, 2022), aligning the research question with appropriate methodology (Karunathilake, 2022), and effective use of mixed methods and action research (Krishnamurthy et al 2022; Kotur & Kotur, 2022).
5. The quality of MER relies heavily on formulating a focused research question, following ethical norms as applicable for education research, using appropriate method or study design, ability to appraise published literature, adopting a systematic approach to the collection and analysis of data, all culminating in to a scholarly publication.

Dialogues that will shape up MER in future

The future of MER in India depends upon several on- going dialogues: We will discuss four of them and argue that we need a balancing act. (Figure. 1)

- The dialogue between Research versus Scholarship (Identity issue).
- The dialogue between profession-based approach versus inter-professional approach (Scope issue).
- The dialogue between the quantitative and qualitative paradigms (Methodological issue).
- The dialogue between internal and external motivators (Accreditation issue).

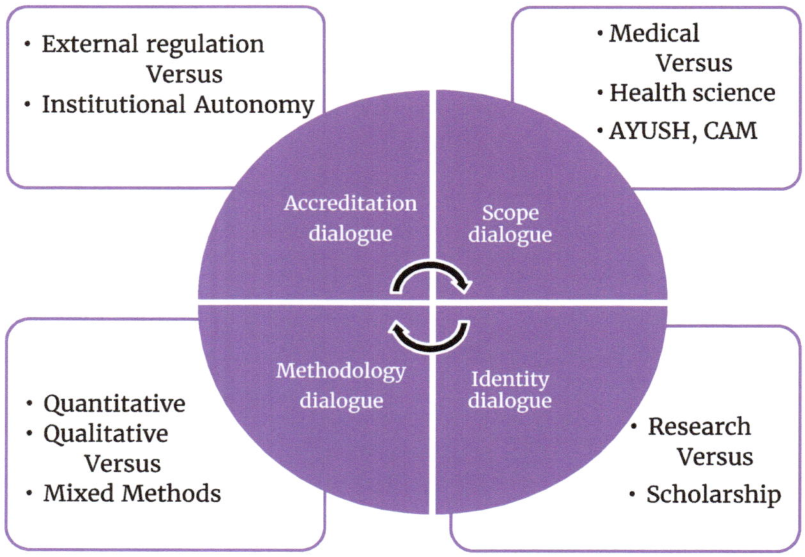

Figure 1: Dialogues in Medical Education Research: Indian Perspective

a) Research versus Scholarship – the identity issue

Conventionally research has played much guarded role in generating new knowledge or applying the same to the benefit of society. However, in health profession education, there has been a dichotomy between education and research. Similarly, service or patient care has been isolated from research. Health profession is a unique case where research for the sake of research becomes defunct. Research becomes an instrument to enhance quality of health care on the one hand, and quality of education on the other. This can happen if MER is seen as an instrument of scholarship, rather than a means for churning out research publications.

Teaching, research and patient care are the trinity of missions of all health care professions. There is a dire need to connect them together. Educational research can bridge education with clinical care (Adkoli & Parija, 2019; Adkoli, 2020)

The National Education Policy (NEP-2020) adopted by Government of India addresses the content and the scope of education at all levels. It seeks to dissolve disciplinary boundaries, foster research and innovation ecosystems to generate Intellectual Property Rights (IPR) so as to drive the economy in a knowledge society. This implies that medical education along-with its partners in health professions education should aim at improving health outcomes, and for this purpose promote innovation and research (NEP 2020).

We therefore see a reason for restating the original four types of scholarship described by Ernst Boyer.

> Restatement of Boyer's Concept: We need to promote research in such a way that all our teaching and assessment becomes more evidence based (SoTL), keeping an eye on their utility and impact on health care delivery (Application), which can be enhanced by making connections among several disciplines and professions (Integration).

The scholarship of integration, which generally means making connections among different fields can also be interpreted as a means of integrating education with patient care. As an example, Sarbadhikari et al (2022) have described how the student assessment system (user driven strategy) can be combined effectively with patient centred approach in bringing about scholarship of integration. We can expect more scholarship of integration in the times to come. However, this leads to the second issue, the future scope of MER.

b) The dialogue between profession-based approach versus inter-professional approach (Scope issue)

Knowledge explosion is the inherent character of a knowledge society propelled by digital technologies, resulting in specialization and super-specialization publications. Specialization gives identity, authenticity and status to the profession. However, the side effect of specialization is creation of silos.

The question arises, do the research protocols applicable for medical education hold good for other health professions? We need to develop and test theories to address this issue. Even within medical education, an intervention proven effective in one discipline may or may not work in the same manner in another discipline. For example, simulation pedagogy in physiology may not be equally effective in another clinical specialty. This brings us to the future need for working towards Discipline Based Educational Research (DBER) which is already felt in science and engineering (National Research Council, 2012).

Some of the upcoming developments in MER across the globe are competency-based medical education (CBME), simulation, online and virtual learning, methods and criteria for selection as well as assessment and international standards and certification (ten Cate, 2021).

In the Indian context, we need to focus on assessment issues, both formative and summative (NEET and NEXT exam), skill building, health team concept and leadership skills to prepare Indian Medical Graduates (IMGs) for working in health teams in diverse settings. Faculty development and assessment as instruments for capacity building have been emphasized by the key regulators (NMC, 2019; NAAC, 2017). Though CBME has been rolled out, the nuances of formative assessment, internal assessment and summative assessment are not yet clear. Program evaluation, development of attitudes, ethics and communication (AETCOM modules) are other areas of interest and concern. Moreover, a sound knowledge base has been created in assessment (Anshu & Singh, 2022). It is time to take a relook at the revised MBBS curriculum with robust research evidence.

While the MER gets a strong foot hold within the profession, the need for it to go interprofessional is equally warranted. Future changes will be influenced by demographic and epidemiological shifts besides disruptive technologies. While a host of high-end diagnostics, imaging techniques, robotics, molecular biology and genomics have already impacted medical science, other technologies such as Artificial

Intelligence (AI), Machine Language (ML), Big Data Analytics, Holomedicine, etc., will have to be applied to MER to bring interprofessional focus.

The COVID- 19 pandemic has further exposed the flaws in the medical care, and its lack of preparedness to deal with psycho-social, economic and cultural issues which at times matter more than biomedical aspects of the disease. We need to balance 'high tech with high touch', technical skills with soft skills (Adkoli, 2020). MER should, therefore, make connection with medical humanities, sociology, behavioural sciences and management. This requires evidence-based approach to be followed by all regulators in a concerted manner.

Thanks to the realization that health care is a holistic concept, integrative medicine needs to be brought into the fold of research and innovation, to address the wider issue of health and wellbeing of the people. (Kligler, 2004; Bansal, 2020)

c) The dialogue between the quantitative and qualitative paradigms; theory versus practice (Methodological issue)

It is now widely acknowledged that conventional designs, viz., experiments, surveys and testing (quantitative approaches) are not sufficient to answer several of the research questions in the field of health professions education. Exploratory methods such as in-depth interviews, focus group discussions, phenomenology and grounded theories are gradually entering mainstream. Authors in this book have vociferously expressed that the choice of methodology depends upon the research question asked by the researcher (Karunathilake, 2022). They can be exploratory, descriptive, evaluative, prescriptive or predictive (Table 1)

Table 1: Type of studies and examples/issues leading to research questions in the future

Type of studies	Likely questions to be asked
Exploratory	Can simulation technology be used effectively to address the problems of slow learners?
Descriptive	What are the best practices in blended learning across health science universities across the world?
Evaluative	What is the impact of 'innovative courses' started by health science universities on skill enhancement or boosting IPR activities?
Prescriptive	What strategies can be adopted for introducing effective peer mentoring programs?
Predictive	To what extent the performance in NEET/NEXT exam predicts the outcomes of IMGs?

Authors have discussed the role of quantitative, qualitative and mixed methods in answering research questions based on evidence (McConnel & Kahlke, 2022; Madalena & Dandekar, 2022; Kotur & Kotur, 2022); The authors have commented on the need for researchers to focus on 'why and how' of an intervention rather than addressing 'what was done and did it work'(Weiss et al, 2022) which is a convenient approach. They have suggested that MER should build on theories, supported by extensive review of literature. They have also noted that integration of several disciplines like health economics, humanities, sociology, ecology, ethnography and ethics can be helpful in advancing knowledge in health care.

While we endorse their views, we also feel that future research should explore from theory to practice and practice to theory. This is necessary in view of the a) urgency of implementation, e.g., CBME, b) the power of grounded theories in generating new hypothesis for boosting innovations and IPR, and c) potential of Integrative Medicine - Yoga/Complementary and Alternative Medicine (CAM) which are time tested. Thus, theory and practice become a moving cycle for development. A mixed methods approach can be seen as bridge. It has been cited as a powerful method for enriching public health research (Krishnamurthy et al 2022) and also holds good for boosting action research (Kotur & Kotur, 2022)

When the methodologies of research change, the way it is taught and learnt will obviously undergo change. The research training is likely to happen following a project-based collaborative approach. It will be supported by diverse professionals, clinicians, biomedical scientists, IT specialists (both hardware and software), behavioural and social scientists who will work with scholars across the health professions. We can expect, therefore, new communities of learning and practice in research.

d) The dialogue between autonomy versus external regulation; internal versus external motivation

The motivation for research is the ultimate determinant that includes individual factors (awareness and motivation) and external factors (recognition, incentives and good governance) to support scholarship (Anshu & Supe, 2022; Henal et al, 2022; Vijayaraghavan, 2022). The issue of internal motivation versus external is also linked with policies adopted by the agencies and authorities. The classical top-down and bottom-up approach have their own strengths and weaknesses. Drawing lessons from the bold initiative taken by the Government of India to reorganize NMC and launch a revised MBBS curriculum, we can infer that centrally directed approach 'works' but at the cost of resistance to change, caused by lack of preparedness. Initiatives from grass root level are slower to come, but easier to implement. Taking in to consideration the complexities of the systems prevalent in India, viz., Central Government versus State Governments, Government versus private; Medical versus other health sciences regulators, etc., we propose that research initiatives should be supported both top down and bottom up. This requires a close dialogue and communication, dialogue and synergy between policy makers and implementers.

Assessment of Scholarship

The need to assess educational scholarship and the justification for assessing all types of scholarship has been echoed by several scholars and some of them have also discussed the criteria (Fraenkel et al, 1993; Glassick et al, 1997; Shulman, 1998; Fincher et al, 2000; Diamond 2002; Sullivan, 2018; Ananthakrishnan, 2019; Santen et al, 2019; Ramani et al, 2020; Cleland et al 2021). The issues are complicated by lack of policy and clarity about different types of scholarship activities, dearth of authentic tools, and shift in the job portfolio from mother discipline to other responsibility such as teaching to research, administration etc (Henal et al, 2022; Anshu & Supe, 2022; Kusurkar, 2022)

We propose that the academic leaders should collectively address this issue by developing a comprehensive credit system based on evidence. The e-portfolio can be used as an effective tool for self-reflection (formative) as well as for deciding the career appraisal for the purpose of promotion (summative), when combined with multi-source feedback. This requires extensive dialogue among academic leaders, followed by pilot studies, and multi-centric trials, to be initiated by the academic community. A suggestive list of metrices for defining the outcome measures for different types of scholarship in a graded manner is shown in table 2.

Table 2: Suggested outcome measures which can be used for deciding credit points for different levels of scholarship activities

Teaching and Learning (SoTL)	Research	Application	Integration
1. Develops and shares innovative teaching practices, educational resources; presents posters.	Completes a project and prepares a report.	Dabbles with innovations, diagnosis, treatment, cost-effective procedures.	Listens, observes the developments happening in other fields.
2. Develops and shares instructional resources with other institutes.	Writes a paper short communication, and gradually, original article.	Developer of SOPs, Clinical Guidelines, Best Practices, and shares with other institutes.	Develops habit of systems thinking; its effectiveness and efficiency.
3. Chairs or moderates in education workshops, conferences.	Makes poster, podium presentation in a conference; engages in peer review activity.	Converts innovations in to IPR (Copy rights, Patents).	Interacts, communicates with other health profession and initiates projects and practices.
4. Resource Person, Guest lecturer.	Conducts Systematic Review, meta-analysis Writes for successful grant.	Establishes a network of innovators; Brings large grants.	Actively becomes a partner in IPE Demonstrates successful interprofessional research outcomes.
5. Publishes papers in peer reviewed journals.	Publishes papers in high impact journal; Editor, lead author.	Engages in Capacity building for IPR activities.	Extends the scope of Inter professional work.
6. Serves as mentor, assessor, Member Curriculum committee or MEU.	Research collaborator in multi-centric studies.	Builds bridge between Academia and Industry.	Breaks the silos and facilitates integrated systems of health, medicine.
7. Advanced course or fellowship, national, international.	Lead researcher Engages in research network.	Demonstrates successful large-scale innovations.	Champions and disseminates interprofessional approach.
8. Policy maker Consultant for SoTL at national level.	Policy maker consultant for Research.	Policy maker for Innovation eco-system	Policy maker for integrated approach to Research & Development.
Note: The outcome of each metrics should be monitored by the mentor based on e-portfolio maintained by the faculty; This can complement the career appraisal, combined with Multi-Source Feedback			

Role of National and International academic communities

In a competitive yet interdependent world, a better future can be found only by a spirit of collegiality and collaboration. It is time for the leaders to introspect and think in what ways they can contribute to the collective good of MER/HPER. With more dialogues, we can better understand each other and bridge the knowledge and communication gap. The Academy of Health Profession Educators (AHPE), various networks, professional/specialty associations, premier medical institutes, centres of HPE located in health science universities should take up interprofessional initiatives by means of organizing conferences, FDPs, sponsoring research studies, and creating forums for publication of books, journals, newsletters, blog posts including social media channels to nurture communities of practice (Lave & Wenger, 1998)

International organizations like FAIMER, SEARAME, WFME, AMEE, are already engaged in supporting scholars directly or indirectly. AMEE undoubtedly positions itself as the largest association with plethora of activities for promoting scholarship. We also need to optimize the flow of expertise from western to non-western countries, and vice versa, leading to a 'win- win' situation. Weiss et al (2022) have suggested possible areas of collaboration, viz., sharing of resources and expertise in research, computing data analysis and specialized simulation equipment. However, they have cautioned that all partners should have equal intellectual contributions. Larken et al (2016) have described the core concepts involved in successful collaboration, viz., focus on shared goals, valuing the culture, equity in sharing, mutual benefit, transparent communication, effective leadership and amicable conflict resolution strategies. It will be interesting to explore why certain innovations work well in certain cultures. The future lies therefore in collective bargain, rather than individual aspirations.

SUMMARIZE

Exploring future pathway for medical education research is a daunting task because of the complexities of the system and the different regulators working in silos. The new vision of India to promote a research and innovation ecosystem demands concerted action by all health professions. The priorities of future research will be based on local and regional needs, driven by accessible technologies, in an interdisciplinary and interprofessional environment. Methodologies should be aligned accordingly. We recommend a balancing act of central leadership connecting with local initiatives supported by autonomy and self-accountability to develop an accreditation culture based on trust. The e-portfolio that documents educator competencies and related scholarship to be maintained by all faculty, establishment of Community of Practice with multi-source feedback will bring synergy into the system. The national and international networks are expected to play a key role in advancing scholarship as a broad-based field of health professions education research (HPER).

EVALUATE

In this chapter, we have thrown suggestions and reforms which are radical and fundamental. Reflect on those issues such as feasibility of giving more autonomy, logistics of introducing credit system and the feasibility of interprofessional approach to research in a conventional set up.

What potential obstacles can you anticipate in implementing these reforms and how do you get prepared for the change?

ROAD AHEAD

The concept of Discipline (specialty) Based Educational Research (DBER) is already felt in science and engineering. Explore more about DBER.

National Research Council. 2012. *Discipline-Based Education Research: Understanding and Improving Learning in Undergraduate Science and Engineering*. Washington, DC: The National Academies Press. https://doi.org/10.17226/13362.

The National Education Policy (2020) is a futuristic document, which deals with all levels of education. A major recommendation is the establishment of National Research Foundation (NRF). The foundation is expected to facilitate, fund and support research across the board. Explore more about National Education Policy (2020)

For more information about the integrative health system health context explore the following resource:

- Bansal P (2020). Medical Education in India: History, current scenario and future perspectives in an Integrative Health System context; Invited paper for NITI Aayog, Government of India
- Explore the possibility of joining a Community of Practice. Engage in reading, browsing, writing or sharing information, books, newsletters, blogs, video, social media, besides scientific publication. A list of forums and journals in MER is available elsewhere in this book.
- MEU India: *http://meuindia.org*
- Academy of Health Professions Educators (India) *www.ahpe.org*
- South East Asia Regional Association for Medical Education*http://www.searame.org/*
- World Federation of Medical Education*http://wfme.org/*
- Association for Medical Education in Europe (AMEE) *http://amee.org*

REFERENCES

Adkoli BV, Parija SC. (2019). Applying systems approach for bridging education, research, and patient care in a health sciences university *Tropical Parasitology* 9(2):77-82

Adkoli BV. (2020). Educational Research: Much Unexplored Pathway to Career Enhancement of Teachers in Health Sciences. *Annals of SBV*;9(1):2–6.

Adkoli B.V. (2020). Post-COVID Mantra for Health Profession: Combine "High Tech" with "High Touch". (2020); *Annals of SBV*.9 (2):34-35.

Ananthakrishnan N. (2019). Perception and assessment of scholarship in health science institutions in India - gap between the existing and the desirable. J Basic Clin Appl Health Sci.;2(1), 32-8

Anshu, Supe A. (2022). Medical Education Research in India: An Overview. In. Adkoli BV and Ray A. (eds). *Medical Education Research: Theory, Practice, Publication and Scholarship.* Chennai, Notion Press (in press).

Bansal P (2020). Medical Education in India: History, current scenario and future perspectives in an Integrative Health System context; Invited paper for NITI Aayog, Government of India

Boyer, E. L. (1991). Scholarship Reconsidered: Priorities of the Professoriate. Princeton, NJ: The Carnegie Foundation for the Advancement. *Metropolitan Universities.*

Buffone, B., Djuana, I., Yang, K., Wilby, K. J., El Hajj, M. S., & Wilbur, K. (2020). Diversity in health professional education scholarship: a document analysis of international author representation in leading journals. *BMJ open*, *10*(11), e043970.

Cleland, J. A., Jamieson, S., Kusurkar, R. A., Ramani, S., Wilkinson, T. J., & van Schalkwyk, S. (2021). Redefining scholarship for health professions education: AMEE Guide No. 142. *Medical Teacher*, 1-15.

Diamond, R. M. (2002). Defining scholarship for the twenty-first century. *New Directions for Teaching and Learning*, *2002* (90), 73-80.

Frenk J, Chen L, Bhutta ZA, Cohen J, Crisp N, Evans T, et al (2010). Health professionals for a new century: transforming education to strengthen health systems in an interdependent world. Lancet. 2010 Dec 4;376(9756):1923-58. doi: 10.1016/S0140-6736(10)61854-5. Epub 2010 Nov 26. PMID: 21112623.

Fincher, R. M. E., Simpson, D. E., Mennin, S. P., Rosenfeld, G. C., Rothman, A., McGrew, M. C., & Turnbull, J. M. (2000). Scholarship in teaching: an imperative for the 21st century. *Academic medicine*, 75(9), 887-894.

Fraenkel, J. R., Wallen, N. E., & Hyun, H. H. (1993). *How to design and evaluate research in education* (Vol. 7). New York: McGraw-hill.

Glassick, C. E., Huber, M. T., & Maeroff, G. I. (1997). *Scholarship Assessed: Evaluation of the Professoriate. Special Report*. Jossey Bass Inc., Publishers, 989 Market Street, San Francisco, CA 94103.

Karunathilake I. (2022). Identifying research problem and Formulating research questions in MER. In. Adkoli BV and Ray A. (eds). *Medical Education Research: Theory, Practice, Publication and Scholarship.* Chennai, Notion Press (in press).

Kligler B., Maizes V., Schachter S, Park CM, Gaudet T, Benn R, Lee R, Remen RN. (2004). Core competencies in integrative medicine for medical school curricula: a proposal. Academic Medicine. 79(6):521-31.

Kotur P., Kotur P. (2022). Action research....... right time to have a look! In. Adkoli BV and Ray A. (eds). *Medical Education Research: Theory, Practice, Publication and Scholarship.* Chennai, Notion Press (in press).

Krishnamurthy J. Mixed Methods Research in Public Health: *From theory to practice.* In. Adkoli BV and Ray A. (eds). *Medical Education Research: Theory, Practice, Publication and Scholarship.* Chennai, Notion Press (in press).

Larkan, F., O. Uduma, S. A. Lawal and B. van Bavel (2016). "Developing a framework for successful research partnerships in global health." Global Health**12**(1): 17.

Lave, J. and Wenger, E. (1998). Situated Learning: Legitimate Peripheral Participation. New York, NY: Cambridge University Press.

MadalenaP., Maladena P., and Dandekar S. (2022). The Process of Writing a Systematic Review in Medical Education Research (MER): Way to Impact Practice and Research. In. Adkoli BV and Ray A. (eds). *Medical Education Research: Theory, Practice, Publication and Scholarship.* Chennai, Notion Press (in press).

McConnel M. & Kahlke. (2022). Research Designs and Traditions in Medical Education Research: An Overview. In. Adkoli B.V. and Ray A. (eds). *Medical Education Research: Theory, Practice, Publication and Scholarship.* Chennai, Notion Press (in press).

NAAC (2019) National Assessment and Accreditation Council (NAAC), Bengaluru, Manual of Health Sciences for Universities Available at *http://naac.gov.in/2-uncategorised/77-health-science-manual*

National Education Policy (2020). Ministry of Human Resources Development, GOI. *https://www.education.gov.in/sites/upload_files/mhrd/files/NEP_Final_English_0.pdf*

National Medical Commission (2021). Medical Council of India Competency Based Undergraduate Curriculum for The Indian Medical Graduate 2018 Available at *https://www.nmc.org.in/wp-content/uploads/2020/01/UG-Curriculum-Vol-I.pdf*

Ramani S, McKimm J, Findyartini A, Nadarajah VD, Hays R, Chisolm MS, Filipe HP, Fornari A, Kachur EK, Kusurkar RA, Thampy H, Wilson KW. (2020). Twelve Tips for Developing a Global Community of Scholars in Health Professions Education. Med Teach., Early Online. *10.1080/0142159X.2020.1839034*

Shulman L. S. (1998). Chapter 1, In: P. Hutchings (Ed.) The course portfolio: how faculty can examine their teaching to advance practice and improve student learning (Washington DC, American Association for Higher Education).

Santen, S. A., Peterson, W., & Wolff, M. (2019). Turning Your Educational Work into Scholarship. *AEM education and training*, *3*(1), 79-80.

Sullivan, G. M. (2018). A toolkit for medical education scholarship. *Journal of graduate medical education*, *10*(1), 1. ten Cate, O. (2021). Health professions education scholarship: The emergence, current status, and future of a discipline in its own right (2021). FASEB Bioadvances. DOI: 10.1096/fba.2021-00011

Sarbadhikari, S., Biswas, R., Priyadarshini, B., SimhachalamK., Jodavula, S., Mukherjee, S., et al. (2022). Scholarship of Integration and the future of Medical Education and Research (MER). In. Adkoli BV and Ray A. (eds). *Medical Education Research: Theory, Practice, Publication and Scholarship.* Chennai, Notion Press (in press).

Singh T., Gupta P. (2021). Can We Consider Scholarship of Teaching Learning Rather than Focusing Only on Publications for Recognition of Medical Teachers by National Medical Commission? Ann Natl Acad Med Sci (India):2021; 57:1–2

Weiss P., Najjar M., Bansal P., Gruppen L. Medical Education Research from an International Perspective (2022). In. Adkoli BV and Ray A. (eds). *Medical Education Research: Theory, Practice, Publication and Scholarship.* Chennai, Notion Press (in press).

www.ingramcontent.com/pod-product-compliance
Ingram Content Group UK Ltd.
Pitfield, Milton Keynes, MK11 3LW, UK
UKHW061032310726
14089UKWH00009B/204
* 9 7 9 8 8 9 5 1 9 1 1 9 4 *